Outbreak Alert

Responding to the Increasing Threat of Infectious Diseases

JASON EBERHART-PHILLIPS, M.D.

New Harbinger Publications, Inc.

Publisher's Note

This publication is designed to provide accurate and authoritative information in regard to the subject matter covered. It is sold with the understanding that the publisher is not engaged in rendering psychological, financial, legal, or other professional services. If expert assistance or counseling is needed, the services of a competent professional should be sought.

Distributed in the U.S.A. by Publishers Group West and in Canada by Raincoast Books.

Copyright © 2000 by Jason Eberhart-Phillips
        New Harbinger Publications, Inc.
        5674 Shattuck Avenue
        Oakland, CA 94609

Cover design by Blue Design
Edited by Jueli Gastwirth
Text design by Michele Waters

Library of Congress Catalog Card Number: 99-75296
ISBN 1-57224-201-9 Paperback

All Rights Reserved

Printed in the United States of America

New Harbinger Publications' Web site address: www.newharbinger.com

02   01   00

10   9   8   7   6   5   4   3   2   1

First printing

For Donna

The more ingenious and clever people are,
the more strange things happen.

—Tao Te Ching

Contents

Preface

During the final weeks of writing this book, "mosquito mania" was reigning supreme in and around New York City. At the time, seven people had died and dozens of others had fallen ill from a virus never before seen in the Western Hemisphere. For New Yorkers accustomed to congested subways and the other indignities of big city life, the arrival of the West Nile virus touched off an uncharacteristic fear and loathing. Many wondered if a seemingly innocent mosquito bite might be the kiss of death. As helicopters and roving trucks doused the city's concrete canyons with insecticides, and health officials sought to calm frazzled nerves, it became clear to everyone in America's largest city that new and dangerous enemies from the microbial world can turn up anywhere.

New York's West Nile outbreak wasn't the only headline news on emerging diseases. At the same time that downstate New Yorkers were keeping away from mosquitoes, nearly one thousand people who attended a fair in upstate New York became ill with diarrhea from a pugnacious strain of *Escherichia coli*. Nearly simultaneous outbreaks were occuring globally on an almost daily basis. A large outbreak from the same organism also occurred in Illinois. Nearby in Iowa, public health officials had to track down hundreds of people who may have been exposed to rabies after they handled an infected bear cub at a petting zoo. Flu broke out among tourists and tour operators in Alaska. Dengue fever erupted in southern Texas. New recommendations were issued on avoiding raw sprouts. North American blood banks started to turn away donors who once lived in Britain because of concern that they may have the human form of mad cow disease. Malaria was reported near an airport in Luxembourg. Infectious diseases are the stuff of late-breaking news.

This book begins where the front-page news stories and eyewitness television reports leave off. It aims to help readers understand how and why diseases caused by new and exotic microorganisms are arising so frequently today, and why certain old diseases are coming back. We are privileged to live at a time when far more is known about the infections that challenge us than ever before. But recent changes in the ways that people live, mingle with each other, and interact with nature are also creating new opportunities for infections to emerge, including some infections that are impossible to cure. The race to comprehend how these emerging diseases arise and how they may be prevented is a first-order priority for science and medicine at the threshold of the twenty-first century. It's a race that none of us can afford to lose.

The pages that follow represent a major revision of a book I recently wrote for New Zealand readers. That book, titled *Plagues on Our Doorstep*, had the same aim as this book, and followed roughly the same outline. Because so much has been learned about emerging infectious diseases since I wrote the New Zealand book, a complete overhaul was necessary for this edition. In addition to the many outbreaks that have occurred in the past year, there has been a flourishing of scientific literature on the topic of emerging infections. This book samples some of the important new discoveries in that literature and shares some of the most fascinating episodes in the recent history of disease emergence. In the introduction of *Plagues on Our Doorstep*, I said, "The stories of how new diseases suddenly appear in unexpected places by unexpected means are often nothing short of amazing." I still believe this is true, and I hope that when you have finished this book you will agree.

Readers of *Outbreak Alert* require little background knowledge in science. In fact, this book is less a scientific treatise than an easygoing discussion about some of the fundamental trends shaping the lives of human beings and their microbial predators at the turn of the twenty-first century. This volume is written for North Americans, but like the diseases themselves, the book knows no boundaries. In the following chapters we'll be traveling to nearly one hundred different countries to see disease emergence at work. If you aren't sure of your international geography, a globe or an atlas might help.

Although it is my name that appears on the cover of this book, many others helped bring it to completion. I am greatly indebted to a number of busy people who kindly read drafts from this edition, or the earlier version, and offered helpful comments. They include Claire Beynon, Nigel Dickson, Denise Koo, Bill Mac Kenzie, Laurene Mascola, Charlotte Paul, David Skegg, Megan Tschannen-Moran,

Antje van der Linden, and Bob Womack. I especially wish to thank my father, Jason Eberhart, for his interest in my work and his discerning critique. Finally, I wish to acknowledge Donna, Luke, and Paul, without whose support I would not have the urge to write.

Chapter 1

Introduction to Emergence

*Not so long ago, many thought the era of communicable
disease would soon be over. But viruses, bacteria, and
parasites have now proved more formidable and adaptable
foes than we had once thought.*

—Sang Tae Han, Western Pacific Region,
World Health Organization

On the sixteenth of August 1945, only a few news stories in American
newspapers were unrelated to Japan's unconditional surrender the
previous day or to the spontaneous celebrations that marked the end
of World War II. Under headlines that read, "Nations Give Thanks"
and "Crowds Go Mad With Joy," news items on page after page
brought home good tidings to Americans everywhere that a terrible
war finally had been won. After six grim years of sacrifice and struggle, the last and most dreaded enemy had surrendered. A new era,
promising peace and prosperity, was beginning that day. "This is the
day when fascism and police government cease in the world. This is
the day for democracies," President Harry Truman told a jubilant
crowd on the White House lawn. His Majesty King George VI
thanked God for this "final victory" over tyranny in his message to
the British Parliament.

One little news story that came over the wire that day seemed
unconnected to the accounts of revelry in the streets or to the
speeches of presidents and kings. Yet the brief article that found its
way into the back pages shared the optimism of the moment. It said
that scientists in Illinois had developed a new drug, different from

penicillin, for use in treating infections. Preliminary experiments with the new medication, using animals, were described as "almost sensational." Although pleased with the results, the scientists predicted that their new antibiotic, streptomycin, would "probably never supplant penicillin" which, at that time, was completely effective against a wide array of infections and was very inexpensive to produce.

In hindsight, the little article about the new infection-fighting drug was an apt footnote to the triumphant headlines of VJ Day 1945. Atomic science and modern military technology had just defeated the menacing armies of foreign aggressors. Now, biological science and modern medical technology appeared ready to subdue the microscopic insurgents behind a host of age-old human diseases. For the first time in history, the conquest of infectious diseases appeared to be within reach.

The Honeymoon Years

There was good reason to believe that infectious diseases were in retreat during the first three decades after World War II. Penicillin, streptomycin, and other new antibiotics were performing like invincible "magic bullets" against a panoply of fatal and debilitating bacterial diseases. DDT and other chemical pesticides were remarkably efficient in ridding industrialized countries of mosquitoes and other pests that transmitted disease. Vaccines were reinventing the experience of childhood, emancipating children from epidemics of whooping cough and measles, and protecting them from the paralyzing effects of polio. Sanatoriums for tuberculosis and leprosy were closing down for lack of patients. Smallpox, traditionally one of humanity's most fearsome afflictions, was well on its way to being wiped off the Earth. It was an exultant time for public health, as one miracle seemed to follow another.

Older doctors who practiced in those heady days could still remember the epidemics of diseases like diphtheria and typhoid fever that had periodically devastated communities large and small throughout America and beyond. The so-called Spanish flu of 1918 had killed more than twenty million people worldwide, most of them young and otherwise fit. In the southern United States, malaria had been an ever-present danger. Sudden outbreaks of cholera and yellow fever had appeared in Europe and North America repeatedly during the previous century. Scarlet fever had ravaged Victorian society, claiming the lives of five of the Archbishop of Canterbury's six daughters. Bubonic plague had erupted in Hong Kong in 1894, and by 1900 was creating havoc in cities as dispersed as Rio de Janeiro, Sydney, Cape Town, and San Francisco. Syphilis and other venereal diseases haunted European and American societies. During the 1930s, at least one million American women were thought to be infected with syphilis, and sixty thousand infants were born each year with malformations and disabilities due to the disease. As late as the 1950s, epidemics of polio and measles sometimes forced schools to suspend classes, theaters to close, and churches to cancel services. In the four years before Jonas Salk's first polio vaccine was licensed in 1955, more than 65,000 American children and young adults were paralyzed in recurrent polio epidemics and 7,516 died.

During the early years of the twentieth century, the three leading causes of death in the United States were still diseases of infection: pneumonia, tuberculosis, and gastroenteritis. Heart disease was a distant fourth, and cancer barely made the top ten. In England, one in five children did not live to their fifth birthday. Nearly all deaths during childhood, adolescence, and early adult life were due to unstoppable infections. In Canada, Australia, and New Zealand the picture was similar. The threat of death from acute infection was woven into the fabric of everyday life. Hospital patients were on average much younger than today and they had fewer underlying health problems. For those sick enough to require a hospital bed, however, the chances of recovery from most infectious diseases were not good. A sudden onset of bacterial pneumonia, or a wound infection that spread to the bone, was as much a death sentence for a twenty-five-year-old father in 1930 as disseminated lung cancer is for a sixty-five-year-old grandfather today.

Within only a few decades, however, infection's oppressive grip on human health changed radically, at least in developed countries. An explosion in scientific knowledge, a burgeoning of new medical technologies, and significant advances in sanitation began to reverse humanity's mortal subjugation to its ancient microbial enemies. The preface to the 1953 edition of Macfarlane Burnet's popular medical textbook reflected this upbeat view: "It is hardly too much to say that infectious disease has now ceased to have any serious social significance in the advanced countries of the world." As early as 1944, Charles E. A. Winslow concluded in his book, *The Conquest of Epidemic Disease*, that rational scientific principles arising from the germ theory had "forever banished from the earth the major plagues and pestilences of the past." By the late 1970s, prominent medical scholars jauntily spoke of revising the disease control agenda for "the post-infection era."

As serious infections withdrew, life expectancy increased. Childhood mortality became increasingly rare. Chronic diseases, such as coronary artery disease, cancer, emphysema, and stroke, that tend to affect older people, became the leading causes of hospitalization and death. Doctors increasingly turned their attention to treating and preventing these conditions. By the 1970s, few medical school graduates had ever seen patients with polio, syphilis, or diphtheria during their training. Few would know how to diagnose cholera in someone with diarrhea, and hardly any would consider malaria when approaching a patient with fever. Clinicians who specialized in infectious diseases were a dying breed. The Surgeon General of the United States spoke for the medical profession at large when he testified before Congress in 1969 that it was time "to close the book on infectious diseases."

For the first time in centuries, most mothers did not have to worry if their children would survive infancy. Lovers could be less troubled about their partners' sexually acquired infections. Bites from ticks or mosquitoes had become only a minor nuisance. Blood was thought to be safe, and so were most of the foods we ate and the water we drank. For better or worse, we had begun to take for granted our apparent mastery over the microbial world.

Awakening to Reality

The honeymoon was short-lived. Humanity's enemies in the microscopic world were not about to accept an unconditional surrender. Postwar expectations for the demise of infectious diseases were naïvely premature. By the 1990s, more than thirty new infectious agents had been identified in humans, and most were proving difficult or impossible to cure. Infectious diseases remained the single largest cause of premature death worldwide, and were still among the leading causes of disability. It was obvious that society could ill afford to close the book on human pathogens, the microbes that cause disease. In 1996, Ronald St. John, director of Canada's Office of Special Health Initiatives, asked rhetorically, "If nature spent over a billion years evolving and perfecting microorganisms, do we really think that we will succeed in conquering them with fifty years of antibiotics?"

Clearly we don't speak of conquest any more. Although some diseases have been amenable to control, others have been far more resistant than anyone would have dreamed a half-century ago. Still other diseases—some of them previously unknown—have thrived in the face of striking social and environmental changes in recent years. Today, the death toll from infectious diseases has reached about fifteen hundred an hour; more than half of these deaths are in children under the age of five. "Infectious diseases are flourishing, and so are those who chase them, study them, and treat them," notes John G. Bartlett of Johns Hopkins University School of Medicine (1997).

Of the "new" diseases thriving in the modern marketplace, AIDS is probably the best known. AIDS came into public view during the summer of 1981 when reports appeared from Los Angeles, New York, and San Francisco describing clusters of unusual infections and cancers in otherwise healthy, young, gay men. At first, the cause of the strange new syndrome was unknown, but there were early indications that it was due to an unrecognized infectious agent that slowly dismantled the immune system. That agent, the human immunodeficiency virus (HIV), was isolated in 1983. Since then, the number of people infected with HIV worldwide has grown to thirty-four million or more, and the death toll has begun to exceed 2.5 million per year.

More than 90 percent of people with HIV infection today live in developing countries, and almost half are women. Gay men and injecting drug users still account for most AIDS cases in industrialized countries, but worldwide the vast majority of HIV infections arise from heterosexual transmission. In a band of African countries stretching from southern Sudan to South Africa, nearly a quarter of the adult urban population is infected with HIV, almost entirely as a result of heterosexual intercourse. Were it not for AIDS, life expectancy in Zimbabwe today would be sixty-five years, instead of just thirty-nine years (Stanecki and Way 1999). By 2010, deaths from AIDS will single-handedly reduce life expectancy in Botswana from sixty-six to thirty-eight years. Life expectancy will drop from sixty-nine to forty-four years in Kenya, and from sixty to thirty-eight years in Zambia. Recent advances in drug therapy have lifted hopes that the unremitting progression of HIV infection into end-stage AIDS can be slowed down. In the United States, deaths from AIDS dropped by two-thirds between 1995 and 1997, in large part thanks to the new therapies. In the desperately poor countries of Africa's "AIDS belt," however, such drugs are having virtually no impact, because their cost—about $12,000 a year per patient—is simply beyond reach.

Until recently, the origin of HIV-1, the main type of HIV responsible for the global AIDS epidemic, was clouded in mystery. Now, due to an elegant genetic analysis by Feng Gao and colleagues, published in 1999, it is almost certain that HIV-1 evolved from a closely related virus that silently infects a subspecies of African chimpanzees. Exactly how certain variants of the chimpanzee virus crossed into humans is anyone's guess, but the custom of slaughtering wild primates for food in many remote areas of equatorial Africa appears to have played a role. A splash of blood when butchering an infected chimp may have been sufficient to transmit viral particles to the first human hosts. Sporadic human infections with such early strains of HIV may have been occurring in isolated African villages over decades, or even centuries, without drawing attention from the outside world. Even within such villages, a small number of premature deaths from an AIDS-like disease probably would have passed unnoticed. Moreover, where HIV might have gained a foothold among human hosts, tribal customs proscribing sexual infidelity may have contained the spread of disease to only a handful of cases. If this scenario is correct, AIDS may have coexisted with humanity for a very long time before science discovered it. "Biologically, the AIDS virus isn't 'new' even though we talk as if it were," said Stephen S. Morse, a virologist and immunologist at Columbia University. Speaking in a 1990 interview, he added, "The virus was there all along."

How AIDS advanced from being a local disease affecting remote African villagers to a full-blown pandemic (worldwide epidemic) is easier to determine. The end of colonization during the 1950s and 1960s ushered in a period of unprecedented social and economic change throughout the African continent. Foreign investment and international aid allowed the construction of an extensive network of new highways, opening up vast expanses of African veldt. Many once-remote villages now found themselves beside the rugged gravel thoroughfares where convoys of long-distance trucks plied their way between coastal ports and interior cities. In time, the traditional rural economy declined as young adults in search of work departed for the continent's teeming urban centers, or settled in the roadside towns that had sprung up to look after the relatively well-paid truck drivers and other travelers who passed their way. Rapid urbanization eroded traditional tribal values and, for many, encouraged greater sexual license. At the same time, the realignment of Africa's work force around cheap migrant labor undermined opportunities for stable sexual relationships and stimulated the demand for prostitution. Truck drivers, modern Africa's answer to the American cowboy, may have been among the first to spread HIV on a large scale, transporting it from wayside brothels around its isolated epicenter to the outside world.

Once HIV gained entry into Africa's major cities, it was able to tap into an ever-growing pool of sexually active hosts. With HIV's long incubation period, an infected person could transmit the disease for a decade or more before symptoms appeared. Tragically, the use of unsterilized needles in vaccination campaigns during the late 1950s and early 1960s may have hastened the spread of the virus. We now know that HIV had reached Leopoldville, the colonial capital of the Belgian Congo, at least forty years ago. Tiny fragments of genetic material from the virus were recently uncovered from a blood sample collected there as part of another study in 1959 (Zhu, Korber, Nahmias, et al. 1998). The specimen came from a Bantu man whose subsequent fate remains a mystery. His death, like that of other Africans with symptoms of AIDS at that time, typically would have slipped past the region's hard-pressed public health system without a second glance. But during the 1970s, sporadic cases of the unusual ailments that would later signify AIDS were beginning to surface in Norway, Denmark, Belgium, France, Germany, and the United States. By 1980—before anyone even knew what AIDS was—transmission of HIV was well under way on three continents. During this time, when talk, of a "post-infection era" was rife, it is likely that one hundred thousand people were already infected with HIV: Air travel had efficiently conveyed an obscure African virus into the bars, back streets, and bedrooms of the industrialized world.

More than any other emerging disease, AIDS has shaken the medical profession out of its complacency over humanity's collective threats from infectious organisms. In retrospect, the only surprise is that HIV did not surface sooner than it did. To Nobel laureate Joshua Lederberg, the global eruption of AIDS was "a natural, almost predictable, phenomenon." Lederberg, the president emeritus of Rockefeller University, is the pioneer microbiologist who coined the phrase "emerging infectious diseases" during the 1980s. In his considered opinion, AIDS may just be the first in a series of new plagues to emerge from hiding and sweep the world during our lifetimes. "Some people think I am being hysterical, but there are catastrophes ahead. We live in evolutionary competition with microbes: bacteria and viruses. There is no guarantee that we will be the survivors," he said in a 1990 interview for the journal *Science*.

The Concept of Emergence

By the time AIDS was discovered, a melancholy parade of other novel pestilences was already in full stride. Table 1 lists just a few of the major "new" human infections to thrust themselves into the global spotlight during the past twenty-five years. Most are now well-known to doctors and specialists in infectious disease control.

Many have gained household recognition through intensive media coverage, and a few would already make the short list of major public health problems of our time. Seven of the best-known plagues to emerge recently are introduced in detail in chapter 2, along with a number of familiar diseases of the past that have lately staged unwelcome comebacks. Their stories depict the variety of threats we face.

Table 1
Significant Infectious Diseases Identified since 1976

Year	Agent	Disease
1976	*Cryptosporidium*	Profuse watery diarrhea
1977	Ebola virus	Ebola hemorrhagic fever
1977	*Legionella pneumophila*	Legionnaires' disease
1977	*Campylobacter jejuni*	Most common bacterial cause of food poisoning
1979	Ross River virus	Ross River fever, arthritis
1981	*Staphylococcus* toxin	Menstrual toxic shock syndrome
1982	*Borrelia burgdorferi*	Lyme disease
1982	*Escherichia coli* O157:H7	Bloody diarrhea, hemolytic uremic syndrome
1983	HIV	AIDS
1983	*Helicobacter pylori*	Peptic ulcer disease
1989	Hepatitis C virus	Hepatitis C
1991	*Ehrlichia chaffeensis*	Human ehrlichiosis
1992	*Vibrio cholerae* O139	New strain of epidemic cholera
1993	Sin Nombre hantavirus	Hantavirus pulmonary syndrome
1993	*Cyclospora cayestanensis*	Epidemics of diarrhea
1996	Prion of bovine spongiform encephalopathy (BSE)	Variant Creutzfeldt-Jakob disease (vCJD)
1997	H1N5 Influenza A virus	"Chicken flu"
1999	Nipah virus	Febrile viral encephalitis

Concern about these diseases, and about dozens of others that have escaped news media attention, has stimulated a new research focus on "disease emergence" among microbiologists, public health professionals, and others. A widely read report commissioned by the Institute of Medicine (IOM), an advisory body to the United States National Academy of Sciences, heightened interest in emerging infections when it was released in 1992. The IOM report affirmed that infectious diseases will not be conquered any time soon, and it predicted confidently that new and sometimes dangerous microbial plagues would continue to emerge well into the future. Since then, papers on emerging diseases have become increasingly common in medical journals and other scientific publications. A new medical journal, *Emerging Infectious Diseases,* was launched by the United States Centers for Disease Control and Prevention (CDC) in 1995. It is available both in hard copy and electronically on the World Wide Web, in an effort to keep doctors and other infection specialists "ahead of the curve" in this rapidly changing field.

Within this growing body of literature "emerging infectious diseases" have been defined as those diseases whose incidence or geographic range has been increasing in recent years, or those diseases that threaten to increase in the near future. The term originally applied only to newly discovered microbial threats, such as those listed in Table 1. But the concept has since broadened to include many well-known diseases that have recently reemerged after years of decline. The study of emerging infections today extends well beyond the fields of medicine and microbiology to include the social and behavioral sciences, as well as ecology and various earth sciences. It is taken for granted that infectious diseases do not emerge simply by chance, but for reasons that can be understood and by mechanisms that can be explained. By definition, all infectious diseases involve invasion by microscopic organisms, that is, pathogens that initiate disease after taking up residence in the bodies of appropriate hosts, such as humans. But, as AIDS taught us, the emergence of infectious diseases on a global scale cannot be explained simply by considering the innate properties of human pathogens to acquire new hosts. The environment in which pathogens and their potential hosts interact is generally much more important in triggering emergence. As we will see in this book, nearly all the changes that favor emergence in the agent-host environment are brought about today by human activities.

According to Columbia University's Morse, who contributed to the IOM report, disease emergence is essentially a two-step process. As he explained in a 1991 paper, it begins with the introduction of an infectious agent into a suitable new host at a given place and time. On rare occasions such agents might evolve de novo. More often—as we suspect for the introduction of HIV into humans—the agent already exists in a different natural reservoir. It arises in a new host as a result of the inevitable "microbial traffic" that occurs over time between species, or between geographically isolated groups of the same species. In the second step, the agent disseminates across the new host population. The two steps can occur almost simultaneously, but, as we saw with AIDS, they are more often separated by long periods of time. Human activities can facilitate either or both steps, first by enhancing the opportunities for cross-species transfer of new agents into human hosts, then by precipitating the epidemic spread of such agents within human populations. It is these epidemics that ultimately herald the emergence of previously unknown diseases.

Emergence is not a new phenomenon. More than twenty-four hundred years ago a mysterious new disease emerging from Africa descended on the city-state of Athens at the height of its cultural enlightenment. One-third of the population died, and ancient Greek society never fully recovered. During the second and third centuries A.D., measles and smallpox emerged with epidemic fury across the Roman world. Mongol armies heading west during the mid-fourteenth century brought bubonic plague across the steppes of Central Asia to Europe's doorstep. After 1492, the emergence of smallpox, measles, typhus, influenza, and other European diseases decimated the native cultures of the Americas, thus facilitating the Spanish conquest. Soon malaria and yellow fever arrived in the New World from Africa, while syphilis landed in Europe from parts unknown.

What is new about emergence today is the speed and intensity with which it can occur. New diseases no longer roam the world by horseback or sail the seas in schooners. Now they travel by jet aircraft and enormous container ships. They take advantage of new, high-volume technologies, unprecedented global changes in climate and land use, unchecked population growth, and massive human population movements driven by war and poverty. Today's mingling of peoples and microbes has no historical precedent. A shared vulnerability to emerging infectious diseases is drawing people of every nation into a single global village, whether we like it or not.

Factors of Emergence

Anyone attempting to understand the emergence and reemergence of microbial threats must acknowledge that interactions between

The Downside of Globalization

As anyone who has noticed the plunging price of telecommunications knows, Americans living in the year 2000 are better connected to the outside world than ever before. Positioned as we are at the vortex of an ever-more-integrated world economy, no country has opened its arms wider to embrace the Internet and other globalizing technologies than the United States. But the revolution in communications is just one sign that we have begun to live in a very different world, a world in which local, regional, and even national perspectives are giving way to a new global identity. For many, the social and material benefits of our headlong push toward a single world society seem limitless. The evolving global market for goods and services is already beginning to meet our needs in ways no single national economy ever could. We are starting to reach across old boundaries and participate like never before in a truly cosmopolitan culture. New friends in far-flung places are as close today as the click of a computer mouse.

But globalization has at least one darker side that all its boosters would rather forget: the easy spread of infectious diseases. Once upon a time Main Street America could afford a degree of complacency about exotic new infections emanating from remote tropical jungles or crowded, unsanitary megacities in the developing world. But our new global society has changed all that. The 1992 IOM report opened with the memorable words that "in the context of infectious diseases, there is nowhere in the world from which we are remote and no one from whom we are disconnected." The human and ecological factors that are facilitating disease emergence today have global reverberations that reach into every community. Today the economy of nearly every state and metropolitan area is increasingly dependent upon international trade and travel, especially from countries less developed than our own. Air travel and modern international shipping have collapsed the barriers of time and space throughout the planet. It is an inescapable fact that a deadly new human infection may appear almost anywhere in the world one day, and be carried silently through an airport near you the next.

Given that most American communities have trouble enough with homegrown infections, no one can afford to ignore the global threats arising here or beyond our shores any longer. If AIDS has taught us anything, it is that we need to acknowledge the dangers we face from emerging infections, wherever we live. Other unrecognized but potentially fatal agents of human disease are almost certainly lurking about in nature's vast microbial reservoirs. When these pathogens emerge from their present obscurity, national boundaries will mean nothing. Today, any community that remains apathetic to new diseases in distant places does so at its peril. "The microbe that felled one child in a distant continent yesterday can reach yours today and seed a global pandemic tomorrow," wrote J. Lederberg in 1988. "Never send to know for whom the bell tolls; it tolls for thee."

pathogens, hosts, and the environment in which they live are often too complex to fit a simple model. There is rarely a single identifiable reason why a new disease has appeared or an old one has returned. Usually a combination of factors is at work, some of which may not be known at the outset. Notwithstanding the likely pitfalls, the authors of the IOM report attempted to classify the specific forces that shape emergence into six broad categories: international travel and commerce, human demographics and behavior, technology and industry, ecological change associated with economic development and land use, microbial adaptation and change, and breakdown of public health measures. These "factors of emergence" had to be somewhat arbitrary, but they have proven so useful in explaining past and present plagues that they now comprise the most widely accepted framework for understanding emerging infections.

   This book adopts the IOM framework, modified by the division of two categories into smaller units, and the addition of biological terrorism; the intentional use of infectious agents has become a greater concern since the IOM report was published. Starting with chapter 3, each chapter will examine in-depth one of the factors responsible for emergence. Significant microbial threats from throughout the world will illustrate the key points, including one primary example for each factor, as shown in Table 2.

Table 2
Factors Related to Emerging Diseases

Factor	Chapter	Primary example
Travel and commerce	3	*Cyclospora* outbreaks from imported raspberries
Human demographics	4	Resurgence of dengue fever in growing urban centers
Human behavior	5	Epidemic of hepatitis C linked to injecting drug use
Technology and industry	6	Bovine spongiform encephalopathy and adulterated cattle feed
Ecological change	7	Human monkeypox and deforestation
Microbial adaptation	8	The Spanish flu pandemic of 1918 following antigenic shift

Antimicrobial resistance	9	Vancomycin-resistant *Staphylococcus aureus* emergence
Breakdown of public health infrastructure	10	*Cryptosporidium* outbreak in a city water supply
Biological terrorism	11	Anthrax outbreak downwind from a weapons research facility

Before we examine the factors causing emergence, it is important to get acquainted with the sorts of threats we face. The study of emerging infectious diseases is grounded in a short but spectacular history, a history of real events played before an attentive news media and a worldwide audience. It is fair to say that a serious student of infectious diseases today grasps a newspaper with one hand and a microscope with the other. The next chapter visits some of the ailments, new and old, that have made the front page and have ignited public interest in infectious diseases in recent years.

What You Can Do To Prevent Emerging Infections

As you read this book and become familiar with the factors responsible for today's emerging infections, you will undoubtedly begin to consider a number of commonsense actions you can take to help yourself and your family avoid these diseases. To encourage your thinking along these lines, each chapter will end with a box offering practical advice from the experts on how to lower infection risks. Each box will highlight simple ways to prevent a disease, or group of diseases, that has been discussed in that chapter.

By the end of the book you'll be well versed in ways to prevent tick-borne diseases, food-borne diseases, diseases of the tropics, sexually transmitted diseases, blood-borne diseases, rodent-borne diseases, and influenza. The boxes will also discuss ways to reduce the spread of antibiotic resistance and will outline the arguments in favor of childhood immunization. Individual responses are important to counter the threat of emerging infections. But be forewarned: Many of the diseases discussed in this book cannot be prevented or controlled by applying self-help techniques. As you will discover in the pages ahead, the forces behind today's epidemics are often beyond the reach of our control as individuals. Solutions will require much more than individual responses.

Chapter 2

Examples of Emergence

The twentieth century has seen unprecedented scientific progress, and so it is ironic that as the century draws to a close, scientists and clinicians must learn to deal with emerging new infectious agents whose existence in human beings was proved only in the past few years.

—Samuel Broder,
National Cancer Institute

We have seen how the resurgence of infectious diseases has caught the worlds of science and medicine by surprise. In 1980, no one in the United States would have thought that deaths from infectious causes would increase by more than 50 percent by 1992, or that an unheard-of virus from Africa would become the leading killer of Americans aged twenty-five to forty-four, as HIV was by the mid-1990s. Few would have thought that infectious diseases would still account for a quarter of all deaths worldwide—and nearly two-thirds of deaths in children under four years of age—at the start of the twenty-first century.

But our thinking has changed. Even before the advent of AIDS the writing was on the wall. By the mid-1970s outbreaks of unusual infections were already refuting the fantasy that the microbial world had been defeated, but, at first, such episodes were treated only as exceptions. Eventually, the accumulation of such "exceptions" forced a new awareness, as Richard Levins of the Harvard School of Public Health points out. He says, "Diseases rise and fall, evolve and spread, and retreat and spread again" (1994).

This chapter profiles some of the most celebrated "exceptions" of the past twenty-five years, diseases that gnawed away at the wishful view that infections were no longer significant threats to public health. AIDS was introduced in the first chapter. Here we begin with the stories of seven other previously unknown diseases that emerged seemingly from nowhere, but soon gained international attention from health professionals and the public alike. Sidebar boxes highlight the latest tick-borne disease emerging in the United States, and the Nipah virus epidemic that rocked Malaysia in 1999. We then consider three important reemerging diseases: cholera, malaria, and diphtheria, and look briefly at the disquieting resurgence of meningococcal disease in the Pacific Northwest and elsewhere.

Finally, we show how infectious agents have sometimes been found to cause diseases that had previously defied explanation. Such discoveries do not constitute emergence in the truest sense, but they are mentioned briefly here because they highlight medicine's growing respect for infectious organisms as causes of human disease.

Seven Modern Plagues

Legionnaires' Disease

During July 1976, the American people were in celebration mode. It was the bicentennial summer, the 200th anniversary of American independence. Tall ships from around the world sailed into New York harbor. Bostonians relived Paul Revere's midnight ride, as Washington was decked out in banners of red, white, and blue. In cities large and small, parades and fireworks displays were the order of the day. But nowhere was the spirit of 1976 felt stronger than in Philadelphia, the place where the founding fathers had signed the Declaration of Independence two centuries before. Philadelphia, "the city of brotherly love," was the cradle of American liberty, and, during the summer of 1976, it would be the focal point of the country's biggest ever birthday bash. So it was no surprise that the Pennsylvania chapter of the American Legion had chosen Philadelphia for its annual convention. Starting on July 21, some forty-four hundred legionnaires and their families descended on the city for four days of spirited camaraderie and patriotic revelry. Convention headquarters was the grand old Bellevue-Stratford Hotel, whose eighteen floors overlooked Broad Street in the center of the city. By all accounts at the time, the convention was a rollicking success.

But within days of returning home from Philadelphia, many of the legionnaires fell ill with an abrupt high fever, cough, and chest pain. X-rays showed a patchy congestion in the lungs, suggesting pneumonia, but none of the usual bacterial or viral pathogens turned up in diagnostic tests. Cases of the strange illness began appearing in hospitals all around Pennsylvania, and some of the victims were dying. No one made the connection to the legionnaires' convention until July 30, when Ernest Campbell, a physician in the country town of Bloomsburg, found himself treating his third case of the mysterious disease. All three patients were legionnaires who had returned from Philadelphia earlier that week. Campbell immediately notified the state's public health authorities that something unusual was going on, and by the following week, "Legionnaires' disease" had become the biggest media spectacle of the summer.

As the cases mounted, and nightly television news programs showed sorrowful legionnaires lowering the coffins of fallen comrades, an élite cadre of state and federal scientists began the five-month investigation that eventually led to discovering the cause of the mystery epidemic. After excluding more than forty known pathogens and dozens of toxic chemicals, scientists from the United States Centers of Disease Control and Prevention (CDC) announced in January 1977 that Legionnaires' disease was due to a previously unknown bacterium. They dubbed the new bacterium *Legionella pneumophila*. Air pumped through the hotel's air-conditioning system had somehow become contaminated with tiny water droplets—aerosols—that contained the bacteria. The source may have been a cooling tower on the roof of the hotel, which fed water to an evaporative condenser in the subbasement, although this was never proven (Lattimer and Ormsbee 1981). By the time the epidemic subsided in mid-August, Philadelphia's bicentennial party was over. The new disease had affected 221 people, of whom thirty-four had died. The Bellevue-Stratford Hotel eventually went out of business, although the building has since reopened as a hotel, office, and retail-shopping complex.

Legionnaires' disease has since been recognized as a relatively common cause of lung infections, particularly for smokers and those with compromised immunity. It is believed to account for up to one-tenth of community-acquired pneumonia in adults in the United States. *Legionella pneumophila* turns out to be an ubiquitous inhabitant of man-made aquatic environments, and it is resistant to chlorine. Since 1976, aerosols containing the organism have caused numerous outbreaks linked to air-conditioning cooling towers and evaporative coolers. Other outbreaks have been traced to whirlpool spas, showerheads, humidifiers, hospital respiratory devices, decorative fountains, and even an ultrasonic mist machine in a grocery store. In February

1999, more than 230 visitors to the world's largest indoor flower-bulb show in Bovenkarspel, Holland, were taken ill with the disease. Twenty-three people died. Investigators traced the source of infection to the fine aerosol spray given off by a whirlpool spa that was on display in a consumer-products exhibition at the show.

Toxic Shock Syndrome

Anyone who listened to the radio or watched American television during 1979 and early 1980 would not have missed the marketing blitz extolling the latest breakthrough in the science of feminine hygiene: the Rely tampon. No longer would active women have to worry that heavy menstrual flow might slow them down. Proctor and Gamble researchers had developed a tampon with twice the fluid-absorbing capacity of conventional products. The message for the modern woman was simple, and it worked: "You can rely on Rely."

Then in January 1980 the state health departments of Minnesota and Wisconsin reported that nine adult women in their states had recently developed toxic shock syndrome (TSS). A high fever, a drop in blood pressure, a diffuse rash with subsequent peeling, and multiple abnormalities in various organ systems mark this potentially severe syndrome, first described in 1978. By May, a total of fifty-five cases of TSS had been reported nationwide. All but three cases had occurred in otherwise healthy young women, and, for most, the illness seemed to strike during menstruation. By September, numerous epidemiological studies had implicated tampons in TSS, particularly super-absorbent brands such as Rely. In one study, women who used Rely tampons were seven to eight times as likely to develop TSS as women who did not (Schlech, Shands, Reingold, et al. 1982). In fact, nearly three-quarters of the first three hundred American women reported with TSS were Rely users. On the basis of this evidence, Proctor and Gamble voluntarily withdrew Rely tampons from the market on September 19. An intensive public education campaign was launched to inform women about TSS and urge them to avoid super-absorbent tampons.

In 1981, two laboratories independently proved that TSS was due to a potent toxin produced by certain strains of the bacterium *Staphylococcus aureus*. Some observers wondered if TSS emerged because *S. aureus* had recently acquired the genetic apparatus to produce the toxin. But analysis of historical strain collections showed that toxin-producing *S. aureus* had been around at low levels for decades. It is more likely that TSS emerged when it did because of changes in tampon technology, marketing, and use. How Rely tampons actually caused TSS is still not fully understood, but it appears that a surfactant used in their production may have enhanced the ability of *S. aureus* to produce its deadly toxin. An industry-wide return to tampons with significantly lower absorbencies than those manufactured in 1980 has resulted in a steep decline in TSS incidence. Unfortunately, this change came too late for more than fourteen hundred women in the United States, and an unknown number in other countries, who suffered from menstrual TSS linked to tampons.

Lyme Disease

In November 1975, a mother from the rural district of Old Lyme, Connecticut, informed the state health department that twelve children in her community, including four who lived on the same road, were suffering from recurrent attacks of swollen and painful joints, most often in the knees. Local doctors had diagnosed juvenile rheumatoid arthritis (JRA), but the mother knew that JRA is a rare disease, too rare to be turning up so frequently in a community of only five thousand residents. The clustering of cases made the mother wonder if the disease was due to an infection. During the next six months, a team led by Allen Steere of Yale University sought help from doctors, school nurses, local health officers, and patients themselves to locate anyone else in the area having repeated bouts of joint pain and swelling with no obvious cause. In all they found thirty-nine children and twelve adults whose symptoms fit the pattern. Some cases dated back to 1972, and one woman claimed her joint pains had started in 1967. Curiously, a number of patients recalled seeing an expanding, red, ring-like mark on their skin a few weeks before their joint problems set in.

The features of the syndrome really did not fit JRA or any other known disorder affecting the joints. Perhaps the mother who tipped off the authorities was correct: this was an infectious disease. But laboratory tests for all imaginable viruses and bacteria were negative. What could this be? Steere carefully considered the evidence. The communities where the victims lived were sparsely populated and heavily wooded. Most residents, particularly those with the disease, lived in large, forested blocks. The illness tended to begin during the summer months, when people spent more time outdoors. Cases were clustered along certain roads, but there was no evidence of person-to-person spread, as the onset of symptoms, even within families, was usually in different years. These facts suggested that the disease was transmitted by a vector, an insect or other living carrier that spreads infectious agents from one host to another. Steere thought about the intriguing mark on the skin that sometimes preceded the joint symptoms. The mark seemed identical to one described in 1913 by an Austrian physician named Lipschutz, whose report linked the mark to the bite of a tiny *Ixodes* tick. By the 1970s these blood-feeding insects were common in the forests around Old Lyme, although their bites were rarely noticed. It seemed likely that the strange new disorder in the bucolic Lyme region of Connecticut—soon to be known as "Lyme disease"—was due to a pathogen transmitted in the bite of a tick.

By the early 1980s, it became obvious that the new disease was not limited to a few residents of rural Connecticut. Today, Lyme disease is by far the most common vector-borne disease in the United States, striking twelve thousand or more people each year. Although the disease has been reported in forty-five states, about 90 percent of cases occur either along the Atlantic seaboard between Maine and Maryland or in the upper Midwest, especially in western Wisconsin. Lyme disease is also widely reported in Europe, Russia, China, and Japan, wherever *Ixodes* ticks are common. We now know that people stricken with Lyme disease can suffer debilitating effects apart from their joints, including heart problems and neurological disturbances. A portion of cases become chronic, and might involve memory loss, drowsiness, or behavioral changes, in addition to prolonged joint pains. The bacterium that causes the disease, *Borrelia burgdorferi*, was identified in 1982. Most cases respond to antibiotics, but sometimes drugs are ineffective. So-called "Lymies" have become a vocal lobby group in several American states, demanding better services for victims of the disease and increased funding for research. One hopeful sign is that a safe and effective vaccine against Lyme disease was licensed in the United States in 1998.

Escherichia coli O157:H7

During the first half of 1982 a fierce intestinal illness of unknown cause suddenly appeared among at least forty-seven otherwise healthy adults and children in Oregon and Michigan (Riley, Remis, Helgerson, et al. 1983). Patients complained of a rapid onset of severe abdominal pain and cramping, followed a day or two later by

Son of Lyme Disease?

Just when the new Lyme vaccine has made it seem safe to go back in the woods, along comes another new tick-borne disease: human ehrlichiosis. Known for decades to cause ailments in dogs and other animals, bacteria in the *Ehrlichia* group were first linked to human disease in Japan in 1954. There, and later elsewhere in Asia, patients would occasionally develop an illness marked by a high fever and enlarged lymph nodes after eating raw fish infested with infected flukes. Then, in 1986, a fifty-one-year-old man bitten by a tick in Arkansas developed a severe febrile illness that required a prolonged hospitalization. It was later shown that he had been infected by a new species of *Ehrlichia*, which was given the name *E. chaffeensis*. Soon it became clear that these bacteria are spread by the bites of two tick species commonly found in the south-central and southeastern United States: the lone star tick and the American dog tick.

Since then more than seven hundred cases of human disease from this organism have been reported among residents of nineteen states. Not all states monitor the disease, but among those that keep track of it, more than half of all cases have been reported from North Carolina, Virginia, Arkansas, Missouri, and Oklahoma. Usually the illness is mild, but sometimes there are severe headaches and muscle aches together with a fever. Unfortunately, the range of ticks infected with *E. chaffeensis* is expanding, and the number of disease reports is increasing each year. Another form of the disease, which caused a third *Ehrlichia* species, was first identified in humans in 1994. Since then it has affected another 450 people in ten states scattered from New England to California. This type of erhlichiosis is transmitted by the same *Ixodes* ticks that spread Lyme disease, and case reports are concentrated in the states where Lyme disease is common.

The real incidence of ehrlichiosis is probably many times greater than the official figures suggest. Most doctors don't know about the disease, and those who do find it difficult to diagnose, as the symptoms can be very nonspecific. Increasingly doctors are being urged to consider ehrlichiosis in patients who are feverish following a tick bite, as some cases are life-threatening without prompt and appropriate treatment. In the latest twist in this evolving epidemic, Richard Buller and his colleagues (1999) found yet another species of *Ehrlichia* in four Missouri patients stricken with fevers and headaches. Until now, this species was thought to infect only dogs.

repeated bouts of bloody diarrhea. Routine laboratory tests yielded none of the usual causes of diarrhea, but investigators soon linked the strange new illness in both states to consumption of undercooked hamburgers from the McDonald's fast-food chain. Specialized tests performed on stool specimens and meat patties finally revealed that the outbreak was due to an unusual strain of *Escherichia coli*. Microbiologists had called the strain *E. coli* O157:H7, because the so-called 'O' protein on its surface was the one hundred and fifty-seventh one identified, and its 'H' protein was the seventh type to be found.

E. coli is a normal inhabitant of human and animal intestines, but certain strains, defined by their 'O' and 'H' serotypes, can produce diarrhea. *E. coli* O157:H7 causes disease by releasing a powerful toxin that damages the lining of the bowels and causes bleeding. In up to six percent of infections the toxin can also initiate a mass destruction of blood cells and acute kidney failure. This complication, known as the hemolytic uremic syndrome (HUS), is particularly common in young children and the elderly, and is the major cause of death from *E. coli* O157:H7 infections. The primary reservoir, or natural habitat, for *E. coli* O157:H7 is the intestines of cattle. Most human infections occur from eating undercooked beef that was accidentally contaminated during the slaughtering process. Other modes of transmission include the consumption of untreated drinking water, unpasteurized milk, or foods contaminated by raw meat products during preparation. Person-to-person spread is also important, especially in child care centers and nursing homes for the elderly. Investigators in the Oregon and Michigan outbreaks were surprised to find O157:H7, because at that time it was such a rare type of *E. coli* to cause disease. The strain had been seen only once before, in a single case of bloody diarrhea occurring in a fifty-year-old California woman in 1975.

Since then, *E. coli* O157:H7 has become one of the leading bacterial causes of diarrhea and a major cause of food-borne outbreaks. It has been reported on every continent, and is thought to cause at least twenty thousand infections in the United States annually, including 250 deaths. In 1993 more than five hundred diners at the Jack-in-the-Box fast-food chain in Washington state contracted the disease, including fifty-six who developed HUS and four who died. Three years later, several outbreaks of *E. coli* O157:H7 struck Japan, affecting nearly ten thousand people and causing twelve deaths. In the largest outbreak, more than six thousand children in Sakai City, Osaka prefecture, developed the disease after eating school lunches. Later that year an outbreak in Lanarkshire, Central Scotland, was linked to meats sold by a single butcher. In all, 490 cases were reported and eighteen people died.

Back in the United States, *E. coli* O157:H7 was behind the largest food recall in history, when a 1997 outbreak in Colorado forced the maker of frozen ground beef products to recall six lots of potentially contaminated beef burgers that had already been distributed to all forty-eight contiguous states. In 1999, more than eighty thousand pounds of ground beef sold in Illinois, Indiana, and Michigan had to be recalled after *E. coli* O157:H7 was detected by federal meat inspectors. Later that summer, the organism turned up in water supplied to a county fair in New York, where sixty-five people had to be hospitalized and two died. It then sickened more than three hundred people who ate contaminated beef at a big Labor Day party in Illinois, and put twenty-two guests in the hospital. Paul Mead and Patricia Griffin (1998), food-borne disease experts at the CDC, recently summed up the problem with *E. coli* O157:H7 this way: "In one country after another, this once obscure pathogen is challenging clinicians, alarming food producers, and transforming the public's perception about the safety of their food."

Hantavirus Pulmonary Syndrome

The Four Corners is the only place in the United States where the boundaries of four states intersect at one point. Here the states of Arizona, Utah, Colorado, and New Mexico come together on a high desert plateau that is home to many well-known Native American tribes, including the Navaho, the Hopi, the Zuni, and the Ute peoples. This colorful region of rocky outcrops and steep canyons might be the last place to expect a new and terrible disease to emerge. But during the spring months of 1993, it was at the Four Corners that a previously unknown illness appeared in epidemic form, causing acute respiratory failure in twenty-four people and claiming twelve lives. Within a year, Hantavirus Pulmonary Syndrome (HPS) had been diagnosed in seventy-two people from seventeen states, including forty-eight who died.

The first cases that caught the attention of local doctors were those of a twenty-one-year-old woman and nineteen-year-old man; each died from the disease within a few days in mid-May. Both had previously been in good health. The man was a marathon runner. They had planned to marry and were living together in a trailer home at a rural location in New Mexico. At the time of the woman's death, her brother and sister-in-law, both aged twenty-five, moved into the trailer. By the following week the brother had developed the same illness, and five days later his wife was stricken as well. In treating these cases and others occurring around the Four Corners that spring, doctors began to recognize a pattern. Typically, the disease would begin innocently, with no obvious signs of distress. But after a few days the chest would suddenly fill with fluid. Breathing would become increasingly difficult, as if the victims were drowning in their own secretions. In the worst cases, blood pressure would drop so low that the heart would slow down and eventually stop. Even with prompt hospitalization, death could not always be averted (Duchin, Koster, and Peters 1994).

Laboratory tests on clinical and autopsy specimens were negative for all suspected viral and bacterial agents, including *Yersinia pestis*, the bacterium that causes the Black Death, also called plague. The new disease did not bear the usual hallmarks of plague, but doctors had to consider it. Since the importation of the disease from China at the start of the twentieth century, rodents in the American Southwest have become well-known carriers of plague. Rodent numbers had reached unprecedented levels in the spring of 1993. Tests on serum from the Four Corners victims then showed that they had been infected with a previously unknown member of the hantavirus group. At first, the new pathogen was named the Muerto Canyon virus, after the locale where it was first recognized; but when some local people challenged the name it was changed, and has since been called the Sin Nombre ("without name") virus.

By 1993, hantaviruses were already known to cause fever, bleeding, and kidney disease in East Asia and Europe, particularly in Korea and Scandinavia, but they had never been associated with acute illness in the Western Hemisphere. The first known hantavirus, the Hantaan virus, had been isolated from a Korean field mouse in 1977 by researchers seeking to explain an outbreak of fever with hemorrhage that had affected more than three thousand United Nations troops during the Korean War in the early 1950s. Hantaviruses find their natural reservoir in rodents, causing human infections only when people accidentally inhale infected aerosols of rodent urine. Not surprisingly, the trailer where the young couple had lived before their deaths that May was heavily infested with deer mice, rodents known to scientists as *Peromyscus maniculatus*.

Since 1993, the CDC has confirmed 217 cases of HPS in thirty states. Of these, more than 40 percent have died. Not surprisingly, high rates of infection among deer mice surveyed in the Four Corners area during the first five months of 1999 coincided with an upsurge in cases there that spring. Another novel hantavirus that causes HPS has been identified in southern Argentina (Lopez, Padula, Rossi, et al. 1996). This virus may be transmitted person-to-person, and is thought to be expanding its range northward. It is also likely that other unknown hantaviruses are circulating today among isolated rodent populations.

Ebola Hemorrhagic Fever

In 1976, when the CDC asked Joel Breman to investigate the first outbreak of Ebola hemorrhagic fever in Zaire, he knew two things: "First, an outbreak of a severe unknown disease was spreading rapidly into all the villages in a remote area of northern Zaire," he recalled. "Second, all the people in the epidemic area had died" (1995). It was a frightening assignment, but one of great scientific interest. Before Breman left for Zaire, a maximum-security laboratory at CDC had identified a new virus in some blood specimens sent from the field. They named the virus Ebola, after a small river in the epidemic zone. During his travels in Africa, Breman always carried a photograph of the virus, as seen by an electron microscope, and showed it wherever he went. "This assured prince and pauper alike that we were dealing with a disease caused by a microbe, and not a scourge triggered by supernatural forces," he said.

When Ebola virus emerged in Africa that year it may well have seemed like a supernatural event. Outbreaks erupted almost simultaneously in the tiny villages around Yambuku, Zaire, and in Nzara, Sudan, five hundred miles away. In all there were 602 recognized cases, of which 88 percent died in Zaire and 53 percent died in Sudan. After an abrupt onset of fever, victims would become weak and disoriented. Soon they would begin to bleed easily and, some time during the second week, death would ensue from shock and multiorgan dysfunction. Caretakers of the sick and dying typically became victims themselves as the epidemics spread. Breman and his colleagues determined that the first patients in each outbreak had become infected by contact with sick animals living nearby. But the virus' natural reservoir eluded them. The epidemics then disappeared as inexplicably as they had surfaced. After 1976, sporadic cases and relatively small outbreaks surfaced now and again in equatorial Africa, and a closely related virus turned up in a shipment of monkeys imported from the Philippines to Reston, Virginia, in 1989. But it seemed as if Ebola virus had returned benevolently to its primordial hiding place—until 1995.

In January 1995, the Ebola virus came back, this time to Kikwit, an impoverished city of half a million situated on the main road four hundred miles east of Kinshasa, the capital of Zaire. Here there were at least 315 cases and 244 deaths, starting with a forty-two-year-old man who worked in the nearby forest. He passed the disease to twelve family members who cared for him at home or handled his body when he died. Other cases in Kikwit included at least ninety health care professionals exposed to the bodily fluids of dying patients. Among these were members of a surgical team, who were drenched in blood when they attempted to operate on the distended abdomen of an infected hospital worker. By the time the epidemic peaked in May, the city's ramshackle, 350-bed hospital was virtually deserted for lack of available staff. The Kikwit outbreak was especially disquieting because it was the first time the Ebola virus had appeared in a large and densely populated urban center. The odds for uncontrolled spread were alarming, and the city was placed under a strict quarantine until the epidemic passed. By now the world had become familiar with the dangers of Ebola virus through books, magazine articles, and the popular movie *Outbreak*. Television cameras rolled as international investigators donned protective suits and respirators to study the "killer virus."

Ebola virus has since returned twice to the Ogooué-Ivindo province of Gabon, a country straddling the equator on Africa's Atlantic coast, where it has claimed at least sixty-four lives. The first outbreak was linked to the butchering of infected chimpanzees for food, but extensive research since the Kikwit and Gabon outbreaks has failed to locate the definitive hosts of Ebola virus in nature. Monkeys and apes are considered unlikely candidates, as the virus is just as rapidly lethal for them as it is for humans. The real reservoir species must be one that can sustain the infection for long periods, but as yet its identity remains an enigma.

Variant Creutzfeldt-Jakob Disease

At three o'clock in the afternoon on March 20, 1996, Stephen Dorrell, the British Secretary of State for Health, read a terse statement to the House of Commons. He said that a government-appointed committee of scientists had discovered a possible link between bovine spongiform encephalopathy (BSE) in cattle and a devastating brain disease that had recently stricken ten people in the United Kingdom. "The committee has concluded that the most likely explanation at present is that these cases are linked to exposure to BSE," Dorrell said.

Despite years of official assurances that a runaway problem with BSE in Britain's cattle posed no threat to human health, the Tory government was now obliquely admitting that people who had eaten meats produced from British cattle risked developing a human form of "mad cow disease." As some experts speculated that there might eventually be a million human cases, a stunned British public learned the stories of the ordinary people who had died merely because they had eaten hamburgers. "My son is lost. Now we must get to grips with this problem before more lives are lost," the mother of a twenty-year-old victim told news reporters. At the time of his death the young man was a vegetarian, but as a boy he had a fondness for beef burgers, his mother said.

The new disease was a distinctive variant of the rare degenerative brain disorder known as Creutzfeldt-Jakob disease (CJD). Like traditional CJD, the new variant form of the disease (vCJD) would start insidiously, before it swiftly progressed to undermine memory, thought, movement, and balance. Like traditional CJD, it did not respond to any treatment, and death was inescapable. But unlike traditional CJD, which typically affects those aged sixty and above, the victims of vCJD were young. Three of the cases made public that afternoon occurred in teenagers. Five victims were in their twenties, and the oldest was only thirty-nine. Psychiatric symptoms were a distinctive early feature, and microscopic examination of brain specimens from those with the new variant yielded a picture quite dissimilar from traditional CJD.

Soon after the initial announcement, the European Union imposed a worldwide ban on exports of British beef. Many British schools banned beef from their cafeterias, and a mass slaughter of cattle over thirty months of age was begun across the United Kingdom. To date, the dire predictions of a massive epidemic of vCJD have not eventuated. By the end of July 1999, only forty-three cases had been detected in Britain, one in France (a country that once consumed large amounts of British beef), and one in Ireland. There is hope that vCJD will remain a medical oddity, but it is too early to know for sure. Future trends in the new disease will depend on the length of its incubation period, which is the time between exposure to the infectious agent and the onset of disease symptoms. The average incubation period for vCJD is unknown, but there is reason to believe it could range as high as thirty years or more (see chapter 6 for more details).

If so, the cases we've seen so far are just statistical outliers, early arrivals in an unfolding saga of misery and death. As Jeffrey Almond and John Pattison (1997), two scientists on the British government's advisory committee on BSE recently noted, "It may take several years before we can be confident that this is not a period of comparative calm before a storm."

Pigs in the Middle: Malaysia's Nipah Virus Outbreak

The newest of the world's new microbial foes came to light in the early months of 1999, when a severe febrile illness affecting pigs in Malaysia was found to jump the species barrier to sicken the people rearing them. In humans, the disease caused fever, severe headaches, and inflammation of the brain, leading frequently to death. At the height of the epidemic, a steady stream of patients filled the beds at University Hospital in Kuala Lumpur, Malaysia's capital. Families of victims crowded the corridors as doctors did what they could to help the victims. "The mortality was very high, sometimes three deaths a day," said Patrick Tan (1999), who helped run the hospital's intensive care unit. "You would see a son die at seven in the morning and his father pass away at noon. We were clearly dealing with something unknown and very threatening."

In September 1998, the disease had surfaced first among pigs in the northern state of Perak. The infection gave the pigs a terrible cough. Farmers called it "one mile cough" because it could be heard a mile away. By December, shipments of infected pigs had brought the disease to the state of Negri Sembilan, just south of Kuala Lumpur. It spread rapidly among pigs throughout the state, and by March had inundated the major pig farming districts around the city of Bukit Pelandok. By April, more than 250 cases had occurred in humans, of whom one hundred had died. As the death toll mounted, the Malaysian government ordered the slaughter of more than one million pigs, a massacre that devastated the country's $400 million pork industry. Eventually the epidemic waned, but sporadic cases in pigs and people alike continued for much of the year.

The first human cases looked like Japanese encephalitis, a viral disease spread by mosquitoes in many rural areas of Southeast Asia, China, and the Indian subcontinent. But field investiations showed that the mystery illness couldn't be one that was spread by mosquitoes.

Instead, nearly all the cases seemed to result from touching or handling pigs, especially pigs that appeared to be ill. This suggested that another agent was involved, and in March an analysis of specimens taken from a deceased truck driver showed that the causative virus was in fact something new. Before his death, the driver had lived in the village of Sungai Nipah, and by April, the world would come to know the virus that killed him as the Nipah virus.

It is still unclear exactly how the Nipah virus found its way into the pigs of Malaysia, but the encroachment of pig farming into the tropical habitat of local bats is strongly suspected. The Nipah virus' closest cousin, the Hendra virus of Queensland, Australia, is known to circulate primarily among certain species of Australian fruit bats. Humans and domesticated animals are merely accidental hosts. The Hendra virus, which was first identified in a Brisbane suburb of that name, caused an explosive outbreak of respiratory disease among twenty racehorses in 1994. A trainer and a stable hand were infected, and the trainer died. In an unrelated outbreak, the virus killed two horses and a farmer in Mackay, six hundred miles further north on the Queensland coast. Where in the world another relative of the Nipah and Hendra viruses will emerge next is unknown, but it will not be surprising when it does.

Diseases on the Comeback Trail

As distressing as newly identified diseases are for the communities in which they emerge, the return of diseases that once seemed well controlled can be even more perturbing for public health professionals working in the front lines. The contemporary renaissance of leading infectious killers from decades or centuries ago is a frightening testimony to the resilience of our microbial foes. It will not be possible here to introduce all the important infections that are currently rebounding around the world, but they will be discussed in detail in later chapters. Included here are the stories of three major reversals in the control of infectious diseases, together with a sidebar box on the resurgence of meningococcal disease at home and abroad.

Cholera

Cholera is an acute intestinal infection transmitted by food or water contaminated with the bacterium _Vibrio cholerae_. Infections are often mild, but sometimes there is profuse, watery diarrhea, which leads rapidly to death from severe dehydration. Cholera has been known since antiquity in the delta region of the Ganges and Brahmaputra rivers, but it did not spread beyond the Indian subcontinent until 1817. That year, a particularly severe outbreak in the Ganges River valley expanded across Asia and the Middle East. A second cholera pandemic reached Europe and North America in 1831, causing tens of thousands of deaths and untold misery in one defenseless community after another. The disease unleashed near-hysteria in London, New York, Montreal, and other teeming industrial cities along its path. Four more waves of cholera swept the globe until the early twentieth century, when the disease inexplicably vanished in all but a few remote areas of Asia. The seventh great pandemic, which is still ongoing, began on the Celebes Island of Indonesia in 1961. The pandemic strain, _V. cholerae_ O1 biotype El Tor, spread rapidly to the Philippines and the countries of East Asia before reaching India in

1964. By 1970, it had settled in West Africa for the first time in a century, and soon cholera became endemic throughout most of the continent.

Cholera had been absent from Latin America since 1895, but, during 1991, it came back with a vengeance. In late January that year, explosive outbreaks due to the El Tor strain were reported almost simultaneously from cities along an eight-hundred-mile stretch of coastal Peru. At least thirty thousand cases occurred within three weeks, including 114 deaths. By February, cholera had spread to the interior of Peru, and, in March, it was established throughout Ecuador and parts of Colombia. By the end of the year, the epidemic had affected at least 391 thousand people in fourteen Latin American countries. The most vulnerable populations were those living in the region's congested periurban *favelas*, squalid slums that lack reliable supplies of potable water and adequate means of sewage disposal. But as the epidemic unfolded the poor and dispossessed were not the only victims. In February 1992, the cholera threat hit home for North Americans when passengers on a Boeing 747 flying from Lima to Los Angeles came down with the disease after eating contaminated airline food. One passenger died, and at least seventy-four others were sickened, accounting for the highest incidence of cholera in the United States during the twentieth century.

By the end of 1994, the Latin American epidemic had affected more than one million people in twenty countries, causing at least ten thousand deaths. These are official figures; the actual caseload was probably much greater. The epidemic looked like it was slowing down by 1997, but there was an upsurge in 1998 in connection with the El Niño weather pattern. Since then, every country from Mexico southwards has continued to report cases, except Argentina, Paraguay, and Uruguay. During the late 1990s the countries of East Africa have also figured prominently in global cholera statistics, especially Kenya, Mozambique, Somalia, Uganda, Djibouti, and Tanzania. Rwandan refugees residing in temporary camps in eastern Zaire were hit hard by cholera epidemics in 1994 and again in 1997. Outbreaks have also been reported recently in war-torn districts of southern Sudan, northeastern Cambodia, and central Afghanistan. In 1999, Taiwan had its first case of cholera in thirty years, and Madagascar suffered its first outbreaks in more than a century.

As if a resurgence of classical cholera were not enough, a new variant of *V. cholerae* appeared in India in October 1992 and spread rapidly to nine other countries in southern Asia. The new strain, dubbed "O139 Bengal," produces severe, watery diarrhea identical to ordinary cholera, but prior infection with conventional strains like El

Tor confers no immune protection against it. Less than a year after its discovery, the first case of O139 Bengal cholera was reported in the United States (Centers for Disease Control and Prevention 1993).

Malaria

Malaria, a parasitic disease spread by *Anopheles* mosquitoes, is as old as humanity itself. Its high fevers and enlarged spleen were well-known to Chinese physicians writing the Nei Ching Canon of Medicine in 1700 B.C. Hippocrates, the great medical thinker of ancient Athens, clearly linked outbreaks of malaria to the stagnant waters of marshes where mosquitoes breed. A sixteenth-century Italian belief that the disease traveled through foul air gave malaria its modern name, which literally means "bad air." References to malaria can be found in the works of Homer, Chaucer, and Shakespeare, and the disease remained firmly entrenched in much of the Untied States, Canada, and Europe well into the twentieth century. The federal agency that would become the CDC was established in Atlanta in 1942 to coordinate control of the disease. The initial aim was to keep more than six hundred military bases and essential weapons-production facilities in the Southern states malaria-free as the country mobilized for World War II. But with the coming of the miracle pesticide DDT in 1943, it quickly became possible to rid civilian populations of the disease too. Soon DDT was widely applied wherever *Anopheles* mosquitoes lived, especially in developing countries of the tropics where malaria had always been a major impediment to economic and social development. Hopes that malaria would be conquered were coming true during the 1950s. The experience in India was typical: Before DDT spraying began in 1946, India suffered seventy-five million cases of malaria each year, with eight hundred thousand deaths. By 1961, there were fewer than fifty thousand cases and virtually no deaths (Walker 1997).

Today, all hopes of eliminating malaria have vanished. The worldwide incidence of the disease has skyrocketed since the early 1990s. Malaria is now responsible for sickening nearly three hundred million people in more than ninety countries, where 40 percent of the world's population lives. At least a million people are dying from malaria each year, more today than when control programs began fifty years ago. Three-quarters of the dead are young children who are too poor to receive antimalarial drugs. In some villages of The Gambia, one child in twenty will die from malaria before the age of five. Survivors of malaria often have little to be glad about, as the disease can damage the brain and other vital organs, leading to permanent disabilities. For the hundreds of millions who are recurrently infected with any of the four species of *Plasmodium* protozoa that cause malaria, even the ordinary activities of life can become a struggle because of the ravaging anemia brought on by the disease.

In Africa, where up to 90 percent of cases occur today, the comeback of malaria is a far bigger public health problem than the Ebola virus. In some areas it is much more threatening than HIV. "Malaria keeps Africa down, and down is where the rest of the world wants us to be," notes Mamadou Kasse (1997), medical editor of a Senegal newspaper. Poverty, civil strife, drug resistance, and a disintegration of routine disease control measures have all contributed to the resurgence of malaria in Africa, India, Brazil, and other tropical areas. But problems with malaria are not limited to poor countries of the developing world. The disease is frequently encountered by Western travelers to malarial areas, with more than one thousand cases reported in Americans returning from overseas trips each year. Of even greater concern is the possibility that intercontinental travel and commerce will reintroduce malaria transmission within industrialized countries, including those where the disease has long been eradicated. For the first time in decades, outbreaks of locally acquired malaria have been recently reported in the United States and Europe. (See chapters 3 and 4 for more information.)

Diphtheria

Diphtheria is a bacterial disease that can rapidly lead to death from suffocation and heart failure. Its name is derived from the Greek word for "leather," referring to the tough, gray membrane that forms in the throat in reaction to a potent toxin released by the causative agent, *Cornebacterium diphtheriae*. Outbreaks of diphtheria have been reported since Roman times. A major epidemic in New England during the 1730s caused panic in many communities and threatened the survival of British colonies in North America. The dreaded contagion moved from town to town, striking down up to 40 percent of the region's children under ten years of age, typically within twelve hours of the onset of symptoms. It was not unusual for large families to lose all their children in a matter of days. An anonymous poem from that time, titled "A Lamentation," put words to the helplessness that many parents felt (Anonymous 1987):

> What tears apace, run from our Face,
> to hear our Children crying

For help from pain, but all in vain,
we cannot help their dying.

Diphtheria remained common in industrialized countries during the first decades of the twentieth century. More than 147 thousand cases were still reported in the United States as late as 1920, and, in Canada, diphtheria prevailed as the leading killer of children aged two to fourteen from 1921 to 1924. From the 1940s, the incidence of diphtheria plummeted in most countries thanks to childhood immunization with a purified derivative of diphtheria toxin. By the 1980s, the disease had become rare in Western countries, with fewer than four cases reported per year in the United States. By this time, diphtheria was also well controlled in the Soviet Union. Universal childhood vaccination had brought the annual incidence as low as 198 cases per year among a population of nearly three hundred million.

Then, in 1990, just as Communism was collapsing, diphtheria reemerged in Moscow and rapidly spread to other urban centers of Russia and the Ukraine (Hardy, Dittmann, and Sutter 1996). Each year, the epidemic escalated, until more than 140 thousand cases were reported throughout Russia and each of the fourteen other newly independent states by 1996. Of these, about four thousand cases were fatal. Investigators blamed the epidemic in part on the failure of the crumbling public health infrastructure to maintain adequate levels of immunity against the disease during a time of massive social and economic upheaval. Large populations of unimmunized children, and ever-increasing numbers of adults overdue for routine booster vaccines, sustained transmission of the disease across thirteen time zones from the Baltic states to eastern Siberia. Shortages of vaccines and ineffective control measures at the start of the epidemic compounded the catastrophe. The diphtheria crisis in the former Soviet Union has now subsided, but it was a reminder of how forgotten scourges of the past can suddenly reappear.

Emergence through Better Understanding

Front-page stories about infectious diseases are not always bad news. Advances in biomedical technology sometimes allow the discovery of microbes that have been around for a long time. Such newly recognized agents are not really emerging: It is only our understanding that has changed. Occasionally these newly detected microbes can be

The Savage and Mysterious Ways of Meningococcal Disease

Meningococci are bacteria that turn up harmlessly in the back of the throat or nose in about ten percent of the population. They cause disease only rarely, but, when they do, the illness is sudden, severe, and sometimes fatal. Early signs of meningococcal disease include fever, an intense headache, nausea and vomiting, a stiff neck, an aversion to bright lights, and sometimes a telltale rash. Delirium and coma are also seen. Commonly, the disease results in meningitis, an inflammation of the meninges, the soft tissues that cover the brain. Most fatal cases occur when the bacteria inundate the bloodstream, causing septicaemia. Immense epidemics of meningococcal meningitis periodically sweep across a belt of sub-Saharan Africa stretching from Senegal in the west to Ethiopia in the east. In the most recent epidemic, in 1996, more than 187 thousand people became ill in a region centered on Mali, Burkina Faso, Niger, and northern Nigeria, and up to 20 thousand victims died. In recent years, the territory covered by the African "meningitis belt" has been expanding. This may be due to global climatic changes, or increased population movements, or both.

Large African-style epidemics are not seen in the United States, but since 1993 sporadic cases of meningococcal disease have been on the rise in the states of the Pacific Northwest. By 1996, the incidence rate for meningococcal disease in Oregon had reached four per one hundred thousand, a level four times greater than rates in the United States at large. Rates in neighboring Washington state have also been increasing, and are now higher than in any year since 1953 (Diermayer, Hedberg, Hoesly, et al. 1999). Worrisome as these rates may be, they dim in comparison to those across the Pacific Ocean in New Zealand. There, a scattered epidemic of meningococcal disease has chalked up more than 2,600 cases, including 121 deaths, since 1991. With a population of just 3.4 million, New Zealand's recent rates surpass those of Oregon by a factor of four. In 1997, the disease struck nearly one in every one hundred children under twelve months of age in New Zealand's large Pacific Island ethnic groups.

Most cases in each epidemic are due to distinct bacterial strains belonging to a class of meningococci known as serogroup B. The Oregon strain is very similar to one that caused a prolonged epidemic in Norway starting in 1974. Other related strains have caused smoldering outbreaks in Cuba, Chile, and Brazil in recent years. It is unclear why these particular organisms appear when they do and extract such a heavy toll, although exposure to second-hand tobacco smoke and living in damp, overcrowded housing are known to exacerbate the risk of disease. Unfortunately, strains from serogroup B are the only epidemic varieties of meningococci for which there is no proven vaccine. The only way to limit these organisms' heart-breaking effects is to educate the public about the signs of infection and to ask doctors to commence antibiotic treatment as soon as they suspect meningococcal disease. Reducing cigarette smoking around children and improving living conditions for poor families may also help.

linked to age-old human diseases of unknown cause, including some never thought previously to have infectious origins. Increasingly, infectious agents are now suggested to cause, or at least contribute to, many of humanity's most common and severe chronic diseases. Such emerging understandings have revolutionized medicine, creating exciting new opportunities for the treatment and prevention of several refractory diseases. No discovery has caused more excitement than the association of a previously unknown bacterium with peptic ulcer disease.

Until recently the major causes of peptic ulcers were thought to be excess stomach acid, diet, smoking, and psychological stress. Ulcers, which cause prolonged episodes of gnawing pain and occasionally disastrous complications, were a common problem of middle-aged to older adults, especially men. Up to 10 percent of the population would be stricken at some time during their lives, and relapses were common. Daily medications aimed at reducing stomach acid offered the only hope of relief, and, by the 1980s, acid inhibitors like Zantac and Tagamet had became the biggest-selling prescription drugs in the world. Then, in 1983, two doctors from Perth, Western Australia, suggested that the spiral-shaped bacteria they had begun to observe in tissue biopsies from ulcer patients were actually causing the disease (Marshall and Warren 1984). The bacteria, which came to be called *Helicobacter pylori*, could be eradicated with a brief course of antibiotics, eliminating ulcers once and for all.

At first the Australians' proposal seemed preposterous, but, after hundreds of experiments, it was proven correct. Today it is generally accepted that *H. pylori* causes almost all cases of ulcer disease, except the small proportion due to drugs such as aspirin. How *H. pylori* is transmitted is unknown, but poor sanitation and crowded housing clearly facilitate spread. The organism is also a strong risk factor for cancer of the stomach, a common disease in developing countries where two-thirds of children are infected with *H. pylori* by the age of ten. In industrialized countries, children rarely harbor the organism, but the prevalence of infection increases with age. In Western Europe and the United States more than half the population over the age of sixty has the organism. Most will never develop ulcers, but for those who do, up to 90 percent can now be cured with a cocktail of inexpensive and effective antibiotics.

H. pylori is the only kind of bacterium thus far linked to cancer, but several viruses already share that distinction. On a global scale, viruses may account for as many as 15 percent of cancer deaths, particularly those due to cancers of the liver and cervix. Chronic infections with either the hepatitis B virus or the hepatitis C virus are responsible for up to 80 percent of liver cancers worldwide. Liver cancer is relatively rare in most Western countries, but it is among the most common cancers diagnosed in parts of sub-Saharan Africa and Southeast Asia. For example, liver cancer accounts for 70 percent of all cancers reported in Mozambique. Among men, the risk of death from liver cancer is twenty times higher in that East African country than in the United States, largely because of the increased likelihood of viral hepatitis early in life. More than 90 percent of cervical cancers show evidence of infection with certain types of human papillomavirus (HPV). HPV is the cause of most genital warts, one of the most common sexually transmitted diseases. Before Pap tests became a routine part of medical care, cervical cancer caused more deaths among American women than cancer at any other site. Globally, the disease remains a leading cancer killer, especially in certain countries of Latin America and Eastern Europe.

Other chronic diseases recently attributed to infectious agents include ischemic heart disease, the leading cause of death in virtually all industrialized countries. The suspect here is a bacterium known as *Chlamydia pneumoniae,* a common respiratory pathogen that infects more than half the population at some time in their lives. Evidence thus far is not conclusive, but it is possible that infection with *C. pneumoniae* somehow induces inflammatory changes in the arteries that supply the muscles of the heart. Such inflammation might set in motion the formation of atherosclerotic plaques, which upon rupture would cause heart attacks and sudden death. If this hypothesis turns out to be right, antibiotics may one day be dispensed to treat and prevent heart disease. Infectious causes and cofactors have also been proposed recently for insulin-dependent diabetes mellitus, asthma, multiple sclerosis, rheumatoid arthritis, obesity, and even various mental illnesses, such as depression and schizophrenia. Modern medicine is looking increasingly to the microbial world to explain many of humanity's most puzzling diseases.

The rest of this book looks beyond such puzzles to consider the underlying factors causing the emergence and reemergence of diseases that are obviously of infectious origin. In the next chapter we begin with international travel and commerce. People and commodities on the go have a long and lamentable history of introducing infectious agents and disease vectors into new territories. The speed and volume of traffic moving around the globe today has no precedent. Regrettably, the rapid growth of air travel and the globalization of trade are giving many unwanted microbial passengers a free ride to distant places.

What You Can Do to Prevent Tick-Borne Diseases

Lyme disease and erhlichiosis don't have to spoil your enjoyment of the great outdoors. A few routine precautions can greatly reduce your risk, according to the CDC and state public health departments:

- When planning to enter areas likely to be infested with ticks, wear light-colored clothing, so that ticks can be spotted and removed before they attach.

- Create a barrier by tucking your pants into your socks or boot tops, and wear a long-sleeved shirt.

- If you use an insect repellent, carefully follow the directions on the container.

- When in a tick-infested habitat, walk in the center of the trail to avoid picking up ticks hiding in the moist, low-lying vegetation around you.

- When you return from your outing, check and recheck yourself and fellow travelers for ticks. Check your dog or cat before allowing the animal inside your home.

- If you spot a tick, don't panic. Grasp the tick close to its mouth parts with tweezers and pull the tick's body away from the skin with a steady motion.

Transmission of tick-borne diseases does not generally occur until the tick has been attached for at least twenty-four hours. Cleanse the area of the tick bite with an antiseptic, and seek medical attention if any signs or symptoms develop over the ensuing days or weeks. If you live, work, or have recreation in areas with a high or moderate risk of Lyme disease, and have frequent or prolonged exposure to tick-infested habitats, you may consider receiving the new Lyme disease vaccine. The vaccine is given in three doses, and is currently licensed for people aged fifteen to seventy years. See your doctor for more details.

Chapter 3

Travel and Commerce

The journey of microbial agents from one country to another, often shorter than the incubation period of the disease, is rendering border controls futile.

—Bruce J. Plotkin and Ann Marie
Kimball, University of Washington

The nonstop movement of people and goods over vast distances is a hallmark of our global economy. Our growing mobility and our daily exposure to people and products from faraway places is enriching and adding variety to our experience of life. It is gradually dissolving our insular attitudes and drawing us into closer relations with countries very different from our own. For humans, there are still many barriers to forming a single-world community. But for the microbes that travel in our ships and airplanes, the world today is truly a global village.

More than half a billion travelers cross international borders every year. Of these, more than 110 million change continents to reach their destinations. Visitors passing through a region can have a pivotal role in disease emergence and spread. We have already seen how truck drivers and other travelers in East Africa probably hastened the dissemination of HIV from its remote jungle habitation. Any city in the world with an airport or a seaport will today play host to visitors whose microbial "baggage" includes some unwanted pathogens. Very few American communities are isolated from the global travel flow. Nearly five hundred thousand scheduled flights now arrive from foreign countries at some 102 international airports in the United States every year.

Today's unprecedented transit of human passengers is dwarfed by the movement of material goods, primarily by container vessels at sea. World trade has increased by 1,500 percent since 1960. Trade in food alone is worth more than $500 billion worldwide, four times more than it was twenty years ago. Thirty years ago foreign trade represented just 13 percent of United States gross domestic product (GDP). Today it has surpassed 30 percent of GDP, with a value exceeding $2.3 trillion. Advances in trade liberalization are rapidly creating a single global market that no country can afford not to join. Tariff reductions negotiated under the General Agreement on Tariffs and Trade (GATT) and new international accords creating open markets for capital investment have dramatically accelerated the free movement of money, goods, and services among signatory countries. In the race to remain competitive in a unified world economy, governments are becoming more reluctant than ever to regulate trade and impose restrictions at the border on imports and exports.

The impact of the global trade is most easily seen at America's commercial ports. More than 665 million metric tons of imported cargo are now unloaded there annually, up from 308 million metric tons in 1970. By the year 2020, the volume of imported goods coming into the United States will triple again, according to the United States Customs Service (1999). Ships are well-known to carry infectious agents, not just in the foods, animals, or other goods listed on the manifest. They also transport microbes in the rats, mosquitoes, or other vermin that sometimes hitch a ride in the cargo hold.

Even a ship's ballast water can spread infections from one part of the world to another. Stricter checks can be imposed on arriving passengers and goods. But with today's growing bulk, scope, and velocity of international traffic, it may not be realistic to think we can prevent the globalization of all microbial risks. As long as people want to travel and to buy things that other countries produce, emerging infections that are spread by commerce and travel will inevitably diffuse into new populations in new places. In this ever-shrinking world, infectious hazards in far-off lands can no longer be safely ignored, as raspberry consumers in North America recently discovered.

Diarrhea Fresh from the Farm

Before 1996, infections with the protozoan parasite *Cyclospora* were a medical curiosity, of interest only to a few parasitologists and infectious disease specialists. The organism was not fully described until 1993. But the diarrheal illness it causes had first been reported in 1979, when it was seen in two children and an adult in Papua New Guinea. During the next decade, the organism we now call *Cyclospora* was isolated from stool specimens of residents and travelers from various regions, including Haiti, Peru, and Nepal. In one study, *Cyclospora* was found to cause up to 11 percent of intestinal illness among expatriates in Kathmandu, especially during the rainy season (Hoge, Shlim, Rajah, et al, 1993). But the parasite was rarely seen in developed countries, except in a handful of returning travelers. Few doctors in North America, Europe, or Australia had even heard of *Cyclospora*—until 1996.

In spring that year, doctors in the eastern United States and Canada started seeing people complaining of relapsing episodes of watery diarrhea. Other symptoms included nausea, vomiting, bloating, cramping, fatigue, and weight loss. Most clinical laboratories were not routinely looking for *Cyclospora* in stool specimens, so the outbreak went unnoticed at first. When some specimens in New York City tested positive at a hospital that happened to search for *Cyclospora*, public health doctors like Marcelle Layton (1997) of the city's Bureau of Communicable Disease knew that something unusual was going on. She asked all diagnostic laboratories in the city to start testing specifically for *Cyclospora*, and she asked doctors to make sure they collected specimens for testing from all patients with diarrhea. She also issued a news media release, advising New Yorkers with prolonged diarrhea to see their doctors and receive the test.

Layton ended up with 161 confirmed cases, most of whom could be interviewed by telephone. Among the cases, men outnumbered women. They tended to be white, well-educated professionals in their forties and fifties, usually without children. One-third of those who became ill owned a second home. Almost all were otherwise healthy, but 6 percent had to be hospitalized because of their illness. When Layton compared what the patients had been eating in the week prior to their illness with the foods reported by a control group, she found a striking association between *Cyclospora* and fresh raspberries. How ironic! Here was a nutritious fruit that doctors would zealously recommend as a "heart-healthy" snack or dessert. Here was a food valued by New York chefs as a sweet and colorful garnish for a range of popular gourmet concoctions. But here was the first food ever shown to transmit *Cyclospora*, an emerging disease.

Layton's findings were confirmed that spring around North America, where 1,465 cases of *Cyclospora* infection were reported from twenty states, the District of Columbia, and two Canadian provinces. Nearly half the confirmed cases involved people attending one of fifty-five social functions held during May and early June. Raspberries were served at nearly all of those functions, and, where the source of the raspberries could be traced, they were invariably imported from Guatemala. In fact, all the contaminated raspberries may have been produced at as few as five large farms. These farms picked their berries by hand, packed them in market-ready plastic containers, and shipped them by air to the United States within thirty-six hours of picking. In just a few days, upscale diners in New York could share the same infections as dispossessed farm workers in Guatemala.

Investigators of the 1996 outbreak found that water used in growing raspberries in Guatemala was filtered to remove debris, but not microbes (Herwaldt, Ackers, and the *Cyclospora* Working Group 1997). Many farm water supplies were suboptimally constructed, vulnerable to contamination from nearby deep pit latrines. The investigators even showed that water on the implicated farms was intermittently contaminated with fecal bacteria. To prevent berries from having contact with the water, the farmers used ground-level drip irrigation systems during the dry season. But farm workers routinely used the farm water to mix insecticides and fungicides that were sprayed directly onto the berries. The investigators surmised that the raspberries became contaminated through such spraying. On some occasions the spraying might have occurred as late as the day the berries were picked. The berries remained contaminated until eaten, as they were too fragile and had too many crevices to be washed thoroughly.

Cyclospora outbreaks have returned to North America each spring since the initial epidemic, despite efforts to improve sanitation and water quality at Guatemalan berry farms. In April and May 1997, the disease sickened at least eight hundred people who had attended forty-one catered functions in thirteen states. The only food served at all forty-one events was fresh raspberries. As before, nearly all the berries that health authorities could trace had been imported from Guatemala. This time around, the federal Food and Drug Administration (FDA) suspended imports of Guatemalan raspberries to the United States, but that merely shifted the disease to Canada in 1998. In Ontario that spring, more than three hundred people were infected with *Cyclospora*, and for the third year in a row investigations of case clusters showed that Guatemalan raspberries were to blame. "It is clear that the control measures instituted after the 1996 outbreak were inadequate to address the actual source of contamination," notes Michael Osterholm (1999), the lead consultant on emerging infections for the Council of State and Territorial Epidemiologists.

Unfortunately, Guatemalan raspberries have not been the only transgressors behind recent *Cyclospora* outbreaks. Two clusters of the disease in Florida in 1997 were associated with eating mesclun, a mixture of baby lettuce leaves. An outbreak among forty-eight people attending a luncheon in Virginia that year was linked to contaminated basil used to prepare a cold basil-pesto salad. In 1999, Guatemalan raspberries were judged not to play a role in another highly publicized outbreak. This incident involved at least ninety-four people from twenty-eight states who were attending an insurance convention at a famed hotel in Palm Beach, Florida. While there was no evidence that Guatemalan raspberries had transmitted the infection in this instance—no source could be proven beyond doubt—one or more other imported ingredients in a fresh fruit platter served at the convention were the likeliest culprits.

The World on Your Dinner Plate

Raspberries are not native to Guatemala. The first raspberry vine was planted there in 1987 with the aim of supplying North American consumers. The fruit is well suited to the Guatemalan climate, and the cost of growing berries there is lower than in California and other areas that traditionally served United States markets. By May 1996, 20 percent of the raspberries sold in the United States, including 40 percent of those sold in New York, were air-shipped from Guatemala.

Changes in the raspberry business are indicative of a quiet revolution taking place at the corner supermarket. First, health-driven changes in diet are increasing the demand for fresh fruits and vegetables in industrialized countries. In the United States, the average consumption of fruits and vegetables has risen by 50 percent since 1970, and public health programs are aiming for even greater consumption to reduce the risk of major killers like heart disease and cancer. Secondly, overseas suppliers are playing a larger role in meeting the year-round demand for fresh produce. Imports of fruits and vegetables to the United States have doubled since 1990.

Until recently, most foods consumed locally were produced locally. Outbreaks of food-borne disease usually had a local source, and public health authorities acting locally could resolve the problem. Not today. The globalization of food, particularly fresh foods that are served uncooked, has conveyed infectious agents from distant corners of the world into the family kitchen. Ingredients for a single meal may originate from many different countries, sources well beyond the reach of the local health department. It is especially worrisome that many of the new suppliers in the global food market operate from countries with inferior sanitation. Today, up to 70 percent of selected fruits and vegetables sold in the United States are grown in developing countries. Doctors advise patients visiting these countries to reduce their risk of traveler's diarrhea by only eating foods that can be boiled or peeled. With so much food imported today from developing countries, "one does not need to leave home to contract travelers' diarrhea caused by an exotic agent," says Osterholm (1997a).

Guatemalan raspberries are not the only imported foods recently linked to the sudden appearance of emerging infections. "It is now possible to produce a food product anywhere, process it for distribution anywhere, for consumption anywhere," says David Swerdlow (1998), a food-borne disease expert at the CDC. Often the foods implicated in outbreaks can be traced back to sources in developing countries, but only after they have caused substantial disease. For example:

- Frozen strawberries supplied to government-sponsored school lunch programs in six states of the United States were found to be contaminated with hepatitis A virus after more than 150 children developed the disease in Michigan during March 1997. The strawberries had been grown in Mexico before they were processed, packed, and frozen in California. Thousands of children who ate lunches made with the strawberries had to receive injections of immune globulin to prevent more cases of the disease.

- Raw green onions, also called scallions, were behind an outbreak of dysentery due to *Shigella fiexneri* in Illinois and Indiana during 1994. The implicated onions were traced to various California-based shippers, all of whom obtained their green onions from a single farm in Mexico. Migrant workers at the farm were reportedly ill with dysentery at the time the onions were harvested.

- Frozen fresh coconut milk imported from Thailand was responsible for four cases of cholera in Maryland during 1991. Imported coconuts also figured prominently in a 1996 outbreak of paratyphoid fever in Singapore. A total of 167 cases of paratyphoid were reported over three months, mostly among ethnic Indians. Investigators determined that some of the one hundred thousand de-husked and de-shelled coconuts imported each day into Singapore had been contaminated in their various Asian countries of origin (Teoh, Goh, Neo, et al. 1997). The de-shelled coconuts were then transported to Singapore and stored without refrigeration, despite the region's tropical heat. This allowed bacteria to multiply to sufficient numbers to cause infection. Cases ceased when the importation of de-shelled coconuts into Singapore was banned.

- Fresh chopped parsley was linked to seven restaurant-associated outbreaks of *Shigella sonnei* during the summer of 1998 in the United States and Canada. In all, at least 486 people developed diarrhea, of whom twenty-two were hospitalized. Parsley implicated in six of the outbreaks was traced to a single one thousand-acre farm in Baja California, Mexico. At the farm, investigators found that water used to irrigate the parsley was not chlorinated, and was vulnerable to contamination (Centers for Disease Control and Prevention 1999a). The same water, which none of the locals would dare drink, was used to chill the parsley after harvest and make the ice in which the crop would be packed for shipment. Cilantro produced at the same farm that summer touched off another outbreak of *Shigella sonnei* diarrhea among more than three hundred patrons of a Mexican restaurant in Northern California. The tainted cilantro was a tangy additive to the restaurant's popular fresh salsa.

Not all international outbreaks of food-borne disease have a developing country at their source. Staphylococcal food poisoning was reported in several European countries in 1984 following the distribution of dry lasagna packets that had been contaminated at a pasta factory in Italy. In 1996, *E. coli* O157:H7 was transmitted by unpasteurized commercial apple juice produced in the United States and sold internationally. Outbreaks of intestinal illness due to *Shigella sonnei* in Britain, Norway, and Sweden were linked to iceberg lettuce that was produced in Spain in 1994. Also that year, *Salmonella agona* outbreaks in Jewish communities in Britain and North America were traced to a ready-to-eat, kosher savory snack manufactured in Israel. *S. agona* had only reached Israel when it was spread around the world in contaminated chicken feed that was produced in Peru.

A Sprouting Food-Borne Disease Problem

One other food item deserves special mention, as it is frequently turning up as a cause of widespread disease: raw seed sprouts. Once a popular homegrown food for hippies, today these crunchy and nutritious newborn plants are eaten regularly by as many as 10 percent of American consumers. Nearly five hundred United States growers produce about 300 thousand tons of alfalfa, clover, and radish sprouts annually, to supply a $250 million market. If seeds used for sprouting are contaminated with even a few organisms of *Salmonella* or other bacteria, they can remain infectious for months in storage. The sprouting of the seeds only enriches the infectious dose for the end consumer. Since 1994, raw sprouts have been linked to at least fifteen large outbreaks, including nine in the United States. In 1996, more than six thousand cases in Japan's epidemic of *E. coli* O157:H7 were attributed to consumption of white radish sprouts. These sprouts gave rise to another 126 cases in Japan during 1997.

Sprout-associated outbreaks often have international repercussions. A massive outbreak of *Salmonella bovismorbificans* in Finland and Sweden in 1994 was traced to alfalfa seeds produced in Australia. In 1995, an outbreak of *Salmonella stanley* affecting Finland and seventeen states of the United States was traced to contaminated alfalfa seeds supplied by a distributor in the Netherlands. The ultimate source of the implicated seeds was unknown, but the distributor was buying seeds from Italy, Hungary, and Pakistan at the time of the outbreak.

Since then, raw sprouts have been implicated in five outbreaks in California, including one in 1996 involving more than five hundred cases. It was due to two *Salmonella* species. In 1997, alfalfa spouts caused a multistate outbreak of *E. coli* O157:H7, in which 108 people were sickened and eighteen were hospitalized. The sprouts had been grown at facilities in Virginia and Michigan, using seeds supplied by farms in Idaho. Several of the farms were found to have deer grazing in the fields, and one farm was adjacent to a cattle feedlot. Both deer and cattle are known hosts of *E. coli* O157:H7.

In 1999, after three large *Salmonella* outbreaks had buffeted four western states, the FDA issued a warning that all people who wish to avoid food-borne illness should not eat raw sprouts. Specifically, the FDA advised:

- When at home, cook your sprouts, as this significantly reduces the risk of disease.

- In restaurants and delicatessens, check that sandwiches and salads do not contain raw sprouts. Request that raw sprouts not be added to your foods.

- Remember that sprouts grown at home also present a risk if eaten raw.

Nightmare of the Iguana: Commerce in Cool Pets

Imported animals are another commercial source of emerging infections. International trading in exotic animals, both legal and illegal, has increased dramatically in the past decade. Although a portion of the trade supplies the growing needs of research laboratories, most animals imported into developed countries are being sold as pets. The public's appetite for strange new animals seems limitless, as pet shops have begun to stock creatures unheard of in previous years, such as African pygmy hedgehogs and Australian flying squirrels. Where laws prohibit wildlife trading, smugglers have entered the market to meet the demand. The profits available to dealers in illegal wildlife may be second only to those made from illegal drugs, according to the United States Fish and Wildlife Service (1998).

The most plausible explanation for the sudden appearance of West Nile virus in New York in 1999 was the smuggling of infected birds, presumably from Africa. Few highly prized parrots and other large tropical birds can be imported legally nowadays. Those that do enter the country lawfully must spend thirty days in a government-approved quarantine station. Smuggled birds bypass this step and go directly to new owners.

Of all the new pet sensations, none other has captured the hearts of the American public like the iguana. Iguana sales in the United States have increased thirty-fold in recent years. They now account for a third of all reptile imports, and the proportion is growing. Children in particular are captivated by the looks and behavior of iguanas. Families might grow so fond of their iguanas that they allow them to roam freely throughout the house. In Los Angeles, iguanas can even be hired for children's birthday parties. Because it is not economical to breed iguanas in captivity, they are usually captured in the wild—in their tropical habitat—and legally imported by the thousands. Border controls are minimal, according to Osterholm (1997b). If the lizards aren't verging on death when they arrive in the United States, they are usually allowed into the country.

The problem with iguanas, as with all reptile pets, is that they silently carry nasty infections, particularly *Salmonella*. An estimated 90 percent of pet reptiles actively shed *Salmonella* in their feces, although they usually show no signs of the disease. In the early 1970s, baby turtles were shown to cause about 280 thousand cases of human salmonellosis in the United States each year. A ban on the interstate shipment of turtles under four inches in length was imposed in 1975. That ban probably prevents at least one hundred thousand cases of turtle-associated *Salmonella* infections in children under age ten each year, including some deaths. But no such controls have been placed on iguanas. Hatchling iguanas typically become infected with *Salmonella* by eating feces. This is a normal behavior for vegetarian lizards, as it establishes bacterial flora for fermentation in the hindgut. Antibiotics given to lizards by iguana wholesalers to suppress *Salmonella* colonization have been largely unsuccessful and are likely to promote resistant strains. *Salmonella* has also been linked to pet pygmy hedgehogs and flying squirrels. Human infections with *S. tilene*, a rare type of *Salmonella*, have migrated across Canada in a pattern mirroring the distribution of pygmy hedgehogs.

The latest pet craze in Japan is the North American prairie dog, the furry brown rodent that lives in large colonies throughout the Great Plains and Rocky Mountain states. More than fifteen thousand prairie dogs are imported annually to Japan with little regulation, despite the fact that they are an important reservoir for *Yersinia pestis*, the bacteria that cause plague. In May 1998, an exotic animal broker in Texas received 356 prairie dogs from a dealer who had captured them in the wild. Within the next eleven days all but seventy-five of the animals died, and the Veterinary Medical Diagnostic Laboratory in Amarillo diagnosed plague. "The diseased prairie dogs had the potential to be shipped around the world," says Jim Alexander (1998), a veterinary surgeon with the Texas Department of Health. "Based on the shipper's protocol, the animals in this incident could have been shipped two days prior to the occurrence of significant death losses, which would have exposed a myriad of people." Alexander added that the whole affair laid open the dangers inherent in removing wild animals from their environment to sell them as pets.

Another exotic pet appearing in people's homes is the bat. The sale of imported bats is usually illegal, but during 1994 a number of improperly issued permits allowed several thousand wild bats to be imported into the United States as pets (Rupprecht, Smith, Fekadu, et al. 1995). Most were the Egyptian tomb bat, although other species were also imported. Bats pose a special risk to human health because they are prime carriers of lyssaviruses, a group that includes the rabies virus. Rabies causes more than thirty-five thousand deaths worldwide each year from an incurable brain disease that follows a bite or scratch from an infected animal. Human rabies is one of the most terrifying diseases that doctors ever witness. In most cases, patients suffer days of extreme agitation, marked by intermittent episodes of thrashing, running, biting, and other bizarre behavior. Spasms in the throat produce choking, gagging, and extreme fear.

Fortunately, human rabies is rare in the United States, but it has been on the increase since 1990, with twenty-six cases reported through 1998 (National Center for Infectious Diseases, Centers for Disease Control and Prevention 1999.) This compares with just ten cases during the decade of the 1980s. Almost all of the recent increase is associated with bats. In several bat-related cases, transmission of the virus occurred without a recognizable wound (Noah, Drenzek, Smith, et al. 1998).

Australia was thought to be free of lyssaviruses, but in 1996 a new virus closely related to the rabies virus was discovered in fruit bats along Australia's east coast. That year, a Queensland woman who cared for injured bats died from encephalitis after she was scratched by an infected bat. Where rabies and other lyssavirus diseases occur, the risk of human cases is reduced when the infection is well controlled in domestic animals, such as dogs and cats. Deliberately bringing bats into homes as pets heightens the risk of human exposure to this life-threatening disease. Other bats imported for scientific reasons have already been found to carry rabies, including a dozen big brown bats collected in Massachusetts during 1994. They had been sold to researchers in Denmark.

Rabid Backyard Bandits

Bats are not the only natural hosts for the deadly rabies virus. In the Eastern United States, the likeliest creature to harbor the organism today is that masked marauder of the suburban night: the raccoon. Raccoon rabies has been slowly spreading north from Florida since the late 1940s. During the 1970s, the epidemic arrived in the Middle Atlantic states when hunters transferred some infected raccoons to Virginia to replenish depleted populations. Since then, it has been expanding northwards at a rate of about forty miles per year. Today, the disease affects raccoons in an area covering about four hundred thousand square miles, a region inhabited by ninety million people.

The epidemic zone crossed into New York State in 1990. During the previous year, just fifty-four rabid animals had been detected through routine monitoring in the state. By 1993, the total had increased to 2,746, giving New York the largest number of rabid animals in the country. Raccoons accounted for 89 percent of the total. Meanwhile, the number of people receiving the prolonged course of vaccines and immune globulin required to prevent rabies after wild animal bites increased in New York from 81 in 1989 to 3,336 in 1993. Given that the average cost of such treatment is nearly $2,400 per person, the increase in preventive therapy for rabies represents a staggering jump in health care expenditure.

By 1998, rabid raccoons had been detected along the southern shore of the St. Lawrence Seaway. This was alarming news for Canadian health authorities, but there was hope that the wide seaway and the fast-moving waters of the Niagara River in western New York would act as barriers to further spread. Then, in July 1999, Canada's first case of raccoon rabies was reported just north of the St. Lawrence Seaway near Prescott, Ontario. The find triggered a massive raccoon eradication campaign in a three-mile radius around the town. In the end, the wide rivers along New York's boundaries proved no match for the raccoons, who are well-known to hitch a ride on boats or trucks. In recent years, at least fourteen tractor-trailers arriving in Toronto from the United States have inadvertently carried raccoon hitchhikers. "It's a miracle we haven't gotten it before," says Rick Rosatte (1999), head of rabies research for Ontario's Ministry of Natural Resources. "We knew it was inevitable."

The Monkey Business

Perhaps no pet can form a stronger bond with its owners than an infant primate. The physical and behavioral resemblance of a baby macaque to a human infant is obvious. Macaques comprise a group of Old World monkeys, including the rhesus species, which are most commonly used in biomedical research. Since 1975, it hasn't been legal in the United States to own a nonhuman primate as a pet, but it is known that many macaques continue to be marketed and kept as pets (Ostrowski, Leslie, Parrott, et al. 1998). Each year, about a dozen nonoccupational macaque bites are reported in the United States, undoubtedly the tip of a large iceberg. One animal recently involved in a biting incident was owned by a couple in Minnesota who considered the monkey a "child substitute." They even hired full-time baby-sitters for it! Macaques no longer wanted as pets have established free-ranging feral populations in Florida and Texas.

The difficulty with pet macaques is that they harbor *Ceropithecine herpesvirus* 1, also known as B-virus, in their saliva. Between 80 and 90 percent of captive macaques are infected with B-virus, although they rarely show signs of illness. Owners who bond with their baby monkeys are often surprised to find that by age two their behavior becomes unpredictable and often very aggressive. Biting is how pubescent macaques establish dominance in their social hierarchy, even if their peers are humans. Human infections with B-virus can be rapidly fatal following a macaque bite, although new antiviral treatments may halt the progression of the disease if given early.

Research monkeys have likewise transmitted B-virus. In the most recent case, a lab worker in Atlanta died from the disease after a monkey splashed her eye with biological material, possibly feces. Lab monkeys have also been involved in two sensational importations of filoviruses, agents closely related to the deadly Ebola virus, described in chapter 2. In 1967, a group of African green monkeys imported from Uganda to a vaccine laboratory in Marburg, Germany, was found to carry a lethal new virus that killed many of the monkeys and spread to twenty-five of their human caretakers. Seven people died from infection with the "Marburg virus," including some having no direct contact with the monkeys. In 1989, a group of macaques imported from the Philippines to a research facility in Reston, Virginia, were found to carry another new filovirus. Four workers were infected, but none had overt symptoms. Quarantine measures devised after the Marburg incident prevented further spread of the "Reston virus" in the United States, but, in 1992, other macaques sold in Italy by the same exporter were found to be infected with the virus.

At present, there are no simple and reliable diagnostic tests to screen incoming laboratory monkeys for filoviruses, B-virus, and other potentially serious pathogens. The ongoing commercial trade of these animals leaves importing countries vulnerable to new and dangerous infections that otherwise would remain removed from human contact in isolated environments. The underground pet market carries even greater risks, as an outbreak spread by illegally imported monkeys would be much more difficult to control.

Rats and Mice: See How They Run!

Where humans travel, rodents are never far behind. Rats and some species of mice thrive on close relations with *Homo sapiens*. They are remarkably adaptable, happy to live off our refuse, and resistant to all our attempts to destroy them. "Rats have piggy-backed on our success and followed us around the world," says James Childs of the CDC in a 1996 interview for *New Scientist*.

In his classic 1934 book *Rats, Lice and History*, Hans Zinsser suggested that rats are "amazingly human" in the ways they live and interact. Like humans, they are omnivorous, they breed year-round, and they even make war on their own kind. "In following man about all over the earth, the rat has—more than any other living creature except man—been able to adapt itself to any conditions of seasonal changes or climate," Zinsser wrote. He surmised that black rats (*Rattus rattus*) arrived in Europe between A.D. 400 and 1100 on the heels of marauding tribesmen who periodically invaded from the east. The rats then spread across Europe so fast that they had become a ubiquitous pest by the time the legend of the pied piper of Hamlen appeared in the thirteenth century.

Europe's infestation with *Rattus rattus* had disastrous consequences for human health in the mid-fourteenth century with the sudden arrival of the Black Death, a disease known today as plague. *Yersinia pestis*, the bacterium that causes plague, is transmitted to humans from infected fleas whose usual hosts are rodents. In 1331, a devastating outbreak of plague hit China, after fur trading extended the range of plague-infected fleas from their endemic focus in marmots inhabiting the steppes of Central Asia. During the next fifteen years, plague spread west from China along the "Silk Road," infecting humans and rodents alike along the route. It reached the trading port of Caffa in the Crimea when Mongol invaders laid siege to the city in 1346. The epidemic compelled the Mongols to retreat, but not before rats in the city became infected. Some of those rats inevitably became stowaways on the many merchant ships departing that summer for Italy.

Upon landing in Italy the diffusion of plague throughout Europe was swift and unremitting. Infected fleas passed from rat to rat, and from rats living within the walls and roofs of houses to humans. Many people bitten by these fleas died from the form of the disease called bubonic plague, in which the infection causes grotesque enlargement of the lymph glands. In countless other cases, the disease invaded the lungs of its victims, from which the infection could be spread from person to person. This form of the disease, called pneumonic plague, produces explosive epidemics. Within four years, the Black Death had spread across France, had reached Britain, and had penetrated Scandinavia. At least twenty million people died, a quarter of the continent's population. In some regions entire communities perished. Plague epidemics would continue to haunt Western Europe until the late seventeenth century. By that time, a shortage of wood for building houses led to more stone and brick construction. Thatched roofs were replaced by tiles, especially after London's Great Fire of 1666. These changes provided fewer habitats for rats in close proximity to humans, making it less likely that an infected flea would come across a human host. The arrival of the Asian brown rat (*Rattus norvegicus*) in the early eighteenth century, which virtually wiped out Europe's black rats, also reduced the risk of plague for humans. Although brown rats make ready hosts for plague-infected fleas, they tend to be more shy around humans than black rats, so the likelihood of contact is reduced.

How Travel Roused the Sleeping Giant

While plague retreated from Western Europe, it remained active in Russia and parts of Asia. Human movements, particularly commercial shipping, then repeatedly introduced the disease to new populations. The present plague pandemic began in China in the 1860s. It reached Hong Kong in 1894. From there infected rats carried the infection by ship to virtually every major seaport in the world. Within a decade, epidemics erupted in one port after another, in Asia, South Africa, Latin America, and beyond, stoking fears that the Black Death of the fourteenth century had returned. After its arrival in Bombay in 1898, plague broke into the interior of India and claimed six million lives. The disease continued to haunt India during the twentieth century, most recently in 1994 when outbreaks centered on the city of Surat caused fifty-six deaths.

When plague landed in Sydney, Australia, in January 1900, more than five hundred people became ill in New South Wales, and 192 died. Later that year an Asian merchant ship brought plague to San Francisco, igniting a small outbreak in the city's Chinese community. Although the human epidemic was quickly contained, the disease gained a foothold in Northern California's ground squirrels and other burrowing rodents. Over the next few decades, rodent plague radiated from San Francisco like ripples across a pond, until the disease became firmly established among a wide array of wild animal hosts inhabiting thirteen western states and parts of Canada and Mexico. Bites from the fleas of infected rodents continue to cause about a dozen human cases of plague in the western United States each year, including a few fatal cases when treatment is begun too late. Signs warning about the hazards of plague have become a common sight for hikers and campers in the West, even at facilities close to major cities like Los Angeles and Denver.

During the 1970s, Vietnam and a few other Asian countries accounted for the most cases of plague, but today the burden of the disease is greatest in Africa. Since the early 1980s, Tanzania has experienced almost nonstop outbreaks of plague, with seventy-four deaths reported in 1995 and sixty-four deaths the following year. This dreadful situation arose after a period of thirty years without any cases of the disease. In 1999, plague also erupted in the Ohangwena region of northern Namibia, causing at least nine deaths. Nomadic herding of farm animals may have helped spread the infection from village to village. Other outbreaks have been reported recently in Malawi, Mozambique, and the Democratic Republic of the Congo.

But the country facing the biggest problem with plague today is Madagascar, which has accounted for nearly half of the world's cases in recent years. Plague was brought to this island of thirteen million people by steamboats from India in 1898. By the 1950s, plague seemed well controlled with improved housing and public hygiene. But since 1989, Madagascar has suffered between one hundred and sixteen hundred cases per year. In the interior plateaus, where most human cases occur, domestic rats are common. A survey of 625 rats trapped at a village marketplace in 1995 found that 10 percent were infected with *Y. pestis* (Chanteau, Ratsifasoamanana, Rasoamanana, et al. 1998). Many carried fleas resistant to available insecticides. The first multidrug-resistant strains of *Y. pestis* are also now emerging, not surprisingly in Madagascar. How long will it be before rodents departing by ship from this island nation provide passage for antibiotic-resistant plague to other countries?

Unfortunately, rodent stowaways aboard the world's commercial ships can spread other diseases besides plague across the globe. Hantaviruses, the family that includes the Sin Nombre virus that caused the 1993 outbreak of severe pulmonary disease in the southwestern United States (see chapter 2), have spread far and wide when their natural rodent hosts have utilized modern human transport. The first identified hantavirus, the Hantaan virus, is transmitted by inhaling viral aerosols arising from the dried urine of the striped field mouse of East Asia. Hantaan virus causes an acute, life-threatening illness typified by fever, hemorrhaging, and renal failure. Several other viruses in the group are now known to cause similar illnesses, but they are transmitted from the urine of their own unique rodent hosts. The Seoul virus, which makes its home in the familiar brown rat (*Rattus norvegicus*) is now found worldwide, wherever brown rats are poorly controlled. It undoubtedly radiated from its Korean home because of international commerce.

Tired Mosquitoes

Rodents are not the only infectious pests to hitch a ride on the world's shipping lanes. International commerce has opened new territories for insect vectors of disease at the same time that it has opened new markets for trade. Mosquitoes accidentally exported from their ancestral habitats often have little difficulty establishing themselves on new turf. With the high volume of traffic moving between continents and across latitudes today, widespread dissemination of potentially dangerous mosquitoes may be unavoidable.

The inadvertent introduction of the Asian "tiger mosquito" to the United States illustrates the risks. Established populations of *Aedes albopictus* mosquitoes were first discovered in Houston, Texas, in August 1985. This was alarming news because tiger mosquitoes are capable of transmitting at least twenty-two viruses known to cause human disease, including all four serotypes of the dengue fever virus, the yellow fever virus, and a range of viruses that cause inflammatory diseases of the brain, including the La Crosse virus. Authorities quickly realized that the mosquitoes had arrived in shipments of used tires from Korea and Japan, where they are a common biting pest. Millions of discarded tires are imported into the United States every year to be retreaded and resold. Unfortunately these tires are ideal incubators for larval tiger mosquitoes. Tires collect rainwater and hold it regardless of the position in which they are placed, and they accommodate none of the predators seen in natural breeding sites, such as fish or frogs.

Two years after their discovery in Houston, tiger mosquito infestations were reported from ninety-two counties in fifteen states. Dispersion of the mosquitoes during those years followed the movements of trucks involved in the domestic used-tire trade (Moore and Mitchell 1997). In fact, the distribution of infested counties in December 1987 could be superimposed on a map of the interstate highway system, forming necklace-like patterns linking major population centers from the Gulf of Mexico to the Midwest. Tiger mosquito populations then expanded outward from each center. By 1998, the infestation had spread to 866 counties in 26 states, stretching from New Jersey to the Texas panhandle, and as far north as Chicago.

Everywhere they've settled, tiger mosquitoes have become a public nuisance, although it is not yet clear if they are causing any human disease. But one worrisome find in 1997 suggests they may soon become a significant threat to health in Middle America. That summer, health officials in Peoria, Illinois, a well-known hotbed for human La Crosse virus infections, found numerous tiger mosquito larvae in tires and other containers at several sites. La Crosse virus finds its usual hosts in chipmunks, foxes, squirrels, and woodchucks of the upper Mississippi and Ohio River valleys. But humans in those regions can be infected inadvertently by mosquito bites during the warmer months of the year. Laboratory studies have shown that Asian tiger mosquitoes are actually more effective at transmitting the La Crosse virus than its natural, local vectors. In Peoria, investigators suspect that tiger mosquitoes have already begun to transmit the disease among local chipmunks (Kitron, Swanson, Crandell, et al. 1998). Now it seems likely that they will spread it to humans.

Mosquitoes That Love to Fly

Since 1980 more than fifty episodes of "airport malaria" have been reported in Western European countries that have been otherwise free of malaria for decades. In these incidents, none of the infected people had traveled to malarious regions of the tropics, and none had received a blood transfusion that might have contained malaria parasites. Often they were aircraft mechanics, baggage handlers, customs officers, or others who had spent long hours at international airports. Sometimes, as was the case for an outbreak in Luxembourg in 1999, the victims merely lived near the country's main airport, or had visited it only briefly. The only plausible explanation for how the people in any of these outbreaks contracted malaria is that they were bitten by tropical anopheline mosquitoes that had traveled to Europe by jet.

The possibility that aircraft might disperse insect vectors of disease was first considered in the 1930s. For that reason, insecticide spraying of aircraft passenger compartments and cargo holds following stops in tropical countries is practiced routinely in many countries, and can be required for aircraft arriving in the United States when health officials demand it. But these procedures are by no means completely effective, and some mosquitoes may be resistant to the insecticides that are used. Aircraft might even disseminate insecticide resistance genes across the world. Searches of 592 treated aircraft landing at Trinidad, West Indies, yielded some 967 mosquitoes (Le Maitre and Chadee 1983). At London's Gatwick Airport, live mosquitoes were detected in twelve of sixty-seven aircraft arriving from tropical regions (Curtis and White 1984).

It is likely that fertilized female mosquitoes looking for a blood meal are attracted to the artificial lights of open hangars at tropical airports. They may also be drawn toward the carbon dioxide given off by jet engines during nocturnal stopovers. Experiments have shown that mosquitoes that cling to the inner wheel bays of Boeing 747 aircraft can survive flights of more than nine hours, despite extremely low air pressures and external air temperatures below minus fifty-degrees Fahrenheit at cruising altitudes (Russell 1987). Following such trips, female *Anopheles* would be anxious to secure blood meals periodically to nourish successive batches of eggs. In crowded European airports they need not look far, but some have been carried by winds as far as four miles from airports, and others have procured ground transportation in motor vehicles.

Malaria-infected mosquitoes have also traveled in personal baggage transported from endemic areas. In August 1994, two workers at a sewage treatment plant near Berlin developed *Plasmodium falciparum* infection, the most severe form of malaria. Investigators concluded that the men had been bitten by an infected mosquito brought home from Africa or Latin America in someone's luggage (Mantel, Klose, Scheurer, et al. 1995). *P. falciparum* has also been linked to *Anopheles* mosquitoes imported by ship. During the summer of 1993, two elderly people living near the port of Marseille, France, were stricken by the disease. Modern container vessels can reach Marseille in just six to eight days from malarious ports in Senegal or the Côte d'Ivoire.

Ballast Water Passing in the Night

Since the 1880s, ocean-going ships have filled ballast tanks or floodable holds with ambient water to maintain balance and stability at sea. When this water is released at subsequent ports of call it can introduce aquatic organisms into new marine ecosystems thousands of miles away. With larger vessels and faster transit times, there is now greater risk than ever that viable organisms can survive such journeys and settle permanently in new environments. These invasions can have catastrophic effects on native species in bays, estuaries, and inland waters where ballast water is released. In 1993, James Carlton and Jonathan Geller identified 367 species of plankton in the ballast water of ships travelling from Japan to Coos Bay, Oregon. They surmise that at least forty-five species have become established in new ecosystems since the late 1970s through the transport of ballast water.

Human pathogens can also find their way into the ballast water brew. These include toxic algae, such as those that cause paralytic shellfish poisoning. Epidemic cholera is probably the most notorious disease to be disseminated recently in ballast water. *Vibrio cholerae* bacteria adhere well to algae, and they can survive for long periods in brackish water and estuaries. Shellfish eaten from such waters can expose humans to cholera. Genetic analysis of cholera organisms isolated early in the South American epidemic showed they were identical to strains involved in a cholera outbreak in Bangladesh (Faruque and Albert 1992). It is now presumed that cholera invaded Latin America as a consequence of contaminated ballast water taken on by one or more ships in Asia and discharged into the coastal fisheries of Peru.

Aircraft do not convey ballast water, but they carry human waste over great distances in their sewage tanks. Recently some researchers at the University of North Carolina identified nineteen infectious viruses from samples of sewage pumped from aircraft arriving in the United States from overseas. Human waste from aircraft is usually treated in municipal sewage plants, but such treatment fails to remove up to 10 percent of viruses. That would permit introductions of exotic pathogens into the environment, said Mark Sobsey (1997), one of the researchers. "It was a bit of a jolt for us," he said. "The range of illnesses that can be transmitted by the world's airlines is quite worrisome."

Diseases Delivered in Human Cargo

In this chapter we have examined how disease-producing microbes journey across the globe in contaminated foods, in animals imported as pets, in rodents, in mosquitoes, and even in ballast water or aircraft sewage. Finally, let's see how pathogens can also roam the world concealed inside the bodies of human travelers.

Since 1800, the average distance and speed that people travel have increased one thousand-fold, while there has been no change in the incubation periods of human pathogens. Airline passengers who are obviously ill can be detained upon entering a country, but travelers who are silently incubating infections will pass undetected. Many serious pathogens today are not readily apparent on sight, and they might even be unknown to their hosts. For example, an overseas traveler may silently carry within the ordinary bacterial flora of the intestines segments of genetic material that can interact with the local microbes at the traveler's destination. Occasionally, such genes might confer increased virulence or resistance to antibiotics. International boundaries mean nothing to germs. As long as people are inclined to cross borders, new and potentially serious infections will cross with them.

Worldwide, the number of airline passengers has increased from 2 million per year in 1950 to more than 1.4 billion today. By 2005, the world's airlines expect to carry more than two billion passengers annually. At any given moment there is a veritable city of sixty-one thousand people in flight over North America. Growth in international air traffic is especially strong. Fifty million passengers now arrive in the United States from overseas each year. Among United States residents, international travel has increased by 131 percent since 1977, a jump six times greater than the growth in population during the same period. Of the thirty million trips that Americans are making annually to foreign countries other than Canada, more than half now include tropical or subtropical destinations, places where visitors are more likely to acquire and bring home exotic infections. Similar trends in international travel have been seen in Europe. Nearly one quarter of Norwegians now travel abroad each year, and many are choosing warm destinations in Asia, Africa, and the Caribbean. Thailand has become especially popular, with a 46 percent increase in visitors from Norway noted between 1997 and 1998. Not surprisingly, Norway has recently witnessed sharp increases in reported cases of tropical diseases.

International travel also presents risks to the country that is receiving visitors, as guests can leave behind more than the pleasant memories of a trip abroad. An epidemic of Ross River virus infection in the South Pacific has been traced to the arrival of an Australian tourist at Fiji's Nandi Airport during 1979 (Aaskov, Mataika, Lawrence, et al. 1981). The tourist, who appeared well, passed the blood-borne virus to local mosquitoes, which passed it in turn to Fiji's human inhabitants. Disease due to infection with the Ross River virus ranges from mild flu-like symptoms to debilitating joint pains. The virus is endemic in parts of Australia, but before 1979 Pacific Island populations had no immunity to it. The epidemic quickly spread from Fiji throughout the South Pacific basin, infecting more than five hundred thousand people.

Adding Adventure to Tourism

Tourism has become one of the world's largest growth industries. By 1998, income from tourism had exceeded $444 billion per year, accounting for more than one-third of total world exports in services. In 1950, there were only five million international tourist arrivals worldwide. Today there are more than 625 million per year, and the total is expected to increase to nearly one billion by 2010. Americans spend more than any other nation on international tourism, about 13 percent of the worldwide total.

One of the fastest growing segments of the industry today is so-called "adventure tourism." Tourists in this market comb the world for "extreme" environments in which to climb mountains, raft rivers, jump from airplanes, or simply survive in the face of outrageous odds. Sometimes these modern adventurers discover that no environment is too extreme for unpleasant infections. In 1996, nine of twenty-six participants in a white-water rafting expedition in Costa Rica developed a sudden febrile illness upon return to the United States. Symptoms included headaches, chills, and severe muscle aches. All nine recovered, but two had to be hospitalized. The illness turned out to be leptospirosis, a bacterial disease spread through contact with the urine of infected animals. Investigators surmised that submersion in the river had exposed the rafters to leptospires excreted by local animals (Centers for Disease Control and Prevention 1997a). A severe leptospirosis epidemic had struck nearby Nicaragua the previous year, affecting about two thousand people and leaving thirty-seven dead.

When Visiting Microbes Decide to Stay

Pathogens introduced by overseas visitors or residents returning from abroad can either be short-lived affairs or they can lead to the establishment and propagation of new infections. The outcome depends on how the disease is transmitted and whether the environment in the receiving country can maintain the disease and its agent. Fortunately, most exotic infections carried by human hosts into the United States are transient, affecting only the travelers involved. For example, 3,456 people were reported with malaria in the United States between 1993 and 1995, but only twenty-five had acquired the infection within the country. Prompt treatment of most cases limits the chance that *Plasmodium* parasites will spread to others in the population, even where abundant mosquito vectors are present. Similarly, more than one hundred cases of dengue fever may be reported each year, but virtually all these infections are acquired outside the United States and they spread no further.

Intestinal diseases, like cholera and typhoid fever, are also unlikely to become established here, thanks to our relatively high level of community hygiene. All cases of cholera reported to the CDC lately are associated with travel, except a small number linked to eating unusual imported foods or seafood harvested off the Gulf Coast of Texas and Louisiana. Travelers introduce a few hundred cases of typhoid each year, but usually these spread no further than the immediate households involved. Homeless people and residents of migrant work camps, however, do present special risks for wider spread of such diseases. Such groups require special monitoring whenever exotic pathogens are imported nearby. But even when the diffusion of travel-related organisms to nontravelers isn't a high risk, it is important for health care professionals to be aware of diseases that originate in other parts of the world, to diagnose them quickly, and to provide prompt treatment for those who arrive in the country infected.

The biggest risk posed by incoming travelers to the United States, or any developed country with a temperate climate, is from diseases spread person-to-person. These would include diseases spread sexually, by the respiratory route, by infected needles, or by unwashed hands. If all sexually transmitted infections were eradicated throughout the United States on a given day, new cases would soon appear among travelers arriving from other countries and in their partners here. Infected travelers have brought the DNA segments that code for penicillin resistance in North American strains of *Neisseria gonorrhoeae* to Europe and the world, while it has brought similar genetic strands from Europe to North America and beyond (Handsfield and Sparling 1995). We will see in chapter 8 how readily influenza viruses span the globe through human travel. The spread of antibiotic-resistant strains of pneumococcus has also been tracked along routes of travel and trade (Levy 1998).

The risk that a traveler infected with the wild poliovirus will reintroduce polio to the United States after more than twenty years without cases is the primary reason that the CDC still recommends four doses of polio vaccine for all children. Travelers from Western Europe have twice introduced the poliovirus into Canada since 1978. Travel from countries like Russia and the Ukraine also helps explain why the population must be still vaccinated against diphtheria, even though cases in the United States now average only about three per year. Measles, another vaccine-preventable disease, also spreads readily into new territories through travel. In 1998, a four-year-old visitor from Japan became ill with measles and sparked an outbreak in Anchorage, Alaska. That outbreak, in which thirty-three people were infected, accounted for one-third of all measles cases reported in the United States that year. One reason why United States measles incidence has recently dropped to historically low levels is the remarkable success of most Latin American countries in immunizing their children against the disease. With fewer importations of measles arriving from countries to the south, North Americans are simply less likely to encounter the virus today, whether they are immunized or not.

Short-term travel, for business or tourism, is not the only type of human movement contributing to the emergence of infectious diseases. Contemporary social, political, and economic circumstances are inducing massive human migrations of a more permanent sort, and these are creating new opportunities for emergence. The next chapter will examine the consequences of these movements and other demographic shifts that are favoring new infections.

What You Can Do to Prevent Food-Borne Diseases

By now it should be obvious that some of the foods coming into your home may look fine but are contaminated with harmful microbes. Other foods may become contaminated later when you handle and prepare for them for eating in your home. There are now seventy-five million cases of food-borne illness in the United States each year, according to the CDC. Of these, 325 thousand lead to hospitalization and 5,000 end in death. Reducing the burden of food-borne disease is a top public health priority. Fortunately, there are a number of simple, common sense steps recommended by the CDC, the United States Department of Agriculture, and state health departments that will keep your food safe:

- Wash your hands with soap and water before preparing foods, and after handling raw meat, poultry, and seafood. Wash your hands again before you eat.

- Wash fruits and vegetables thoroughly, especially those that will not be cooked before they are eaten.

- Prevent cross-contamination by scrubbing cutting boards and kitchen surfaces after preparing food. Don't let the juices of raw meats mix with other foods.

- Cook foods thoroughly, especially meat and eggs. When eating out, order meats well-done. Eggs should be firm and not runny. Avoid raw shellfish.

- Keep hot food hot and cold foods cold after they are prepared. Refrigerate leftovers right away. Make sure your refrigerator is set below forty-degrees Fahrenheit.

- If a food might be unsafe, remember this rule: When in doubt, throw it out!

Chapter 4

Changing Human Demographics

The geographic distribution of human populations is shifting very rapidly, owing both to differential population growth and migration. The most dramatic demographic phenomenon of our times is in distribution rather than in numbers. Whereas the world population was predominantly rural and dispersed at the beginning of this century, we will be living in an urbanized world by the next century.

—Lincoln Chen, Harvard University

People living at the close of the second millennium have seen profound changes in the size, density, and distribution of the world's human populations, transitions that would have been unimaginable only a few generations ago. We have witnessed sweeping changes in our social and economic environments, alterations in traditional lifestyles, and a mixing of diverse peoples on a scale never known before. Such turbulence in the life of the human family has facilitated the emergence and reemergence of many infections.

In just fifty years, the number of people living on the planet has increased from 2.5 billion to just over 6 billion. Although the annual rate of population increase has declined slightly since it peaked in 1989, births still exceed deaths worldwide by more than 75 million per year. Of all the humans who have ever walked the earth, 6 to 10 percent are alive today. In developed countries like the United States, much of the growth in numbers is due to improved survival into old age. Life expectancy at birth now exceeds seventy-six years in North America; it tops seventy-eight years in Western Europe. The aging population base of these regions has added to the cost of health care and has increased the risk of opportunistic infections, those infections that prey on people with weakened immunity.

But the spearhead of population growth today is in the developing world, in countries that have experienced a decline in mortality thanks to marginally improved living conditions without a commensurate drop in fertility. Fully 96 percent of the world's population increase is now occurring in the developing countries of Africa, Asia, and Latin America. In the next quarter-century, as the world's population approaches eight billion, that percentage will continue to rise. Recently, many European nations have actually witnessed declines their in populations, as births have failed to keep pace with deaths. All but two central and eastern European countries lost population in 1997, and massive decreases are predicted in the first half of the twenty-first century for Italy, Germany, Spain, Russia, Japan, and others.

By contrast, several countries in sub-Saharan Africa are on track to triple their populations in the next fifty years. In Kenya, where the population has been growing by almost 4 percent a year, births outnumber deaths by four to one. There, and in many African countries, families with six or more children are typical. No wonder Africa's population surpassed Europe's in 1996 for the first time in recorded history. The pressure such growth is exerting on dwindling natural resources is immense, and it can have disastrous outcomes, as witnessed in the Rwandan genocide of 1994. Rwanda, one of the poorest and most crowded countries on Earth, is caught in what Maurice King (1990) calls a "demographic trap." Its population far exceeds the carrying capacity of its ecosystem, so its people are unable to survive without outside aid. Unless there is a sharp reduction in fertility, Rwanda's choices for the future will come down to starvation or continued slaughter.

The most important aspect of population growth for disease emergence is the astonishing increase in the size and density of cities. In 1985, there were 225 cities in the world with more than one million people. Today there are about four hundred such cities. Fourteen cities can claim more than ten million people. By the year 2015, up to twenty-seven cities will belong to the ten-million club. Of the world's twenty largest cities, only two are in North America and just one is in Europe. Most of the other megacities are in developing countries. They include Mexico City, São Paulo, Rio de Janeiro, Cairo, Karachi, Mumbai, Delhi, Calcutta, Shanghai, Jakarta, and Manila. London has slipped from being the second-largest city in the world in 1950 to twenty-third place today, with a mere 6.4 million people.

In 1800, fewer than 2 percent of humans lived in urban communities. Two-thirds of humanity was still dwelling in rural villages and remote farms in 1970. But some time early in the twenty-first century more than half the world's population will reside in cities. That proportion could reach 65 percent by 2025, according to the United Nations. The expanding population of cities is partly fuelled by high birth rates among those who already live there, but much of the growth is due to migration out of the countryside. Today the world is experiencing an unprecedented mass movement of workers and their families from rural districts to burgeoning urban centers, especially in the developing world.

Migrants are abandoning rural areas for many reasons. Triggers include droughts, famine, conflicts, or simply a lack of productive farmland. They are attracted to cities by the promise of jobs, as well as social services, such as schools and health care. In short, they are coming to cities in search of a better life. Many find it there, but life in the city can expose them to new risks of infectious diseases. Countless other migrants find themselves unwanted in the cities and end up living in vast slums at the margins of established urban centers. These densely populated settlements, called *favelas* in Latin America, lack the infrastructure that city dwellers in developed countries take for granted. Without adequate sanitation and access to clean water, these ghettos become breeding grounds for introduced infections.

This chapter is about how today's colossal demographic shifts, particularly the shift toward urbanization and the worldwide growth of an urban underclass, are promoting infectious disease emergence throughout the world. To look at the impact of modern urban development on the emergence of disease, and to see how hopes for controlling major infections depend on collective community involvement, the problem of dengue fever in Singapore is a good place to begin.

Dengue Fever Comes Knocking

It was after 10 P.M. when Steven Wrage heard five sharp knocks on his Singapore apartment door. The American political science professor had arrived home from work an hour earlier, and had noticed that the fern on the balcony beside the front door looked thirsty. "I watered it thoroughly, really soaking the thing," he recalled in an article for the *Atlantic Monthly* (1996).

When he scrambled to answer the knocking at his door he was startled to see two police officers standing there shoulder to shoulder, pointing at his sickly fern. "Is this your plant?" the senior officer asked. "It is," Professor Wrage stammered to reply. He wondered what the problem could be. Was his wilted plant obstructing traffic? Was it a public eyesore?

"You are subjecting the neighborhood to the danger of dengue hemorrhagic fever," the officer said, pointing to the pool of water in the saucer under the plant. "That saucer is a magnet for lethal disease. Standing water is precisely what pregnant female mosquitoes are searching for."

When Professor Wrage quickly removed the saucer and emptied it in his bathtub, the officers looked pleased. No citation would be issued this time. "I'm glad you understand," the senior officer said. "We all need to work together to do our part to keep Singapore safe and secure and healthy for all." On returning inside his apartment, Professor Wrage realized that one of his neighbors must have turned him in. Every apartment in his building had a plant by the door, but none had a saucer under the pot. Shaken by his brush with the law, the American professor felt both protected and threatened. "Big brother cares about me, and he knows exactly where I live," he wrote.

Singapore has good reason to be concerned about standing water and the mosquitoes that might breed there. This island city-state of 2.9 million at the equatorial tip of the Malay Peninsula sits squarely in the middle of a region that is now undergoing a resurgence of dengue fever. Singapore's high population density and rapid urban development have made it especially vulnerable to dengue. Despite intensive efforts to eradicate the mosquitoes that transmit dengue virus, Singapore has witnessed an upsurge in cases of dengue fever, from about three hundred cases per year in the late 1980s to more than four thousand cases per year by 1997.

But Singapore's problem with dengue pales in comparison to the growing crisis posed by dengue in more than one hundred other tropical countries, many of which lack Singapore's public health resources. As many as eighty million people are infected with dengue each year in Southeast Asia, Latin America, the South Pacific, and parts of Africa and the Middle East. The disease is characterized by an abrupt high fever, severe headaches, muscle and joint pains, and a rash. There is no specific treatment. An increasing proportion of dengue today is the severe hemorrhagic form of the disease, dengue hemorrhagic fever (DHF). In these cases, patients rapidly develop shock due to abnormal leakage from their blood vessels, and death is common without prompt intravenous fluid replacement.

Since 1997, record-setting outbreaks of dengue and DHF have been reported from Vietnam, Malaysia, Thailand, Indonesia, Honduras, Venezuela, and Brazil. Dengue returned to Cuba for the first time in sixteen years, and Argentina had its first cases since 1916. A dengue outbreak also swept the South Pacific, starting in French Polynesia in late 1996. From there it moved to the Cook Islands, Samoa, Tonga, Vanuatu, New Caledonia, and Fiji. In Fiji alone, more than twenty-five thousand dengue cases were reported, affecting 3 percent of the country's population in just five months. At least ten thousand cases of dengue occurred in Puerto Rico during 1998, including eighty-eight cases of DHF and five deaths. In August, at the peak of the epidemic, the number of reported cases was six times higher than usual for that time of year. Dengue imported from Thailand also struck northern Queensland, Australia, in December 1997. Nearly 240 confirmed cases were reported from Cairns, prompting the fumigation of every building and house along the resort city's famous waterfront.

The reasons behind the terrible upsurge of dengue in the world today are complex. To some degree, the growing menace of dengue is related to each of the factors of emergence examined in this book. Modern travel and commerce have played a big role in spreading the virus and its *Aedes* mosquito vectors into new territories. This chapter is looking closely at dengue because it illustrates well how the changes wrought by urbanization have fostered the recent emergence of a serious disease.

Dengue Virus: The Ultimate City Slicker

Classic dengue fever and DHF are caused by four distinct serotypes of the dengue virus (DEN-1, DEN-2, DEN-3, and DEN-4). Although dengue originated in jungle primates, today it is primarily an urban disease affecting only humans. Its preference for city dwellers relates to characteristics of the virus and the behavior of its principal vector, the *Aedes aegypti* mosquito. The dengue virus is present in human blood for just a short time, usually only for the six or seven days that the victim is stricken with fever. That short infectious period doesn't give the virus much time. During that interval it needs a hungry *Aedes* mosquito to find the infected person and carry off the virus in a blood meal. More importantly, the virus then needs the infected mosquito to locate and feed off of at least one other person who is susceptible to the disease. In sparsely populated rural areas propagation of the dengue virus is much less likely to be successful than in large and crowded cities where susceptible human hosts are concentrated. An infected mosquito has a much better chance of locating new hosts in a bustling city apartment block than in a remote farming village.

A bout of dengue fever will drive most people indoors for bed rest during the time the virus is circulating in their blood. But indoors is exactly where people in the tropics today are likely to encounter the chief vector of the disease. *A. aegypti* relishes close contact with humans, its favorite prey. It dwells primarily in and around people's houses, and it is loath to fly more than a few yards to obtain a blood meal. More than two hundred years ago *A. aegypti* began to spread from its African home to virtually every community in the tropical Americas and Asia, exploiting the slave trade and other commercial shipping. Unless there are persistent eradication programs, *A. aegypti* mosquitoes will thrive in the urban landscape of warmer countries, where 2.5 billion people now live. Surveys of houses in Thailand, for example, have uncovered an average of twenty female *A. aegypti* mosquitoes in every room (Yasuno and Tonn 1970).

Uncontrolled urbanization in many parts of tropical Asia and Latin America have created prime conditions for rapid proliferation of *A. aegypti*. In 1985, *A. aegypti* could be found in only ninety-one of Brazil's five thousand cities. Ten years later it was a confirmed pest in nearly 1,800 cities. The urban environment in the developing world today is littered with ideal habitats for mosquito larvae, such as discarded tires, drink bottles, and plastic containers that collect rainwater. Millions urban dwellers today who receive no piped water into their homes must store their household water in open cisterns. This water provides an ongoing nursery for larval mosquitoes within the domestic environment where *A. aegypti* prefers to live.

Even where urban development has accompanied new prosperity, as in certain countries of Southeast Asia, dengue has recently emerged. "From the mid-1980s and the 1990s, Thailand and Malaysia have undergone a boom period in their economies, leading to a feverish building boom," says Subramania Aiyar (1998), a microbiologist at the Universiti Sains Malaysia. "This created fertile breeding grounds for the *Aedes* mosquito at construction sites, etc. This was compounded by the rapid demographic change of increased urban migration." Aiyar notes that in Thailand the highest rates of dengue are in Bangkok, and that areas of the most intense new development in Malaysia—Kuala Lumpur and the Klang Valley—account for most of that country's dengue fever.

Construction sites seem to present special risks for the breeding of *Aedes* mosquitoes. Despite a recent downturn in several Asian economies, many of the largest construction projects since the pyramids have recently been started in the urban centers of Southeast Asia. In June 1998, twenty workers at the site of the unfinished Mega Exhibition Centre in Singapore developed dengue, including one who died. The outbreak forced the Korean construction company to stop work on the project and remove all the discarded building materials where *A. aegypti* mosquitoes had been breeding. Work teams were set up to fog the site with insecticides three times a day to keep it mosquito-free.

Dengue Hemorrhagic Fever

Urbanization is not only making dengue more common, it is also helping to make dengue more deadly. The ongoing movement of people into overcrowded cities in the developing world has hastened the emergence of DHF. This new disease was first recognized in 1953, when it erupted in the Philippines. It then spread to other Asian countries. In 1981, it emerged in the Western Hemisphere during an outbreak in Cuba, before spreading to Venezuela and Brazil. Since 1956, more than 1.3 million cases of DHF have been reported in Vietnam alone.

Dengue Hemorrhagic Fever is thought to occur when a person is sequentially infected with two different dengue virus serotypes. Prior infection with one serotype, such as DEN-1, leaves an individual immune to that strain upon subsequent exposure; but such people are at increased risk of DHF if exposed later to a different dengue serotype. Antibodies from the previous infection seem to enhance dengue virus replication in a host who is reinfected with a novel serotype. In recent years, dengue serotypes have extended their range because of human travel and migration, and in most large cities of Asia all four serotypes now overlap. The mixing of serotypes in these cities means that people are more likely than ever before to acquire new infections from distinct strains. Some of those who are repeatedly infected this way will develop DHF.

The impact of overlapping serotypes on the risk of DHF can be seen in Fiji's recent history of dengue. An outbreak caused by DEN-2 in 1971 and 1972 resulted in no cases of DHF, but left thousands of people with immunity to that serotype. When a DEN-1 outbreak erupted there in 1974 and 1975, a large proportion of hemorrhagic cases occurred among those infected previously with DEN-2. All four dengue serotypes have since circulated around the South Pacific. With every new outbreak, the DHF risk for certain individuals increases. Waves of ordinary dengue fever and DHF have also followed introductions of new dengue serotypes to the Western Hemisphere in recent years. The 1981 emergence of DHF in Cuba resulted from the arrival of a new strain of DEN-2 only four years after an outbreak of DEN-1 in that country. The introduction of an Asian strain of DEN-3 into Central America in 1994 resulted in a severe outbreak of DHF in Nicaragua.

The spasmodic emergence of new serotypes into Latin America and the Caribbean helps explain why DHF often affects adults in the Americas, while DHF is primarily a disease of children in Southeast Asia. An adult pattern is seen when there are long periods between introductions of new serotypes, as happened in Cuba. During the epidemic of DEN-2 there in 1997, all but one of the 205 cases of DHF occurred in people over twenty years of age. Only adults over twenty had been alive during Cuba's 1977 outbreak of DEN-1, so only they carried antibodies that would put them at risk of DHF during a DEN-2 epidemic. In many tropical Asian cities all four serotypes are now so well established that a child is much less likely to reach adulthood before having a second infection with a different serotype; so in these urban centers DHF is usually a pediatric disease. In fact, many adults in Southeast Asian cities today may no longer be susceptible to dengue, as they have already been infected with all four serotypes.

Dengue Control: Search and Destroy

Ultimately, the control of dengue and DHF will depend on the development of a vaccine. Research into dengue vaccines is complicated by the virus's four serotypes, and it is unlikely that a vaccine will be commercially available for mass immunization for several years. Another approach may be to genetically alter *Aedes* mosquitoes so they are incapable of replicating dengue virus and cannot transmit it to new hosts. A promising low-tech tactic, currently under trial in parts of Vietnam, employs a microscopic, one-eyed crustacean to devour *Aedes* larvae wherever it can find them in standing water. So far the voracious, shrimp-like crustacean appears to have wiped out the larvae in much of the northern province of Phan Boi (Kenyon 1999). But while research on dengue prevention continues, the key public health responses to the disease still involve traditional methods of mosquito eradication, particularly the elimination of *Aedes* breeding sites in urban environments.

No tropical country has become more vigilant about annihilating mosquitoes than Singapore, as Professor Wrage discovered at his door late that night in 1996. "The public is constantly reminded to keep their homes mosquito free by adopting a routine system of checks for *Aedes* breeding habitats within and around their homes," says K.T. Goh, of Singapore's Ministry of the Environment (1997). "Health education and publicity through all possible channels, including the use of videos, are continued throughout the year and stepped up whenever there are signs of an impending outbreak." The ministry works with grassroots organizations to promote neighborhood sprucing-up projects, and to apply insecticide paint to roof gutters and other places where water collects. "Without sustained community participation, the war against dengue cannot be won and outbreaks will continue to occur," Goh says.

The Uneasy Wait for Dengue in the United States

Outside of Puerto Rico, the Virgin Islands, and certain United States territories in the Pacific, the war against dengue has yet to settle permanently on American soil. Since 1945, the only documented, locally acquired cases have occurred in the southernmost counties of Texas, during periods of intense dengue activity in neighboring Mexico in 1980, 1986, 1995, and 1999. But as the global ordeal with dengue intensifies in coming years, it remains a real possibility that homegrown infections will also arise in American communities away from border areas.

Transmission of dengue, like any vector-borne infection, requires three elements to succeed: an infectious host, a susceptible population, and a competent insect vector to spread the virus around. So far, the missing ingredient for the spread of dengue in the United States has been large numbers of infectious hosts. The other two requirements are here in abundant supply: Virtually the entire United States population is susceptible to dengue infection, and vectors to spread the virus are plentiful in most southern and eastern states every summer. We have already seen how the Asian tiger mosquito, *Aedes albopictus*, is well established in twenty-six states. Tiger mosquitoes have little difficulty transmitting dengue, but they aren't as comfortable around humans as *Aedes aegypti* is, so they aren't as efficient as dengue vectors. That's the good news.

The bad news is that *A. aegypti* is also here in large numbers, readily available to spread the disease among Americans today. Despite repeated attempts to eradicate it, this bloodthirsty pest is now entrenched across a region stretching from Texas to South Carolina. Recent sightings have also been made in Maryland, New Jersey, and Arizona (Engelthaler, Fink, Levy, et al. 1997). Large dengue outbreaks in the United States are unlikely. But it seems only a matter of time before returning travelers, or visitors from endemic areas, provide the missing piece for sporadic transmissions in America's heartland and provoke significant public alarm.

Tuberculosis: The Real "Millennium Bug"

Dengue is not the only infection to emerge on the back of modern urbanization trends. Migration to the teeming cities of the developing world has also played a large part in the recent resurgence of humanity's leading microbial predator: tuberculosis (TB). After a century of slow decline, TB started roaring back during the late 1980s. In 1993, the World Health Organization (WHO) took an unprecedented step and declared TB a global emergency. The disease burden of "the white plague" today defies exaggeration.

Fully one-third of the world's population is infected with the mycobacterium that causes TB. In most cases, the body's normal immune response walls off the infection and keeps it under check for life. But in 5 to 10 percent of infected people the organism breaks free at some time in their lives and makes them chronically sick. In most cases, the disease strikes the lungs, which helps spread the infection to others. People with active pulmonary TB can propel the organism into the air around them whenever they cough, sneeze, or simply talk. Infection can result from inhaling a single organism.

Left untreated, someone with active TB will infect on average ten to fifteen other people. Someone in the world is newly infected with TB every second. That means that each week a population as large as that of Boston, Cleveland, or New Orleans acquires TB infection. At such rates, between now and the year 2020, one billion more people on Earth will be infected with TB. More people will die from TB this year than in any previous year, and next year is likely to set another new record. TB is the single largest infectious cause of death, and the sixth largest cause of death overall. It accounts for 26 percent of all preventable deaths in adults. TB kills more women than all causes of death associated with pregnancy and childbirth. In fact, TB is the largest single killer of young women in the world, accounting for 9 percent of deaths in women between the ages of fifteen and forty-four years. Only war comes close, causing 4 percent of deaths in these young women.

No country in the world is free of TB, but the biggest burden is undoubtedly in South Asia, where there are about three million new cases of active TB per year, and in sub-Saharan Africa, where there are about two million new cases per year. India leads the world in TB incidence and mortality, accounting for about 40 percent of all cases. Someone dies from TB in India every minute. Half the adults of India are infected with TB and one of them, on average, develops active disease every thirty seconds. Because treatment is usually lacking, there are 3.5 million people in India with active pulmonary TB at any moment. This group—larger in number than the city of Chicago—is highly infectious and is likely to pass the disease on to susceptible contacts.

The economic turmoil in the former Soviet Union has prompted a resurgence of TB there in recent years, after more than forty years of decline. There are now about 250 thousand TB cases per year in Eastern Europe. Russia has seen TB incidence increase by about 10 percent per year since the collapse of the Soviet Union, and there is now a shocking 25 percent mortality rate from the disease. Besides Russia, the WHO in 1998 identified fourteen other countries that are falling behind in controlling TB. In Asia they are Afghanistan, Pakistan, India, Burma, Thailand, Indonesia, Iran, and the Philippines. In Africa they are Ethiopia, Sudan, Uganda, and South Africa. In Latin America they are Brazil and Mexico. There are also "hot spots" of TB in other countries, including some wealthy countries like the United States. In the early 1990s New York City experienced a sudden upsurge in TB cases, a 150 percent increase from the previous decade.

Urbanization and the "White Plague"

The recent resurgence of TB is partly due to the interaction between HIV and TB. Of the thirty-four million people now infected with HIV, about a third are also infected with TB. In some countries, including India, TB infects about 60 to 70 percent of AIDS patients. TB-infected people with HIV are thirty times more likely to develop active tuberculosis than those without HIV, and TB is now the leading cause of death in HIV-infected people worldwide. Another reason for TB's re-emergence is drug resistance, a problem we will examine in chapters 9 and 10.

But the main reason for the growth of TB today is migration to cities and the poverty that millions of people confront there. As people infected with TB move from sparsely populated rural areas to more densely populated urban environments, their mixing with other people increases, and the chance of spreading TB to susceptible individuals multiplies. A person with active TB living in a remote village will encounter few uninfected people during the course of their illness. Standing on an urban street corner or riding in a city bus, that same person might encounter hundreds of susceptible people in a single day.

Activation of latent TB infection is also more likely in today's urban scene, especially for those condemned to live in the squalid ghettos of modern megacities. The appalling living conditions in overcrowded urban shanty towns, together with high unemployment and malnutrition, create stress and promote a host of respiratory and diarrheal diseases. These combine to weaken the body's immune defenses, leading to the eruption of active TB in infected people. The cramped living space of the slums then allows the easy spread of TB to others, and the cycle of infection continues. Refugees are migrants at special risk of TB. The number of refugees has increased nine-fold in the past twenty years, as a result of wars and natural disasters. Untreated TB spreads easily among the poverty-stricken people who crowd into refugee camps, and treatment is not always available in time. At least half the world's refugees are infected with TB.

Nonrefugee migrants to developed countries, like those in North America and Europe, are also at higher risk of TB. Nearly 40 percent of active TB reported in the United States occurs in people born outside the country. In 1997, foreign-born Americans were about seven times more likely than their United States-born counterparts to develop active TB. Two-thirds of foreign-born TB patients in the United States hail from just seven countries: Mexico, the Philippines, Vietnam, China, India, Haiti, and Korea. Homeless people in developed countries today are also at special risk of TB. Incidence of active TB in such populations sometimes mirrors that seen in developing countries. For example, 30 percent of San Francisco's homeless and 25 percent of London's homeless may be infected with TB (World Health Organization 1998a).

Robert Koch, the bacteriologist who first identified the cause of TB, said in 1882, "If the number of victims which a disease claims is the measure of its significance, then all diseases, particularly the most dreaded infectious diseases such as bubonic plague, Asiatic cholera, etc. must rank far behind tuberculosis" (Koch 1993). More than one hundred years later, TB remains the chief infectious scourge of humanity. It is riding into the twenty-first century on the wave of human urbanization and exploiting the ever-widening maldistribution of human wealth.

The Oppressive Toll of Urban Poverty

Today about 1.5 billion people live in absolute poverty, earning less than $1 a day, according to the World Bank (Abbasi 1999). This rapidly urbanizing underclass now comprises a quarter of the human family. The recent financial crisis in East Asia has only worsened the picture, with tens of millions thrown into poverty since 1997 in Indonesia, Thailand, Korea, and elsewhere. Poverty creates innumerable opportunities for emerging infections. The WHO reported in 1995 that poverty "conspires with the most deadly and painful diseases to bring a wretched existence to all who suffer from it." For many of the world's poorest nations, the burden of unpaid debts compounds the dangers their people face. How can a country like Uganda, which can spend just $2.50 per head each year on health, confront a crisis with HIV, malaria, TB, and other deadly infections when it is forced to spend $15 per head servicing its debts to the wealthy nations of the world?

The impact of poverty on disease emergence is easily seen in Mumbai, the city formerly known as Bombay. With 14.5 million residents, Mumbai is now India's largest urban center, and the third largest city in Asia. Dengue, malaria, TB, cholera, and sexually transmitted diseases are rampant. Every day approximately three hundred rural families migrate to Mumbai in search of work. Housing is in short supply, and most migrants are lucky if they find single room tenements. The city's water supply meets only 70 percent of the demand, and seepage of sewage from corroded pipes is widespread. About one hundred thousand new community latrines are needed immediately to improve sanitation. Villagers who migrate to Mumbai are often accustomed to defecating in open fields, and many would rather not change their habits and use the city's filthy communal toilets. Crime-riddled city streets are inhabited by street kids who have come to work in juice bars, hotels, garages, or for drug dealers. More than two thousand tons of garbage is dropped on the streets of Mumbai every day, and the stench of rotting waste is ubiquitous, especially during the rainy season.

Mumbai's primitive housing and inadequate sanitary standards are sadly typical of urban environments throughout the developing world. During the first months of 1991 such conditions allowed the explosive emergence of cholera in the *favelas* of Peru, Ecuador, and Colombia. For years those communities had received their drinking water from poorly maintained municipal systems that were prone to cross-contamination from raw sewage because of unrepaired leaks, illegal connections to water mains, sudden drops in water pressure, and lapses in routine chlorination. Once cholera was introduced into Peru's coastal fisheries, and had entered the local diet, it was not long before these dilapidated distribution systems became contaminated and spread the disease far and wide. Contaminated drinking water in urban slums also plays a large part in spreading hepatitis A, typhoid fever, and innumerable other diarrheal diseases that cause the most common epidemics in urban centers today.

We have already seen how rainwater collected in discarded containers brings forth the *Aedes* mosquitoes that can carry dengue. Piles of organic refuse that accompany uncontrolled urban growth also provide ideal breeding sites for other insects that carry human diseases and for rodents. In late 1997, newspapers in Beijing, China, reported an explosion in the rat population, particularly in the city's sprawling suburbs and rural margins. Health officials distributed more than 250 tons of poison bait throughout the city, as they urged residents to clean up rubbish-strewn sites where rat densities were at dangerous levels. Poisons were also disbursed around Nicaragua during the summer of 1999 when burgeoning rat populations in Managua and elsewhere sparked an epidemic of leptospirosis, a bacterial disease of humans and animals that typically includes a sudden onset of fever and severe muscle aches.

The expeditious breeding habits of rats permit them to multiply rapidly whenever human negligence gives them an opportunity. A female brown rat will begin to mate at two to three months of age. She can give birth to ten to twelve pups at a time and produce six to eight litters in a year. The larger the rat population becomes, the more likely it is to carry disease. A recent survey of rats trapped in England and Wales found that those from the most overcrowded colonies carried the most human pathogens (Webster and Macdonald 1996).

Urbanized Infections

Migrants to urban areas of the developing world not only bring themselves and the pathogens dwelling within them, they also bring their customs, traditions, and the accoutrements of rural life. Rural practices they bring to the city might include raising livestock, collecting drinking water from rivers and ponds, constructing their own homes from mud and sticks, walking barefooted, and sleeping outdoors. Some of these traditional ways may put the newcomers at risk of new diseases in the urban environment. But the massive transfer of rural people and their cultures into the cities of the developing world has also brought diseases of the countryside to urban settings for the first time.

Kala-Azar

Visceral leishmaniasis, or kala-azar, is a chronic wasting disease marked by fever, diarrhea, weight loss, cough, and lethargy. If untreated it is usually fatal. It's caused by different species of *Leishmania* parasites and is spread between mammalian hosts by the bite of a sand fly. Until the 1980s, visceral leishmaniasis was almost exclusively a disease of rural people, particularly poor and malnourished children of semi-arid regions of South Asia, the Middle East, East Africa, and Latin America. Since then, the disease has produced large outbreaks in urban communities where migrants from rural areas have congregated. During late 1997 and early 1998, a 439 percent increase in visceral leishmaniasis was noted in eastern Sudan following the resettlement of thousands of refugees from *Leishmania* endemic areas. There was also an upsurge of cases in certain cities of Ethiopia and Eritrea.

Recent outbreaks of visceral leishmaniasis among malnourished children in Brazil's urban *favelas* have been linked to the introduction of farm animals to the city and the favorable sand fly habitats they create. The disease can spread easily to large numbers of susceptible people when an infected animal arrives from the countryside. "The habit of keeping domestic animals, such as dogs, chickens, and horses, in the backyard provides an abundance of blood meals for sand fly vectors and raises vector population densities dramatically," notes Jorge Arias of the Pan American Health Organization. He and his colleagues investigated the growing problem of visceral leishmaniasis in Brazilian cities in 1996.

Chagas Disease

Another disease of the countryside, Chagas disease, has lately become an urban problem with the influx of migrants into the cities of Latin America. Chagas disease is caused by a parasite transmitted by the bite of blood-sucking insects called reduviids, also known as kissing bugs. Kissing bugs reside in the cracks and holes of primitive rural homesteads from Mexico to northern Argentina. They emerge at night and acquire the parasite from ingesting the blood of an infected person or animal. The vectors remain infected for life, passing on the disease to new hosts with subsequent feedings. Acute infection causes a fever and malaise. Chronic Chagas disease can damage the muscles of the heart, leading to death.

In recent years kissing bugs have accompanied human migrants from the rural hinterlands to their new homes in urban *favelas*. In metropolitan Santiago, Chile, 60 percent of slum houses have become infested with the insects. In one study, 15 percent of captured kissing bugs were infected with Chagas disease (Mott, Desjeux, Moncayo, et al. 1990). The poorer the construction material, the more likely the dwelling was infested. Up to 45 percent of kissing bugs trapped in urban Tegucigalpa, Honduras, were infected with the disease, as were up to 42 percent of kissing bugs studied in ten Bolivian cities. Tragically, the movement of Chagas disease into urban centers is now extending beyond residents of the *favelas* through the inadvertent transfusion of blood infected with the parasite.

Disease and Demographic Change in Djibouti City

The recent struggles of Djibouti city show how emerging infectious diseases can vex a rapidly growing metropolis in the developing world (Rodier, Parra, Kamil, et al. 1995). Djibouti, a coastal city in the horn of East Africa, was formerly the colonial capital of French Somaliland. With an influx of refugees and economic migrants from Ethiopia and Somalia, its population has swollen to more than three hundred thousand people. This represents a tenfold increase over the 1950 population, with the fastest growth occurring in the past decade. For most residents, living conditions are deplorable. According to the Minister of Urbanism, the city has significant problems with its drinking water supply, sewage system, and garbage collection. Rats are poorly controlled, and, since 1990, hantaviruses have been detected in brown rats around the port. Before October 1991, Djibouti was thought to be free of *Aedes aegypti* mosquitoes. But during that month the city experienced its first outbreak of dengue fever. That epidemic affected twelve thousand people, and further outbreaks have subsequently been reported. An entomological survey in 1992 showed that *A. aegypti* was abundant in many parts of the city (Cope 1993). Discarded plastic water bottles, foil-lined milk containers, metal barrels, and clay water jars were all identified as larval habitats. The extension of Djibouti city into farming districts has also seen the emergence of urban malaria in recent years, through greater human contact with *Anopheles* mosquitoes.

   Rural districts of Djibouti had limited cholera outbreaks in 1973 and 1985, but the disease was not a problem in the city until July 13, 1993 when it suddenly emerged in the Salines area, one of the poorest quarters of Djibouti city. Thanks to the rapid chlorination of all fresh water sources, the outbreak was controlled by September. But at least five thousand people developed cholera, and more than fourteen hundred were hospitalized.

   Tuberculosis (TB) is not new in Djibouti, but its incidence has nearly doubled since the 1980s. Much of the increase is among native Djiboutians. Since the late 1980s, multidrug-resistant TB has also been emerging. In March 1992, a strain of TB appeared that was resistant to eight different drugs. Djibouti's TB predicament stems not only from urban crowding, but from an exploding increase in HIV infection. Serum tests in 1987 showed that 5 percent of street prostitutes and 1 percent of bar hostesses were infected with HIV. Six years later infection rates in these women had reached 57 percent and 23 percent, respectively (Rodier, Parra, Kamil, et al. 1995).

Demographic Transitions in Developed Countries

Recent demographic changes in highly developed countries are also contributing to the emergence of infectious diseases. These changes include the recent acceleration in cross-border migrations by workers and their dependents, realignments in social class because of economic restructuring, and the dramatic growth in the elderly population. We shall consider each of these briefly in turn.

Accelerated Cross-Border Migration

Economic and political upheavals in many parts of the world have lately created millions of displaced people, many of whom seek refuge in industrialized countries. An estimated 70 million people, mostly from developing countries, cross international boundaries each year to sell their labor. Much of the movement is temporary or seasonal, and its direction is determined by the opportunities to pick crops or work in factories. Often today's migrants hope to settle permanently in new countries. Since 1945 the migration into and out of Australia has increased almost one hundred-fold. Immigration now accounts for the majority of Western Europe's population growth, with most new arrivals drawn from South Asia, the Caribbean, North Africa, and the Middle East. Net immigration to the fifteen member states of the European Union was essentially zero in 1984, but by the early 1990s it had exceeded one million net new arrivals per year. Germany, by far the biggest magnet for immigration flows, now hosts some 6.9 million foreign workers and their families. Of these, 2.2 million are Turks. Foreign populations residing in other European countries range from 3.6 million in France, to 2 million in the United Kingdom, to 1.3 million in Switzerland.

Immigration to the United States is also on the rise, recently reaching levels not seen since the tidal wave of European migration during the early years of the twentieth century. About 750 thousand people are legally granted United States residence each year, not including an estimated 275 thousand undocumented aliens. The size of the influx today is more than double the average number admitted each year through the middle third of the century. At current rates, the United States Census Bureau predicts that 65 percent of the country's population growth in the next fifty years will result from immigration. The composition of the immigrant mix is also very different than in the past. Today, more than two-thirds of new United States residents are coming from less developed countries in Asia, Latin America, and the Caribbean. One-fifth of the legal inflow arrives from a single country: Mexico. There are now 25.8 million foreign-born people residing in the United States, just under 10 percent of the total population. That proportion is higher than at any time since 1910, when 14 percent of United States residents were foreign-born. California hosts the largest number of foreign-born Americans, with nearly one-quarter of its thirty-three million residents born outside the country. About eight million United States residents were born in Mexico, and the Mexican government predicts that number will double by the year 2020.

As we have seen with TB, migrants from less developed countries may harbor infections not commonly seen in the United States. One such infection is malaria. Since 1991, three outbreaks of locally acquired malaria have been reported in densely populated areas of Texas, New Jersey, and New York City in people with no history of travel or even close proximity to an airport. In each incident the infections could be traced to immigrants or undocumented laborers living nearby who unknowingly carried malaria parasites in their blood. Transmission in rural settings, which has occurred in nearly fifty distinct episodes since 1957, is also commonly linked to nearby immigrants from malaria-endemic countries.

Since 1980, at least thirteen outbreaks of malaria have occurred among migrant farm workers in California. The largest outbreak, in 1986, involved twenty-six Mexican migrant field workers and two local residents of Carlsbad in coastal San Diego County. California's migrant farm workers, who include undocumented laborers from malarious districts in Mexico and Central America, must often subsist in substandard housing as they move from job to job. Frequently they sleep outside, under bridges or in makeshift cardboard huts, where they end up providing blood meals for local *Anopheles* mosquitoes. If any of these workers carry malaria parasites in their blood, the mosquitoes can transmit the disease to others during their nightly rounds. The United States Office of Migrant Health estimates that there are 4.2 million migrant and seasonal farm workers in the United States. Malaria is just one of the infectious hazards these workers face. The crowded and unsanitary living conditions of many labor camps also predispose them to respiratory infections, hepatitis, and diarrheal illnesses. Compared to other working adults of similar age, migrant farm workers are six times more likely to develop TB.

The cultural practices of new migrants can also present new challenges for infectious disease control. For example, many recently settled Portuguese immigrants in Massachusetts and Rhode Island like to consume imported raw limpets, a molluscan shellfish that they consider a delicacy. This custom has resulted in outbreaks of viral intestinal illnesses not previously seen with the eating of similar mollusks harvested from local waters (Townes, Landrigan, Monroe, et al. 1995). Among Mexicans and Central Americans, capsules made from dried rattlesnake flesh have long been a popular folk remedy for a variety of medical conditions. During the 1980s these capsules were the surprise source of a smoldering outbreak of *Salmonella arizona* infection in Los Angeles (Waterman, Juarez, Carr, et al. 1990). The capsules were widely available at *farmacias* and *boticas* serving the city's Latino communities. Unfortunately, reptiles like rattlesnakes are the primary hosts for *S. arizona*, and the capsules delivered a massive dose of the bacteria to those who ingested them.

Poverty Amidst Plenty

Poverty in the United States is not limited to migrant farm workers. More than thirty-five million Americans—about 13 percent of the population—live below the poverty line, as defined by the Untied States Census Bureau. This total, which hasn't changed despite nearly a decade of economic growth, includes about 20 percent of the nation's children. One in six Americans—forty-three million in all—cannot afford health insurance, and the number increases by one hundred thousand every month. Although America's booming economy has produced unimaginable wealth for a few, life for those on the bottom of the economic pyramid has hardly improved. For black men living in New York's Harlem ghetto, for example, the prosperity promised by the new global market is a cruel joke. They are less likely today to reach the age of sixty-five than men living in Bangladesh, one of the poorest countries in the world.

The widening disparities between rich and poor are obvious today in every American city. The lower 40 percent of American wage earners have seen virtually no real increase in wages since 1967. By contrast, real income for households in the top 20 percent has risen by 55 percent, after adjustment for inflation. Explanations for the growing inequalities in income and opportunity have pointed to the wage-depressing effects of globalized trade for unskilled workers, the decline of American trade unions, the increase in single-parent households, and the erosion of the government's social welfare safety net. For those left on the bottom, serious health risks from infectious diseases loom large, especially respiratory diseases and other illnesses related to overcrowding and damp, dilapidated housing. As long as poverty persists in this country, can it really come as a surprise that "Third World" diseases like TB and meningococcal disease continue to plague us?

Of all America's poor, those who live on the streets of our cities are among the most vulnerable. The number who are homeless for at least part of the year probably exceeds one million, but no one really knows. A lack of adequate shelter exposes homeless people to atrocious physical adversity, social abuse, and mental distress. A recent study of street youths in Montreal found that they were twelve times more likely to die during a given year than youth in the general population of Quebec (Roy, Boivin, Haley, et al. 1998). Drug-taking and prostitution were common behaviors that put these young people at risk of HIV, hepatitis, and sexually transmitted diseases. Homelessness was a major risk factor for developing TB during a recent outbreak in Los Angeles (Barnes, Yang, Pogoda, et al., 1999). Three large shelters for the homeless, including one that housed 595 occupants in three rooms, were determined to be the likely sites of transmission for 55 of the 79 cases in the epidemic.

Besides TB, homelessness is now a recognized risk factor for infection from HIV, syphilis, genital herpes, hepatitis, influenza, and intestinal worms. Sadly, indigent people in some American cities are also coming down with other infections, including those previously unheard of in prosperous countries. One example is the outbreak of trench fever among homeless people in Seattle in 1993. Trench fever was first described during World War I, when it affected more than a million troops in Europe. It is caused by infection with *Bartonella quintana* bacteria, and it is spread to human hosts by lice that reside in the seams of unwashed clothing. Besides a sudden fever, the infection causes a rash and relapsing bone pains. By World War II, trench fever was almost eliminated in American soldiers, and *B. quintana* infections virtually disappeared in the general population. But with growing numbers of Americans forced to live on city streets, trench fever has made a comeback. Recently it was shown that 20 percent of the residents of Seattle's "skid row" had antibodies to *B. quintana*, indicating a prior infection (Jackson and Spach 1996).

The Coming Elder Boom

The color of America's future is gray. The number of Americans over sixty-five years of age has increased eleven-fold since 1900 to more than thirty-three million. This growth compares to just a three-fold increase for the nonelderly population during that time. By the year 2030, when the baby boomers of the 1950s and 1960s have all retired, the United States Census Bureau estimates the number of elderly will exceed seventy million. Today, one in eight Americans ranks among the elderly. By 2030, it will be one in five. The fastest growing group is the "oldest old," those over eight-five years of age. Today they number about four million, almost double their number in 1980. The population in this group, the most demanding for health and social services, will more than double again by 2030. Similar trends have been predicted in Western Europe and Japan. How industrialized countries will meet the needs of their aging populations and avoid intergenerational conflict remains to be seen.

Old age is a strong risk factor for a number of leading infectious conditions. As a group, the elderly have weaker immune defenses, impaired circulation, poorer wound-healing ability, and a diminished cough reflex to keep pathogens out of the lungs. For these reasons they are disproportionately represented in statistics for urinary tract infections, food-borne diseases, and bacterial skin infections. Community-acquired pneumonia is fifty times more common in people over age seventy-five than in those aged fifteen to nineteen years. Pneumonia is the third leading cause of hospitalization in the elderly, and it is a common cause of death. The elderly are also far more likely to experience reactivations of old infections with TB. Recently TB has reemerged in Japan, after nearly forty years of decline. In 1999, Japan declared a TB emergency, as its rates of active disease rose to the top of the standings among industrialized nations. The main reason for the TB crisis is Japan's aging population. More than half of reported cases have occurred in those aged sixty years and above.

Other Factors of Change

Changes in the social environment in which people live can have far-reaching effects on human attitudes and behavior. Human behavior has a major role in transmitting infections. Individual behaviors, such as sexual activity and injecting drug use, have recently contributed to the dissemination of a number of emerging infections. Collective behaviors, such as bringing children together for day care, have also assisted in spreading infections. At the same time, efforts to motivate constructive human behavior have proven to be society's best defense against certain serious pathogens. The next chapter will examine the force of human behavior on disease emergence.

What You Can Do to Prevent Diseases When You Travel to the Tropics

A trip to an exotic destination in the tropics can be one of life's sweetest pleasures. Unfortunately, the tropics play host to a range of infectious diseases that are unfamiliar today to most North Americans. These include malaria, dengue fever, yellow fever, hepatitis A, leptospirosis, rabies, cholera, typhoid fever, and traveler's diarrhea. To keep that dream tropical get-away from turning into a nightmare, travel health experts at the CDC and state health departments recommend a few simple precautions:

- Schedule an appointment with your doctor or a special travel clinic as soon as you know your travel plans. Six months before you leave is not too early.

- Receive the recommended pretravel vaccinations, and if your doctor prescribes a medication to prevent malaria, remember to take it as directed.

- In the tropics, avoid being bitten by mosquitoes by applying insect repellents containing DEET (N,N-diethyl-metatoluamide), as directed on the container.

- While sleeping, stay in an air-conditioned environment, in a well-screened room, or under a bed net. Nets should be impregnated with the insecticide permethrin.

- Unless you are certain the drinking water is safe, limit yourself to beverages made with boiled water, carbonated drinks (no ice!), and beer or wine.

- Do not purchase foods or drinks from street vendors, and remember this simple rule for what you should eat: "Boil it, cook it, peel it, or forget it."

Chapter 5

Human Behavior

When an infectious disease is transmitted or maintained because of attitudes, behavior or surroundings, a purely germ-oriented approach is unlikely to provide effective control.

—Elizabeth Barrett-Connor,
University of California, San Diego

Demographic changes, such as those related to urbanization, migration, and economic restructuring, are inevitably accompanied by changes in lifestyle from one generation to the next. Value systems that had meaning in the past may carry less weight for young people struggling to better themselves in their contemporary social environments. For an urbanized world that is increasingly interconnected in a market-driven global economy, the moral standards of traditional rural life may simply not withstand the bombarding influences of Western mass culture. Even in wealthy, industrialized countries where recent demographic shifts have been less acute than in the developing world, attitudes about acceptable social conduct have been constantly under revision. In all societies, the choices that individuals are making about how they live their lives are undergoing change. Such change can have profound impacts on the emergence of infectious disease.

This chapter will consider the effects of individual behavior on the recent spread of some particularly worrisome infectious diseases. In a few instances, very old behaviors handed down in traditional societies have had unexpected outcomes in spreading infections. More often the diffusion of relatively new behaviors has played a role. Chief among these is the uniquely twentieth-century phenomenon of injecting drugs into the bloodstream to achieve mind-altering effects.

But other new behaviors related to changing family dynamics, our modern "life in the fast lane," and today's career ambitions also deserve mention. One additional human activity that must be examined is sex, an ancient behavior whose uniquely modern expressions have had substantial effects on the emergence of HIV and other significant infections in our time. But let's begin this survey of human behavior and disease with a glimpse at hepatitis C, an emerging infection whose impact may soon begin to dwarf that of HIV in many countries.

The Clandestine Killer

Like most people who find out they are infected with the hepatitis C virus, Dominique Benet was caught unawares. At age thirty-five she was a successful manager of a busy bookstore in downtown Boston. She looked and felt completely healthy, but she had decided it was a good time for a medical check-up. A routine blood test done as part of her physical examination picked up a slight abnormality in her liver enzymes. Her doctor thought it was probably nothing. But the next test revealed antibodies to hepatitis C in her blood, and another detected the ribonucleic acid (RNA) of the virus itself.

"It's hard to believe I'm carrying a potentially fatal virus and yet I don't feel ill," Dominique told her neighbor and friend Jerome Groopman, a hepatitis researcher based in Boston. Groopman featured Dominique's story in a 1998 article he wrote for *The New Yorker* about hepatitis C. The article, in which he changed the names of real people, was ominously titled "The Shadow Epidemic."

As Dominique came to grips with her diagnosis, Groopman helped her ascertain how she might have contracted the hepatitis C virus. This emerging infection is most often spread by direct through-the-skin exposure—from the blood of one person mixing with another—usually through dirty needles. As the two friends considered all the possibilities, Groopman decided the most likely exposure had occurred more than a decade earlier when Dominique was a university student. At that time she had felt she was under more pressure than she could handle, so she began to snort cocaine. It was "to get a buzz, to stay awake, to take away the fear," she said. She had never used intravenous drugs.

Groopman conjectured that by inhaling cocaine repeatedly through a straw Dominique had made the lining inside her nose

liable to pinpoint bleeding. That fragility would have given the hepatitis C virus unimpeded passage into her bloodstream whenever she
inhaled the drug through a straw already contaminated with traces of
another user's blood. Dominique's drug use ended with a successful
detoxification treatment after university, but that was too late to stop
the virus from settling permanently in her liver. Like 2.7 million other
Americans infected with hepatitis C—and more than 170 million people worldwide—Dominique now finds herself facing a very uncertain
future.

"Over the past two decades there has been a hepatitis C epidemic, but it has been overshadowed by AIDS," Groopman wrote.
"As physicians, public health officials and politicians have focused on
HIV, hepatitis C has been silently spreading." Americans chronically
infected with hepatitis C now outnumber those with HIV infection by
three to one. About ten thousand Americans die each year from the
ravaging effects of persistent hepatitis C infection on the liver. Most
cases do not respond well to available treatments. Already hepatitis
C accounts for about half of the four thousand liver transplants performed each year in the United States. Short of a miracle, serious
liver disease due to hepatitis C will triple in developed countries during the next ten to twenty years, and the number of deaths will surpass those from AIDS. "For the community as a whole, hepatitis C is
a viral time-bomb which is slowly destroying the health of large
numbers of the world population," say the authors of the book, *Living with Hepatitis C* (English and Foster 1997). In recent years, new
discoveries have been adding letters to the alphabet soup of hepatitis
viruses. First there was hepatitis A, a relatively common cause of
acute jaundice spread most often by contaminated food or water.
Although the symptoms of hepatitis A can frequently be unpleasant,
almost everyone gets over it within a few weeks. During that time
the body mounts an effective immune response, expelling the virus
from the liver and leaving the patient with lifelong immunity to subsequent infection.

Then came hepatitis B, which is transmitted both by sexual contact and by drops of infected blood left on shared intravenous needles, razors, or even toothbrushes. About one-third of hepatitis B
infections have no obvious source. Unlike hepatitis A, this virus is
capable of long-term infection. Persistent infections with hepatitis B,
lasting many years, can lead to cirrhosis or cancer of the liver, ending
in death. There are probably more than 350 million people worldwide infected chronically with hepatitis B. Most live in East Asia,
sub-Saharan Africa, or among indigenous populations of the Western
Pacific. In these regions transmission of hepatitis B typically occurs at

birth, when infected mothers pass the virus to their babies. For some reason infections acquired by newborn children almost always persist for life. By contrast, more than 90 percent of adults who become infected with hepatitis B will clear the virus, develop immunity, and have no further problems.

In 1989, a third hepatitis virus was identified and was promptly designated the hepatitis C virus. Right away doctors recognized that this virus accounted for most cases of the awkwardly named "non-A non-B hepatitis," a clinically distinct form of hepatitis, transmitted like hepatitis B, that was first reported in transfusion recipients in 1975. Testing for the new hepatitis C virus then revealed that ongoing silent infections were far more common in the general population than anyone had imagined. Unlike the other hepatitis viruses, this one is not easily purged by the adult immune system. It deftly evades all the immune responses the body can throw at it, so that infection becomes lifelong in 85 percent of cases. Once established, it secretly destroys the liver of its host. Usually the illness only becomes apparent after the virus has vandalized the liver for twenty years or more.

In the United States, new infections with hepatitis C have actually declined by more than 80 percent since peaking at about two hundred thousand per year in 1989. But silent infections acquired in the past have left a harsh legacy that millions in the population must now bear. Since 1980, the incidence of liver cancer has risen sharply in the United States, mostly because of the growing pool of Americans with chronic liver infections. Hepatitis C alone now accounts for 40 percent of chronic liver disease in the United States. Medical and work-loss costs due to persistent hepatitis C infections are thought to exceed $600 million per year, not including liver transplant costs. As most people infected with the virus are not yet clinically ill—or even aware of their status—the economic toll of hepatitis C can only increase substantially in coming years as complications from the disease set in. Blood transfusion once figured prominently in the transmission of hepatitis C. Before July 1992, when routine screening of the blood supply began, up to eighty thousand people in the United States became infected from tainted blood every year. Today that risk has dropped almost to zero. By far the most common mode of transmission at present is injecting drug use. The prevalence of hepatitis C infection among America's one to two million injecting drug users (IDUs) ranges from 72 to 86 percent. In this group the infection is acquired quickly, with 50 to 80 percent of IDUs becoming infected during their first six to twelve months of illicit drug use. Hepatitis C can also be transmitted sexually, or from an infected mother to her baby, but these routes appear to be far less efficient in spreading the virus than contaminated drug paraphernalia. Other suspected modes of transmission are nonsterile needles used for body piercing and tattooing. And, like hepatitis B, one-third or more of hepatitis C infections defy easy explanations.

Treatment for chronic hepatitis C is an area of intense research. Until recently, the mainstay of medical therapy has been alpha interferon, a naturally occurring protein that interferes with viral reproduction. When used by itself, interferon helps only about 20 percent of patients. Now it is often given in combination with ribavirin, another antiviral agent, but even this cocktail can halt the destruction of the liver in only about 40 percent of cases. For reasons still unclear, certain strains of hepatitis C respond better to available drugs than others, and the predominant strain in the United States—accounting for three-quarters of infections—is especially difficult to treat. Regardless of the regimen, treatments must be given by injection for six months or more, and relapses after the completion of therapy are common. Interferon alone costs about $700 per month, and many people are unable to tolerate its side-effects.

Given the hard facts about treating hepatitis C, an ounce of prevention would be worth many pounds of cure. Unfortunately, there is no vaccine against hepatitis C, and one is not likely to appear soon. Control of this epidemic will depend on identifying, testing, and counseling those at greatest risk. In 1999, the federal government launched a new public awareness campaign on the disease while it began the onerous task of identifying the one million Americans thought to have been exposed to the virus through blood transfusions before 1992. Reducing the injection of illegal drugs, or at least decreasing the sharing of contaminated drug paraphernalia, would prevent the most new cases today. But no group in society is harder to reach with health education messages than America's IDUs.

The Haystack of Needles

Despite endless media crusades to discourage the misuse of drugs, the habitual and "recreational" use of psychoactive drugs is common and is increasing worldwide, especially among young people. One in seven Americans reports having used cocaine at least once. Consumption of heroin has risen sharply in the United States and parts of Europe since the price of the drug plummeted in the mid-1990s. Police in the United Kingdom are reporting that even in small towns heroin use has become common among disaffected youth. The public health burden of illicit drugs pales when compared to alcohol abuse;

but the widespread use of these drugs, particularly drugs injected directly into the bloodstream, is maintaining a reservoir of people infected with blood-borne viruses like hepatitis C in virtually every American community. A uniquely modern human behavior with complex social and biomedical causes, the misuse of drugs has fueled this uniquely modern epidemic with bleak consequences for those involved and for society at large.

Unfortunately, hepatitis C is not the only infectious disease spread through substance abuse. Up to one-third of IDUs entering drug treatment in New York City are infected with HIV. The movement of HIV into the subculture of IDUs early in the AIDS epidemic significantly accelerated spread of that disease. Of the 688,200 cases of AIDS reported in the United States by the end of 1998, at least 26 percent occurred because of injecting drug use. An additional 6 percent of cases occurred in people with both homosexual contact and injecting drug use. Substance abuse has played an especially important role in exposing women and their children to HIV. Among American females, 43 percent of AIDS cases have occurred through injecting drug use, and an additional 17 percent have resulted from heterosexual contact with an IDU. Exposure of mothers to HIV in these two ways has accounted for more than half of the 8,461 pediatric cases of AIDS reported in the United States by the end of 1998. Moreover, at least 10 percent of hepatitis B infections in the United States are acquired from injecting drugs.

Poor hygiene and nonsterile injecting techniques also put IDUs at high risk of skin infections and subcutaneous abscesses due to antibiotic-resistant strains of *Staphylococcus aureus* and other agents. Staphylococci and other bacteria that gain entry to the bloodstream from needles can rapidly settle upon the valves of the heart. The resulting disease, infective endocarditis, can cause irreparable damage to the valves and requires weeks of expensive hospital treatment. Contaminated injection equipment, adulterated drugs, or an IDU's unwashed skin are likewise potential sources for the spores of *Clostridium tetani*, the bacteria that cause tetanus. These spores will awaken in wounds or other devitalized tissue and release a powerful neurotoxin that paralyzes the host. Patients often require mechanical ventilators to breathe, and one-quarter of cases end in death despite intensive hospital care. Of sixty-seven cases of tetanus reported in California between 1987 and 1997, 40 percent occurred in IDUs, particularly those who injected heroin just under the skin by a technique known as "skin-popping."

Looking beyond the direct disease risks from shooting drugs, the chaotic lives and meager living conditions of most substance abusers increase the chances they will develop food poisoning, hepatitis A, tuberculosis, or meningococcal disease. The exchange of sex for drugs also heightens the risk of acquiring sexually transmitted diseases. Without treatment, IDUs will typically inject illicit drugs about one thousand times during a year. For those who cannot or will not stop injecting, obtaining fresh supplies of sterile syringes is one way to lower the risks. Needle exchange programs have repeatedly shown they can reduce a community's toll from HIV and other infections, but they are illegal in many states. Moreover, Congress refuses to fund needle exchange programs in places where they are legal for fear of appearing "soft" on drugs.

The Needle-Sharing Doctor

In May 1998, the health department in Valencia, Spain, announced that at least 217 patients undergoing surgery during the previous year had been infected with the hepatitis C virus. The source of the outbreak was a forty-year-old anesthetist who for years had led a secret life as an intravenous morphine addict. Immediately after surgery the anesthetist would inject himself with a portion of the pain-killing opioid drugs intended for his patients. He would then administer the rest of the drugs to the patients, using the same syringe. The health department estimated that the doctor had anesthetized more than two thousand people since he developed hepatitis C infection in 1995. While those patients were traced and tested for the virus, a group representing hospital patients in Spain demanded the doctor's immediate imprisonment.

The Facts of Life: Sex and Disease

In most industrialized societies, the last half of the twentieth century witnessed a greater social acceptance of the sexual side of human nature. Today an interest in sex is generally affirmed as a normal, healthy part of being human. As social attitudes about sex have become more relaxed, sexual relations outside marriage have become more open in Western countries. Sex during adolescence, sex before marriage, prolonged cohabitation instead of marriage, and sex with multiple partners are increasingly common. Stigmas associated with homosexual behavior have not disappeared, but they have faded significantly in the wake of the worldwide awakening of gay consciousness. Perhaps there have never been fewer moral restraints on sexual expression for consenting adults.

But society's new sexual freedoms have not come without costs. These would include unwanted pregnancies, unsafe abortions, single parenthood, and sexual abuse, to name a few. The burdens of such costs have not been shared equally, but their social repercussions have been felt by everyone across the community. From a public health standpoint, the most obvious consequence of increased sexual activity is the spread of sexually transmitted diseases (STDs). It is a sad fact of life that at least twenty viruses, bacteria, and other infectious agents are spread among humans primarily by sexual contact. The worldwide burden of STDs is immeasurable, but the World Health Organization estimates that at least 333 million people are stricken each year by just the four main diseases for which there are cures: gonorrhea, syphilis, *Chlamydia* and trichomoniasis. Among those infected, barely one quarter have access to adequate treatment, so the cycle of infection and reinfection rolls on.

Rates of curable STDs are now higher in the United States than in any other developed country. STDs account for five of the top ten diseases notified by law to the CDC, or 87 percent of all reports received for those diseases. Approximately twelve million new cases of STDs are reported each year, three million among teenagers. One in five Americans is now treated for an STD before their twenty-first birthday. Excluding HIV infections, STDs are thought to cost the United States economy about $10 billion every year, or about forty-three times the amount spent preventing them. Public knowledge and awareness of STDs remains low, and efforts to promote condom use and other healthy behavioral changes are generally unfocused and controversial. So the suffering from STDs continues. Prince Morrow once noted, "It is a conservative estimate that fully one-eighth of all human suffering comes from this source" (Gerbase, Rowley, and Mertens 1998). He made this observation in 1912, while chairing a committee examining the problem of venereal diseases in America. Sadly, despite enormous medical advances since then, his words are just as true today.

Concern about STDs has begun to gain momentum, thanks in part to an unsettling report released in 1996 by The Institute of Medicine. The report, titled *The Hidden Epidemic*, called for a radical overhaul of America's STD prevention strategies, including massive new investment in public education, sexual health services, and research. One reason for the renewed interest in STDs is the fact that many of the common infections seen today are caused by viruses, and are not readily curable. Another reason is the growing awareness of the long-term harm that STDs can cause, particularly to women. Cancer, infertility, chronic discomfort, and serious disease in newborn infants are among the grave complications that can result from the more common infections encountered today. Ulcerative and inflammatory diseases of the genital tract have also been shown to facilitate the transmission of HIV, perhaps the most dreaded STD (Cohen 1998). The importance of sex in spreading dangerous new diseases is becoming obvious to all.

In chapter 1 we saw how the emergence of HIV from its jungle reservoir was helped along by the sexual behavior of long-haul truck drivers and other travelers through East Africa's AIDS belt. More recently, India's truck drivers have played a similar role in the diffusion of HIV there. India now has the distinction of leading the world with the largest number of HIV-infected people, about four million. As in the rest of Asia, the AIDS epidemic began slowly in India. But since the mid-1990s it has been expanding rapidly, in part thanks to the hazardous sexual behavior of the country's five million long-distance truck drivers. One study that interviewed fifty-seven hundred consecutive truck drivers at a busy highway check post found that 87 percent had "frequent and indiscriminate change of sexual partners," including sex with roadside prostitutes (Rao, Pilli, Rao, et al. 1999). Among drivers under thirty years of age, more than one-third said they had sex with thirty to sixty different partners during a year. Only 11 percent said they used condoms during commercial sex. Not surprisingly, HIV prevalence among India's truck drivers is about twenty times higher than the national average.

The high-risk sexual practices of a few key individuals may have also played a decisive role in igniting the AIDS epidemic in the industrialized world. When the virus seeped out of Africa during the late 1970s, probably first in Europe and then in the United States, it was able to diffuse as quickly as it did with the help from certain sexually active members of the gay community. In his book *And the Band Played On*, Randy Shilts documented the pivotal early role of a Canadian airline steward known today to epidemiologists as "Patient Zero." The steward, who traveled often to Europe, had been one of the first people diagnosed in North America with the syndrome that would later be known as AIDS. During the next four years, before his death at age thirty-one, he continued to practice unprotected anal intercourse with multiple partners, who in turn spread the virus to others. Many of the first cases diagnosed in New York and Los Angeles could be linked to Patient Zero's traveling sexual exploits. In fact, at least 40 of the first 248 gay men who developed AIDS in the United States had sex with Patient Zero, or with one of his partners.

Giving STDs a Head Start

One of the strongest risk factors for acquiring HIV and the other STDs is the early initiation of sexual experience. There is no doubt that sexual activity is beginning at a younger age today than in previous generations. According to the largest survey of American sexual behavior to date, just 35 percent of men and 19 percent of women born between 1933 and 1952 had begun sexual intercourse by the age of sixteen years (Laumann, Gagnon, Michael, et al. 1994). Among those born a generation later, between 1953 and 1972, the proportions had risen to 48 percent for men and 37 percent for women. Similar generational shifts have been reported in studies from the United Kingdom, Belgium, France, Norway, Sweden, and New Zealand. "In Western countries it is now fair to say that initiation of sexual intercourse in the early to midteenage years has become a social norm for both sexes," says Charlotte Paul, an epidemiologist at New Zealand's University of Otago (Paul, Fitzjohn, Eberhart-Phillips, et al. 1999).

In the most recent survey of sexual behavior among American high school students, approximately 38 percent of ninth graders and 61 percent of twelfth graders reported having sexual intercourse at least once (Centers for Disease Control and Prevention 1998a). This survey, completed in 1997 on a representative sample of more than sixteen thousand students from all fifty states, showed virtually no difference in sexual experience between teenage boys and girls. It also found that 12 percent of ninth graders and 21 percent of twelfth graders had already had intercourse with four or more partners. These figures represent a slight decrease in teenage sexual activity from that reported in previous surveys from 1991, 1993, and 1995. But they still portray a higher level of adolescent sexual experience than in any generation that came of age before 1980, even the generation of the 1960s' "sexual revolution." The 1997 survey also showed improved use of condoms in both age groups, although 40 to 50 percent of sexually active students still reported that they had not used condoms during their last sexual intercourse.

The main reason why early sexual activity is a risk factor for STDs nowadays is its strong correlation with the number of sex partners one is likely to have. The greater the number of partners, the greater the exposure to possible infection. Although the age of first intercourse has dropped in industrialized countries, the average age at which young adults settle into their first "permanent union" has remained fairly constant—about 24 years of age—since the 1950s. Although such partnerships today are less often formalized by marriage, they are generally monogamous for their duration.

Normalizing sexual behavior at a younger age has widened the "risk window" for acquiring STDs, increasing the number of years that a young person is likely to be sexually active with multiple partners before entering a permanent relationship. The fact that the behavior shift has occurred among adolescents, whose sexual relations are more often unplanned or sporadic, increases the risk of STD transmission even more.

The effect of multiple sexual partners on STD risk is evident from a 1992 study by Gavin Joffe and colleagues, in which 467 female students at a large midwestern university were surveyed during their senior year. Overall, 12 percent of the women reported having at least one STD since coming to college. But the risk was not evenly spread. Those who reported having sex with five or more partners were eight times more likely to have an STD than those who reported having only one partner. This trend was confirmed in a study of one thousand New Zealanders surveyed at age twenty-one (Dickson, Paul, Herbison, et al. 1996). Among the women, 39 percent who reported having sex with ten or more partners in their lifetimes could recall having an STD, compared to less than 3 percent whose sexual experience was limited to one partner. The young men in the New Zealand study had fewer STDs overall, but the effect of multiple partners on their STD risk was the same. Men who reporting having sex with ten or more partners in their lifetimes were about nine times more likely to report an STD as those who said they had only one sexual partner.

Heightened sexual activity among adolescents is especially worrisome because of the additional harm that STDs can cause in this age group. For both sexes such infections may bring stigma and embarrassment at a critical time in psychological development. For females there is mounting evidence that sexual exposure to certain infectious agents during adolescence can lead to more serious disease. *Chlamydia trachomatis*, in particular, targets the type of cells found more commonly on a younger woman's cervix. Not surprisingly, this bacterial infection is much more prevalent among teenagers than any other group.

The Covert Operations of Chlamydia and Herpes

As the sexual activity of adolescents has increased, so has the public health burden of *Chlamydia*. Globally there are approximately eighty-nine million new genital infections with *Chlamydia* every year. The largest numbers of cases are in South Asia and sub-Saharan Africa, but *Chlamydia* infections are ubiquitous in all young, sexually active populations. In the United States, *Chlamydia* is by far the most commonly reported infectious disease, with more than four hundred thousand cases notified to the Centers for Disease Control and Prevention (CDC) annually. Assuming that only 10 percent of cases are actually reported, there are probably four million new infections in the United States each year, according to the Institute of Medicine (1997). Genital infections with *Chlamydia* have been detected in nearly 10 percent of female recruits for the United States Army (Gaydos, Howell, Pare, et al. 1998). They are also routinely discovered in 4 to 8 percent of young women attending family planning clinics. A study of publicly financed clinics in Baltimore picked up *Chlamydia* in 24 percent of female patients aged twelve to nineteen years (Burstein, Gaydos, Diener-West, et al. 1998). The highest infection rate, 28 percent, was in girls fourteen years of age.

Much of *Chlamydia's* success as a pathogen relates to its secrecy. Up to 80 percent of *Chlamydia* infections in women and 50 percent in men cause no symptoms. Unless doctors actively search for *Chlamydia* and prescribe antibiotics to all the sexual partners of people who are infected, the epidemic will persist. The reluctance of many adolescents to seek sexual health services compounds the problem. The urgency of treating *Chlamydia* infections stems from their devastating complications, especially for adolescent women. If untreated, *Chlamydia* can readily spread from the cervix into more distant regions of the reproductive tract. Acute infections of the fallopian tubes cause a syndrome of severe lower abdominal pain called pelvic inflammatory disease (PID), an outcome particularly common among adolescents. Smoldering, silent infections of the fallopian tubes can also occur. Either way, scarring from tubal infections can render a woman infertile for life. It is estimated that *Chlamydia* accounts for as much as half of female infertility today. Scarred fallopian tubes also increase the risk of ectopic pregnancy, a potentially life-threatening condition where the fertilized egg implants outside the womb. The incidence of ectopic pregnancy has quadrupled in the United States since the 1960s. Women who have had PID are more than eight times as likely to suffer from ectopic pregnancy than those with no such history.

Another surreptitious STD that is currently causing much apprehension is genital herpes. Infection with either of the two herpes simplex viruses can cause episodes of painful genital ulcers that may recur over a lifetime. Today about five hundred thousand cases of genital herpes are estimated to occur each year in the United States, not counting recurrences. Traditionally, herpes infections around the mouth were caused by herpes simplex virus type 1, while genital infections were due almost entirely to type 2 viruses. Today, the type 1 virus accounts for 20 to 60 percent of genital herpes cases, reflecting changing patterns of sexual behavior. New antiviral medications can diminish the pain of herpes attacks, accelerate healing time, and reduce recurrences, but they are not curative.

Since the late 1970s, specialized laboratories have been able to test blood specimens for antibodies to the herpes simplex virus type 2 (HSV-2). Serum surveys of populations in many countries of the world have shown that silent HSV-2 infections are far more common than clinically recognized cases. For example, 22 percent of Americans over the age of twelve were shown to have antibody evidence of HSV-2 infection in a recent survey of thirteen thousand-plus randomly selected people (Fleming, McQuillan, Johnson, et al. 1997). Less than 10 percent of those with HSV-2 infection could remember having the symptoms of genital herpes. This is worrisome because HSV-2 can be transmitted sexually whether there are symptoms or not. If many millions in the United States and elsewhere are infected with herpes and don't even know it, how many millions of others are being exposed unknowingly to this grim, incurable disease? No one can say.

What can be said is that the number of Americans infected with HSV-2 is immense and appears to be growing. HSV-2 prevalence has increased 30 percent in the United States since 1978. The prevalence among people in their twenties has doubled, while for those aged twelve to nineteen years old it has increased five-fold. A similar picture is evident in most other countries across the globe. In studies conducted on five continents (Mindel 1998), HSV-2 antibodies have turned up in 6 to 53 percent of pregnant women, and 5 to 18 percent of blood donors, on routine testing.

Among patients studied at various STD clinics, the rates have ranged from 8 to 83 percent worldwide. Add to this the increasing incidence of genital herpes due to the type 1 herpes virus, and it is no surprise that herpes has taken center stage as a public health menace. Soon the test to detect antibodies to HSV-2 will become more widely available, and pressure will be on doctors and patients alike to check for the disease. Until there is a vaccine—and none is expected for a decade or more—the spread of herpes is likely to continue.

Sexual Hazards in the Bayou

Men who have sex with other men still comprise the single largest group of Americans who become infected with HIV each year. Prevention of new HIV infections will depend on understanding the sexual behavior of this group and finding acceptable ways for them to reduce high-risk activities. A recent anonymous survey of 3,171 patrons at gay bars in Louisiana suggests that HIV prevention in this population isn't going to be easy (Kohl, Wendell, Farley, et al. 1995-1998)

Among the gay men surveyed, more than one quarter said they had practiced unprotected receptive anal intercourse in the previous thirty days. Receptive anal intercourse is one of the most hazardous sexual activities for HIV transmission, conferring ten times the risk of vaginal intercourse. Of the study's respondents who knew their HIV status, 12 percent were HIV-positive. Among those, 77 percent said they had HIV-negative partners. One-fifth of those with uninfected partners said they had practiced unprotected insertive anal intercourse during the previous thirty days, putting their partners at high risk. Among HIV-negative respondents, 17 percent reported having HIV-positive partners. Of those with infected partners, 28 percent said they had put themselves at high risk through unprotected receptive anal sex during the previous thirty days. Simply knowing one's HIV status, and that of one's partner, does not seem to be enough to prevent high-risk sexual behavior.

Culture and Disease

Although substance abuse and sexual conduct are obvious human behaviors involved in the emergence of infectious diseases, they are not the only human activities worth citing. Sometimes the behaviors leading to disease are culturally determined, as seen with the link between umbilical cord care and neonatal tetanus in many parts of the world. Almost three hundred thousand newborn babies die each year in developing countries because of the powerful neurotoxin released by *Clostridium tetani* bacteria. *C. tetani* spores surround us every day in soil and dust, and they sometimes contaminate unclean wounds, as we have seen with injecting drug users. But the fatal consequences of tetanus infection are extremely rare today in developed countries thanks to hygienic wound care and the protection afforded by tetanus vaccine. For babies born in less fortunate circumstances, however, infections with tetanus acquired at birth are still common, and have an all too predictable course. By the sixth day of life such infants become irritable and feed poorly. Their muscles then stiffen progressively, and by the eighth day they are usually dead. In some cultures, neonatal tetanus is known locally as "eighth day disease."

Babies who succumb to tetanus are typically born at home under aseptic conditions to poor mothers who have never received tetanus vaccine, so they are unable to pass on immunity to their babies through the womb. In such settings, birth attendants often apply locally made dressings to the baby's umbilical wound, after the cord has been cut with a kitchen knife or scissors. Substances applied to the cord stump vary according to culture, but sometimes they can foster tetanus infections. In a recent survey of thirty rural communities in Bangladesh, where neonatal tetanus had caused 34 percent of infant deaths in the previous year, investigators discovered that mustard oil and cow dung were among the substances commonly administered to the baby's cord stump during the first few days of life (Hlady, Bennett, Samadi, et al. 1992). In rural Pakistan the favored dressing is ghee, a homemade butter derived from the unpasteurized milk of water buffaloes. Such substances may be intrinsically contaminated with *C. tetani* spores, or they may physically block out oxygen from the umbilical wound, promoting the germination of spores already present. Strongly held cultural practices will have to be addressed sensitively if the World Health Organization's goal of eliminating neonatal tetanus is to be achieved.

Cultural factors may have also hastened the cholera epidemic in Latin America, starting in 1991. In parts of South America *ceviche* is a popular traditional dish in which uncooked fish or shellfish is marinated in citrus juice. Early in the epidemic it was suspected that eating *ceviche* from contaminated local waters was a risk factor for cholera. But when public health officials in Peru announced that fish should be thoroughly cooked before eating it, many people in coastal areas resisted the suggestion. As a compromise, the public was then urged to marinate the fish for longer periods, in the hope that the acid in the juice would penetrate the meat and inactivate the cholera organisms.

Cholera rapidly has made further inroads in Latin America's urban centers through the custom of purchasing foods and beverages from street vendors. Although they often have little knowledge of food hygiene, thousands of these vendors eke out a living on city streets, hawking such items as peeled fruits, homemade beverages, and flavored ices. Out of necessity, their pushcarts hold the foods they sell at ambient temperatures for long periods. This allows bacterial contaminants like *Vibrio cholerae* to multiply in the foods, increasing the chances of disseminating the disease. Meanwhile, in the

Peruvian Andes, funeral practices have spread the cholera epidemic further. Funerals in the three thousand-meter highlands of the Caja-marca region are lavish, three-day affairs in which guests eat *mote*, a boiled corn dish. Investigators have found that family members who prepare the bodies of cholera victims for burial are often involved in preparing the mote as well (Suarez, Swayne, Castaneda, et al. 1995). This allows transmission of cholera to the guests, perpetuating the cycle of infection.

Cultural influences on disease transmission are not limited to developing countries. In chapter 3 we saw how health-conscious Western diets have turned increasingly to fresh fruits and vegetables. This behavior has had predictable consequences in terms of out-breaks of food-borne disease. People in today's fast-paced Western societies are also increasing their consumption of food outside the home, especially in fast-food restaurants. This trend too may be exposing them to increased risks of food-borne disease. Almost 80 percent of outbreaks of diarrhea in the United States involve food eaten away from home. Mass-produced meals aimed at diners on the go may not be sufficiently cooked to kill pathogens such as *E. coli* O157:H7 (see chapter 2). In a busy commercial setting, one food can easily be cross-contaminated by another. A minor food contamination can be amplified more easily than at home, as when a single egg tainted with *Salmonella* is pooled with other eggs to make a large batch of omelets. Similarly, a harmlessly low dose of *Bacillus cereus* in cooked rice can turn ghoulish at a take-out stand when the rice is held for hours at a temperature that promotes bacterial growth.

When today's time-pressed consumers do eat at home, their provisions are often unlike anything that Mom used to make from scratch. The average number of meals purchased ready-to-eat and consumed at home has doubled in the United States since the mid-1980s. With two-income families demanding more convenience and ever quicker food preparation times, supermarket delicatessens, bak-eries, and other take-out franchises have proliferated to offer an array of ready-made home-meal replacements. The United States Depart-ment of Agriculture (USDA) recently questioned whether consumers know that they should treat such foods as perishable (USDA 1996). Their report warned that hot foods need to be received hot and eaten within two hours to avoid disease from food-borne pathogens. Young adults today may know less about food safety than earlier generations because they grew up spending less time in the kitchen observing their mothers and grandmothers. They may have even fewer opportunities to pass on safe home food preparation practices to their children. With 70 percent of American women aged twenty-

Microbes Made for Leisure

In October 1997, a doctor in suburban Melbourne, Australia, reported that he had recently diagnosed hepatitis A in three school-age boys. The boys, who all belonged to the local junior football club, had complained of fever, fatigue, and poor appetites. One by one their skin had taken on the yellow tint of jaundice. The doctor's report triggered a public health investigation, and four other boys on the team were found to be suffering from the same symptoms (Tallis and Gregory 1997).

Investigators discovered that on August 31 that year all the boys had attended a family barbecue at a team member's home. The boys, aged eight to fifteen years, had enjoyed a dip in the home's heated spa pool, while ten girls attending the affair stayed out of the water. Further queries determined that while the boys were in the pool they had played a game called "whale spitting," in which mouthfuls of spa water were spewed out in a projectile manner. It turns out that one boy who had been playing in the pool had to go home early because he was feeling tired and feverish. You guessed it: He had hepatitis A, and it appears that he shed it into the spa. None of the girls at the barbecue got sick because they didn't play in the water.

For all the health benefits claimed by spa manufacturers, soaking in the whirling, warm waters of these pools can sometimes lead to infection. The risks are reduced when spa owners follow recommended guidelines for pool disinfection, but it is impossible to eliminate all infectious contaminants. The warm waters of whirlpool spas also provide an ideal environment for *Legionella pneumophila*, the bacteria that cause Legionnaires' disease. We have already seen how a spa display in Holland caused a massive outbreak of Legionnaires' disease in 1999 (see chapter 2). In another large outbreak, in 1994, fifty cruise ship passengers developed Legionnaires' disease following exposure to the ship's whirlpool spas. The infections occurred during nine cruises between New York and Bermuda before the outbreak came to the attention of public health authorities. According to investigators, many of those affected had not even entered the spas. As in the Dutch epidemic, they had simply inhaled contaminated aerosol droplets given off by the pools as they walked past them (Jerrigan, Hofmann, Cetron, et al. 1996).

five to forty-four years in the workforce today, children are increasingly preparing food at home on their own.

Recent surveys have confirmed a widespread lack of knowledge about food safety. Only 43 percent of one thousand American adults surveyed during 1996 recognized that fruits and vegetables may contain harmful bacteria (American Meat Institute 1996). In another survey, one in five respondents did not perceive any risks in leaving cooked meat on the kitchen counter for a period of four hours

(Collins 1997). More than 90 percent of adults said in a telephone interview that they always wash their hands after using a public toilet (American Society for Microbiology, 1996). But when 6,330 adults were watched in public rest rooms during 1996, only 74 percent of women and 61 percent of men actually washed their hands. Unwashed hands may be the single greatest cause of preventable infections in developed countries today.

Ring around the Rosie: Infections and Childcare

Demand for out-of-home childcare has risen dramatically in recent years, as more parents have opted for paid employment while their children are young. In 1975, fewer than 40 percent of United States mothers with children under the age of six worked outside of home. By 1995, that percentage had increased to 62 percent, according to the Bureau of Labor Statistics (1998). In today's mobile job market, fewer working parents live close enough to relatives who otherwise might provide help at home with young children during the day. As a result, almost one-third of America's 10.3 million preschoolers with mothers in the workforce now attend organized childcare facilities during working hours. Another 15 percent receive care in less formal settings from someone other than a relative. In most cases, out-of-home care now begins during the first six months of life.

Professional care outside of home offers children many advantages in terms of nutrition, mental stimulation, and activities that promote social development. But infections in childcare settings are rife. Infants and toddlers who attend childcare centers are thought to acquire at least 50 percent more infections than children cared for at home, and on average they suffer more than twice as many days of illness. Factors that promote infections in childcare settings include crowding, poor ventilation, contaminated playthings and food preparation sites, and the unhygienic behavior that is typical of youngsters. "Children are gregarious. They share everything. Coughing and sneezing at close range is common. Fecal contamination of food and toys is frequent. Everything goes in a child's mouth," says Jerome Klein (1986), a pediatrician at Boston City Hospital.

Dr. Klein notes that on average children between the age of two and four years put their hands or another object in their mouths every three minutes. Viruses that cause colds, and pathogens that cause other more serious respiratory infections, can remain infectious

Nursing Homes for the Elderly: Nursing Infections?

Another germ factory awaiting many Americans at the other end of the life cycle is the nursing home or the skilled nursing facility. The number of people over age sixty-five now living out their twilight years in these facilities has risen to more than 1.5 million in the United States. Although the proportion of older Americans choosing to live in the country's seventeen thousand nursing homes has dropped since the 1980s, the sheer growth of the elderly population has continued to push up the number of nursing home residents. Except for inmates in prisons, nursing home residents now comprise the largest institutionalized population in America. The average age of admission to nursing homes is eighty-two years. With the population of octogenarians expected to grow rapidly during the next thirty years, the nursing home industry can look forward to continued expansion well into the twenty-first century.

Nursing homes present special challenges for many infectious diseases. Skin infections, eye infections, and diarrhea are more common in nursing homes than acute care hospitals, and they often arise in outbreaks that spread from one patient to the next. Pneumonia and urinary tract infections are also frequent problems. One reason for high rates of infection in nursing homes is the residents' increased susceptibility to disease, which is due to such factors as their advanced age, underlying chronic illnesses, immobility, and dependence on invasive devices such as urinary catheters. Certain medications can also increase susceptibility to infection, and the heavy use of antibiotics in nursing homes can promote resistance over time, making infections harder to treat.

But the most significant reasons for high infection rates in nursing homes may be organizational. Increased levels of nonprofessional staff, high patient-to-staff ratios, and high staff turnover go with the territory of operating nursing homes today. Together these factors can contribute to an inconsistent approach to infection control in many facilities. Without repeated staff education, basic hygiene practices—such as hand washing after every patient contact—can lose priority. Policies that penalize employees for taking sick leave can also put residents at risk. When outbreaks occur, a limited ability to recognize the problem early and isolate affected patients quickly can magnify the dangers. With nursing home care now costing as much as $35 thousand a year, a professional approach to infection control should not be too much to ask.

on nonporous toys for hours or even days. A recent study in Brazil found that children who attend childcare centers were more than five times as likely to develop pneumonia as those who stay at home (Homewood 1996).

Children in diapers present special risks, and childcare staff must be careful to wash their hands thoroughly after diapers are changed. Surfaces contaminated with feces can remain infectious for weeks, and may transmit such common childhood pathogens as rotavirus, hepatitis A virus, and *Giardia lamblia*. Many familiar infections of young children can be contagious before any signs of disease are apparent. Outbreaks at childcare centers are a frequent consequence. Sometimes the infections that children pick up in group care settings are brought home, spreading to older children and adults. In a massive outbreak of hepatitis A in Phoenix, Arizona, during the first ten months of 1997, household contacts of those attending or working in childcare centers were more than three times as likely as other people in the community to contract the disease (Venczel, Desai, Bell, et al. 1998). It is no wonder that public health professionals sometimes refer to early childhood education centers as "germ factories."

In wealthy countries of the industrialized world, technological advances have created an abundance of material wealth that would have been unimaginable a century ago. The next chapter looks at the role of modern technology and industry on disease emergence. In terms of food production, new technologies have created greater choice with increased efficiency and lower costs. In terms of medical care, technology has prolonged life and improved the quality of life for many people. But we will see that highly evolved technology in both the food industry and the health care system can inadvertently disseminate pathogenic organisms to large numbers of people, facilitating emergence.

What You Can Do To Prevent Sexually Transmitted Diseases

The best protection against STDs is not to have sex, or to have a mutually monogamous relationship with someone who is not infected. If you decide to have sex in other situations, then consistent use of condoms is essential. Sex with condoms is not 100 percent safe, but it is much less risky than sex without them. According to the United States Food and Drug Administration (FDA) condoms can be used correctly if you follow some simple rules:

- Buy only latex or polyurethane condoms where the package states they are for prevention of disease. Store them in a cool place, out of direct sunlight.

- Use a condom for every sexual act involving the penis, including oral sex. Never reuse a condom.

- Put the condom on after the penis is erect and before any contact is made with any part of the partner's body. While pinching the tip, place the condom against the penis and unroll it all the way to the base.

- Water-based lubricants will prevent irritation and reduce the risk of the condom breaking during use. Avoid oil-based lubricants, as they weaken latex condoms and may increase the chance of breakage.

- After ejaculation, hold onto the rim of the condom and withdraw carefully while the penis is still erect.

If you think you should be using condoms but your partner refuses, say "no" to having sex with that person.

Chapter 6

Technology and Industry

Innovative, progressive changes introduced by humans can provide advantages to microbes, which, in turn, threaten the population. In most cases, advantages are provided unwittingly as a by-product of technology.

—Robert F. Breiman, Centers for Disease Control and Prevention

From Paleolithic times to the silicon age, humans have subdued hostile environments and bettered their chances for survival through technology. But technological advances have often come with unintended consequences. In the nineteenth century, for example, the Industrial Revolution created considerable material wealth and opportunity for some, while producing unliveable cities plagued by poverty, pollution, and social disintegration. Modern machines have extended human productivity and provided comfort at the cost of making us sedentary, increasing our risk of heart disease. Increasingly, our everyday lives are bathed in new technologies, but deep down we wonder if the unforeseen by-products of industrialization are not endangering our health.

On balance, technologies introduced in the twentieth century have lowered the risk of infectious disease in humans. Drinking water purification, pasteurization of milk, sewage treatment, vaccines, and antibiotics are all relatively recent technologies that have protected human populations against exposure to dangerous pathogens. But modern technology, especially in food production and medical care, has provided new opportunities for the widespread occurrence of certain infections that might otherwise have remained obscure. And the more technology-dependent a society becomes, the more vulnerable it can become to the emergence of particular infectious diseases. Recently the United Kingdom has discovered just how vulnerable it can be.

Mad Cows and an Irishman

For Maurice Callaghan of Belfast, Northern Ireland, the disease began with difficulty sleeping. "He was very agitated, he felt dizzy, short-tempered, fatigued. He was having pains in the soles of his feet," his wife Clare told John Lanchester (1996) of *The New Yorker* a year after her husband's death. "He was finding it hard to keep up with his work. He wasn't sleeping, so, obviously, he was feeling tired. His short-term memory was starting to go even then." When the disease became evident in February 1995, Maurice and his doctor assumed the problem was stress. At twenty-nine years of age, Maurice, a mechanical engineer with a degree from Queen's University, was working hard as the energy manager for the university's building maintenance department. He had married Clare in 1991, and they had a daughter.

But by his thirtieth birthday party, on the first day of June, it was obvious to his friends and family that Maurice was not himself. His speech was slurred, his balance was impaired, and his responses in everyday conversation were no longer appropriate. Shortly thereafter the hallucinations began. During the Rugby World Cup he was convinced that members of New Zealand's team, the All Blacks, were lurking upstairs in his house. Sometimes he would awaken in the middle of the night and would not know that Clare was his wife. In July he was admitted to the Royal Victoria Hospital, and his condition worsened progressively. By September he was unable to walk or talk. Maurice died on November 4, 1995, ten days before Clare gave birth to their second child. The initial death certificate listed pneumonia and "premature dementia" as the causes of death.

We now know that Maurice Callaghan was one of the first victims of "variant Creutzfeldt-Jakob disease," or vCJD. As we saw in the chapter 2, this neurodegenerative disorder has now claimed at least forty-three lives in Britain, one in France, and one in the Republic of Ireland. At an inquest held nearly a year after Maurice Callaghan's death, the Belfast coroner, John Leckey, said that in all likelihood Maurice died from eating British beef contaminated with bovine spongiform encephalopathy (BSE) (Lanchester 1996). How BSE emerged in Britain and spilled into the human population is a modern tragedy infused with the high-output technology that typifies our age.

Worried Cows

The first case of BSE was identified at a dairy farm near Ashford, East Kent, on April 25, 1985. Colin Whitaker (BBC World Television 1996), the local veterinary surgeon, noted that the cow was acting nervously and appeared rather uncoordinated. The symptoms reminded him of scrapie, a disease of sheep first described clinically in England in 1730. But scrapie had never been seen in cattle. Within eighteen months there were cases in seven more dairy cows at the farm, and other sporadic cases were starting to occur elsewhere in Britain. What began as a trickle in 1985 was evolving into a bovine Armageddon. By the end of 1996, BSE would claim the lives of more than nine hundred thousand British cattle.

It is not fair to say that cows affected by BSE are mad. "That word is an absolute misnomer," says Richard Sibley (1996), a veterinary surgeon in the dairy country of Devon. "These cows are not mad. If you want an easy name, I would prefer to call it worried-cow disease, or anxious-cow disease." By 1986 it was clear to scientists that BSE was a disease like scrapie, part of a family of neurological diseases called transmissible spongiform encephalopathies (TSEs) These diseases include human Creutzfeldt-Jakob disease (CJD) and kuru, a disease spread among the Fore people who once practiced ritual cannibalism in remote areas of New Guinea. These diseases are now thought to be caused by infectious particles unlike any others.

According to a theory first put forth by Stanley Prusiner in 1982, TSEs arise from the transmission of unconventional proteins—*prions*—that can replicate themselves without the help of nucleic acids like DNA or RNA. It turns out that prions are identical to normal proteins found in nerve cells called PrP, except they are twisted into a different shape. When a healthy PrP encounters a prion it can be refolded into the deviant version, which is then capable of transforming other PrP. The result is a chain reaction leading to the buildup of plaques in the brain and spinal cord. These plaques eventually cause the degenerative symptoms of TSEs.

British epidemiologists were quick to locate the likely source of BSE. They said that cows stricken with BSE were probably infected by contaminated meat-and-bone meal (MBM) fed to them as calves. This crunchy, protein-rich feed is derived from the unsellable remnants of animal carcasses, including sheep, pigs, chickens, and cattle.

Prions from a scrapie-infected sheep, or from a previously unrecognized but isolated case of bovine TSE, could have entered the food chain of cattle through MBM. Given that only a gram of BSE infected tissue is sufficient to infect a cow, a contaminated batch of MBM that included the ground-up remains of a kilogram of brain tissue from a single infected creature could theoretically distribute the infection to one thousand other animals. If the remains of those one thousand cattle were likewise recycled into MBM, the epidemic could spread to a million cows in only two generations.

The technology of Britain's rendering industry that was able to produce MBM, together with the unnatural practice of feeding meat products to herbivorous animals, thus resulted in the widespread exposure of cattle to an otherwise rare infectious agent. Accidental contamination of a small amount of the raw product was amplified by the mass technology behind MBM, so that a large amount of the processed product became adulterated. Thanks to a technology designed to improve the growth and conditioning of cattle, a new disease gained an opportunity for emergence. One reason BSE has appeared most often in dairy cows is its long incubation period, usually five years or more. Most cattle raised only for meat would have been slaughtered before the disease had time to express itself.

The emergence of epidemic BSE only in Britain seems puzzling, given that MBM has been fed to cattle throughout the world since the 1940s. Perhaps it was merely a result of bad luck. Remains of a scrapie-infected sheep or a cow with a rare, sporadic TSE could have been randomly introduced into MBM anywhere, and by chance it occurred in one of Britain's forty-six rendering plants. That chance would have been stacked against the United Kingdom with its long history of scrapie and the relatively high proportion of sheep-derived tissue in British MBM—about 20 times as much as in American MBM.

On the other hand, the emergence of BSE in Britain and the timing of the epidemic may not have been simply a matter of fate. Starting in 1985, the BSE epidemic commenced roughly one incubation period after a profound change in British rendering practices. Discarded fat, bones, offal, and other "mixed material" that arrives at rendering plants is treated at high temperatures to separate molten fats called tallow from the protein-rich *greaves* that go into MBM. Tallow is used to make such products as soap, deodorant, linoleum, margarine, and insecticide. Traditionally the greaves, which still contain up to 14 percent fat, underwent further fat extraction by prolonged heating in a hydrocarbon solvent. Residual solvent was then removed with high-pressure steam. But by the late 1970s the market for tallow had softened, and there were safety concerns about using solvents in the workplace, so the second fat extraction step was dropped. In retrospect it appears this second step might have prevented prions from being recycled into MBM.

Unworried Politicians

Unfortunately, knowing the cause of the BSE was not enough to control the epidemic and prevent its spread to humans. The agriculture ministry in Britain is charged with protecting the interests of producers while simultaneously looking after the rights of consumers. With the British cattle industry employing about 136 thousand people and adding $6 billion to the economy per year, there may have been strong incentives for government ministers to downplay the risks of BSE to humans. For ten years the British public was assured that it was simply not possible for BSE to enter the human food chain.

In July 1988, after the diagnosis of BSE had been confirmed in one thousand cattle, the government banned the use of ruminant-derived protein in ruminant feed. Farmers were required to report all affected cattle for compulsory slaughter, although they were offered only 50 percent compensation for the first eighteen months. In November 1989, a ban was imposed on human consumption of specified bovine tissues known to harbor BSE. These "specified offals," which included the brain, spinal cord, thymus and spleen, had often found their way into hamburger, meat pies, and sausages sold in the United Kingdom before the ban. This prohibition came six months after pet food makers had voluntarily stopped putting offal in their products because of the BSE risk.

The 1989 offals ban proved to be too little too late. More than four hundred thousand infected animals had entered the human food chain before the ban was imposed, and with inadequate enforcement of the ban, another 283 thousand animals had probably slipped through by 1995. As one meat inspector told the BBC in 1996, taking the brains out of cows was a messy, uncertain business. Meat picked from the heads of cattle could easily be contaminated with brain material before it was sold as hamburgers or meat pies for human consumption. The government thought it had good reason to be relaxed about the risk of BSE to humans. No human disease had ever been linked to consumption of scrapie-infected sheep in more than two hundred years. An official BSE working party reported in 1989, "From the present evidence it is likely that cattle will prove to be a 'dead-end host' for the disease agent and most unlikely that BSE will have any implications for human health" (Ministries of Agriculture, Fisheries, and Food 1989).

But it became increasingly obvious that BSE was unlike scrapie in its ability to cross into other species. First it turned up in some exotic ruminants fed MBM at British zoos, in such species as nyala, kudu, gemsbok, eland, and Arabian oryx. Then it surfaced in "mad cats," starting in 1990. By 1998 at least eighty-five domesticated cats in the UK had succumbed to feline spongiform encephalopathy, most likely from eating pet food produced before the voluntary offals ban. Feline spongiform encephalopathy also turned up in cheetahs, pumas, ocelots, and a tiger residing in British zoos. Under experimental conditions, BSE could be transmitted to the mouse, mink, sheep, goat, pig, marmoset, and macaque. "The more animal species that became affected the more we worried about the transmission potential of BSE, and the possibility that it would include humans. There is no getting away from that," said Jeffery Almond (1996), a member of Britain's scientific advisory committee on BSE. But the government was not willing to admit any doubts about the effectiveness of its actions. It was gambling with the health of the population, and dissent among government officials was discouraged.

Is vCJD Human BSE?

Since the startling announcement in March 1996 that ten British people had contracted vCJD, evidence supporting a link to BSE has grown. Each of the agents that cause transmissible spongiform encephalopathies (TSE) produce slightly different pathological changes in their hosts. When certain lines of inbred laboratory mice receive different strains of TSE agents, the pathological damage to their brains can be scored, resulting in a reproducible signature for each strain. The signature left by the agent of vCJD is distinct from that of traditional CJD, but it is indistinguishable from that produced by BSE in cattle or any other infected animal. It now seems certain that vCJD is human BSE. The incomplete inactivation of prion-contaminated animal tissue in the manufacture of cattle feed nearly twenty years ago allowed the spread of a rare and deadly infectious agent. Modern cattle feeding processes, and the technology that supports them, amplified the otherwise insignificant risk of exposure to the BSE agent, causing a massive bovine epidemic. Contamination of meat products sold for human consumption, made certain by a slow and blundering government response to BSE, allowed the agent to pass into humans.

Since 1992, very few cases of BSE have been reported in Britain among cattle that were born after the 1988 ban on ruminant-derived feed, and overall BSE incidence has plummeted in the United Kingdom since it peaked at the start of 1993. By August 1999, progress in controlling the disease among cattle allowed the European Union to lift its worldwide ban on the export of British beef. It is worrisome, however, that BSE is turning up among cattle in other countries, including France, Ireland, Belgium, Holland, Portugal, and Switzerland. Cases of vCJD arising from exposures other than British cattle remain a possibility. So far, human cases of the new disease in Britain have fallen far short of the grim prophecies made in 1996. But given the long and variable incubation period of vCJD, no one is yet willing to say the danger of a major epidemic has passed.

New cases of vCJD appearing today would probably be the result of exposures occurring well before the offals ban of 1989, certainly before it was seriously enforced. In one case that came to light in 1996, the victim had been a strict vegetarian from 1985 onwards. This would suggest that vCJD has an incubation period of at least eleven years. The average incubation period for kuru among human cannibals is ten to fifteen years, with some cases occurring up to forty years after exposure. All this suggests to John Collinge, a leading CJD researcher at Imperial College in London, that Britain's epidemic of vCJD may still have a long way to go. Collinge figures that human dietary exposure to the agent of BSE did not peak until about 1990. He notes that if it takes ten to fifteen years, or more, to incubate the disease, then "it would be logical to conclude that many more cases must result" in coming years (Collinge 1999). A new test that detects the prion of vCJD in biopsies taken from human tonsils may soon be available to give advance warning to those incubating the disease. But this begs the question: Who would want to know?

Mad Cows in the Colonies?

As far as anyone knows, there is no BSE in North America. The one reported case was in a cow imported to Canada from Britain. But can we be sure that none of the one hundred million cows on this side of the Atlantic are free of the disease? Most mammals will spontaneously develop TSEs at roughly the same rate that humans develop classic CJD, about one in one million per year. If that's the case for cows, then one hundred cases of BSE may be arising in the American cattle herd each year. It is thought that one hundred thousand cattle per year "go down," meaning they become too ill or too weak to stand and simply lie down. Do any of these "downer cows" harbor the agent of BSE?

We may never know, according to Clarence Joseph Gibbs, chief of the Laboratory of the Central Nervous System at the National Institutes of Health. In a 1998 interview with Ellen Ruppel Shell for *The Atlantic Monthly*, Dr. Gibbs pointed to the lone reported case of BSE in Canada: "That cow was found by a rancher who had gone out on the range to feed his herd because of a severe snowstorm. If there had been no storm, the rancher would have stayed home, the cow would have gone down, a coyote would have eaten it, and no one would have been any the wiser. Do we have BSE in the United States? The real question is, if we do, will we find it?" Several outbreaks of BSE-like disease have already been documented here among ranch-bred mink whose diets included cattle parts and the carcasses from "downer cows." Another American TSE with less clear origins is chronic wasting disease, an illness like BSE affecting wild mule deer and elk in Colorado and Wyoming. In 1999, this disease was detected among elk at an Oklahoma game farm. The elk had been shipped there from a game farm in Montana. Neither state had previously reported the disease.

Since Britain's BSE crisis, federal regulations have banned American farmers from feeding most ruminant-derived products to their cattle and sheep. But United States rendering facilities continue to produce animal-based food supplements labeled as feed for poultry or pigs, species that seem to be spared from TSE diseases. With little regulatory supervision of the rendering industry, there is no way to be certain that "downer cows" or deer suffering from TSE diseases are not finding their way into these feeds, or that these feeds are not still finding their way into cows and sheep. American meats continue to contain bits of brain, spinal cord, and the other "specified offals" banned in Britain in 1989. One million cattle brains are intentionally sold for human consumption in the United States each year. So far no Americans have had to suffer from vCJD. But as Shell notes in her article, "Avoiding this disease may be only a matter of chance."

Hitchhikers on the Technology Highway

Just as the prions that cause BSE would not have found their bovine hosts without the human ingenuity that devised new kinds of cattle feed, other agents of disease would not have a hope of finding a human host if technology did not provide a way. The epidemic of toxic shock syndrome that was discussed in the chapter 2 would not have occurred without the technological breakthrough of super-absorbent tampons. Many massive outbreaks of water-borne disease, like one we will examine in chapter 10, would not occur today without the modern sophisticated network of water systems that delivers drinking water to thousands of homes on demand.

Legionella, the bacterium that causes Legionnaires' disease, is probably an ancient life form. It only emerged as a cause of disease late in the twentieth century when human technologies provided ideal settings for its multiplication and the means for it to disperse to human hosts. As anyone who has attempted to grow *Legionellae* in the laboratory knows, these bacteria have complex nutritional requirements, so they are unable to survive on their own in water. In nature they overcome this problem by tricking much larger single-cell amoebae that live in water to swallow them. There, inside their unicellular hosts, they obtain the nutrients they require to multiply. Eventually the poor amoebae explode, releasing countless new *Legionellae* into the aquatic environment.

It turns out that *Legionellae* can only reproduce in water that is relatively warm—between 75 and 105 degrees Fahrenheit. Few such environments exist in nature, but a number of recent man-made devices provide plenty of inviting habitats for *Legionellae*, maintaining reservoirs at just the right temperature for *Legionella* replication. As we saw in the last chapter, these habitats include the ever-popular whirlpool spas. *Legionellae* are even more commonly found today in rooftop cooling towers and evaporative condensers used to chill the air in buildings without chemical refrigerants. Such technologies typically recirculate water that is rich in organic matter and the microorganisms on which *Legionellae* thrive.

Beyond giving *Legionellae* new aquatic homes, these same technologies disseminate infections by producing aerosols, fine droplets of water in which *Legionellae* can hide. These droplets, which are one to five microns in size, are small enough to drift into the deepest recesses of human lungs. In the lungs, amoeba-like cells at the front line of the immune response swallow the *Legionellae*. But just as before, the *Legionellae* replicate in these cells until they burst, splattering large numbers of bacteria onto host tissue and causing the pneumonia of Legionnaires' disease. Without human technology, the fickle *Legionella* would never have emerged as a cause of disease. Few other pathogens have exploited technology so effectively to gain access to the human respiratory tract. Most microbes adopting a technological strategy today have found their hosts through mechanized food production or through invasive procedures in high-tech medical care. After we look at tuberculosis in airplanes, the rest of this chapter will focus on these technologies.

Tuberculosis at Thirty-Five Thousand Feet

Jet airplanes are one of the most technologically sophisticated environments people today are likely to encounter. The number of people traveling by plane has increased to 1.4 billion each year, a seventeen-fold rise since 1960. Airline passengers today can remain confined in the tight quarters of their pressurized vessels for periods lasting up to half a day or more, awaiting their flight's arrival at its destination. For this reason, aircraft are likely places for transmission of flu viruses, as they are easily spread through the air wherever people are crammed into enclosed spaces. In 1977, a woman who was acutely ill with the flu was able to infect more than 70 percent of her fellow passengers when their Boeing 737 was delayed on the ground for three hours because of engine failure. Investigators concluded that a shutdown of the aircraft's air-recirculation system during the delay may have created prime conditions for transmission of the virus (Moser, Bender, Margolis, et al. 1979).

The closed cabins of modern aircraft also seem favorable for the spread of tuberculosis (TB). In recent years, the Centers for Disease Control and Prevention (CDC) (1999) has conducted seven investigations of possible TB transmission on jet airliners. These investigations, involving more than twenty-six hundred passengers and crew who were exposed in flight to people with highly infectious disease, found evidence of TB transmission in only two circumstances. In one episode a flight attendant spread TB to other crew with whom she had worked for twelve or more hours. In the other case a passenger spread the disease to at least six fellow passengers. In the latter instance, the infectious passenger was a woman from Korea suffering from active disease due to a multidrug-resistant strain. In 1994 her travels between her home country and the United States included an 8.75-hour flight from Chicago to Honolulu, during which the transmissions occurred. Within two weeks of the flight she died from complications of TB (Kenyon, Valway, Ihle, et al. 1996).

All six passengers infected on the flight had traveled in the same compartment as the infected woman. One was a flight attendant who worked in her vicinity, and three others sat within two rows of the woman. The other two affected passengers were seated twelve and thirteen rows away, but they reported having frequently visited friends seated near the woman during the long flight. This suggested that the TB bacilli had not circulated widely through the cabin, but had been transmitted through close contact with the infected woman. Since then, the CDC has collaborated with the World Health Organization to develop guidelines for responding to possible TB transmission on aircraft. These guidelines recommend that people with infectious TB refrain from flying. In instances where TB is diagnosed after a flight has occurred, the guidelines recommend informing just those passengers who were seated nearby about the exposure, advising them to see their physicians for tuberculin testing.

Assembly Line Epidemics

Modern food production technology has made it possible to feed most people cheaply and plentifully, with a wide variety of foods. The concentration of food industries in the hands of a few large producers and distributors has lowered the costs of human nutrition overall. But as we saw with BSE-tainted cattle feed, modern mass production can amplify the effects of an accidental contamination, leading to what the CDC's Robert Tauxe (1999) calls "a new outbreak scenario" for food-borne disease. In today's scenario, instances of food-borne disease outbreaks are no longer restricted to localized groups, where errors in food-handling or other easily traceable causes can be found. Now, thanks to less-obvious, low-level contamination occurring along the industrial chain of commercial food production, outbreaks have potential to become much more diffuse and widespread. Due to the large scale of modern food processing, and the wide distribution of today's food products, a small problem in the production pathway can have wide-ranging effects.

This was the case in the state of Northrhine-Westfalia, Germany, when at least fifty-two people developed trichinellosis after eating a range of processed pork products sold commercially (Centers for Disease Control and Prevention 1999b). Trichinellosis is a potentially fatal disease causing diarrhea, headache, fever, muscle pains, and swelling of the face and legs. In most cases, it is caused by eating improperly cooked pork that is infected with the larvae of *Trichinella* worms. One investigation into the German outbreak linked the disease to ground pork products sold by a single supermarket. The supermarket belonged to a chain that made its ground pork products by mixing meats supplied from nine different slaughterhouses in Germany, Belgium, and Holland. These slaughterhouses received their pigs from approximately forty different farms, any one of which could have supplied the animal or cluster of animals behind the outbreak. No one will ever know.

Another example of the new outbreak scenario is the 1993 epidemic of *E. coli* O157:H7 in Washington State, in which illness was linked to hamburgers sold by the Jack-in-the-Box fast-food chain. Hamburger patties served by the chain throughout the western states were produced at a single patty-making plant in California. Approximately 90 percent of the 255 thousand patties recalled by health authorities to control the outbreak had been produced at the plant on a single day (Bell, Goldoft, Griffin, et al. 1994). Although the O157 bacterium is found in the feces of fewer than one in five hundred cows, it made its way into many thousands of patties prepared at the plant that day. In all likelihood, the infected intestinal contents of a single cow had contaminated the surface of some of the beef during slaughter or processing. Grinding large amounts of the meat into hamburger distributed the bacteria into what became fast meals for thousands of people in Washington State. Inadequate cooking of the contaminated meat at individual chain restaurants then removed the last defense against infection.

Consolidation of the egg industry has seen the average size of hen houses in the United States increase from five hundred birds in 1945 to one hundred thousand hens today. Squalid conditions in these houses have led in recent years to widespread contamination of eggs with *Salmonella enteritidis* (SE). By the late 1980s, SE had become the dominant type of *Salmonella* isolated from infected people in both North America and Europe. *Salmonella* spreads easily among chickens housed in close quarters, often with no obvious symptoms. Eggs are infected when cracks or pores in the shell allow entry of the bacteria after contact with chicken feces. It is also possible that hens can infect the eggs before they are laid. Large outbreaks of SE have resulted when eggs from infected flocks were widely distributed and served undercooked.

The same kinds of conditions on large poultry farms allow the easy spread of diseases among flocks destined for human consumption. According to Tim O'Brien (1997), head of research for Compassion in World Farming, hot weather turns these factory farms into bacterial incubators. "When the temperature rises, bacteria multiply everywhere—on and in poultry, in their feed and water, and in the excrement they're forced to live in," he says. Most retail chicken sold in the United States today is contaminated with *Campylobacter*. Random supermarket surveys have found these bacteria in up to 98 percent of specimens tested (Altekruse, Stern, Fields, et al. 1999). *Campylobacter* infections typically cause several days of nasty diarrhea, fever, and abdominal pain. *Campylobacter* was only recognized as a human pathogen in the late 1970s, but today it is by far the largest bacterial cause of food-borne infection in the United States. Consumption of undercooked poultry is a major risk factor for *Camplyobacter* infection, along with the careless handling of raw poultry at home. Raw poultry is also a likely household source for *Salmonella* and other harmful bacteria, such as *Yersinia enterocolitica*.

As long as humans are involved in food processing, errors will occur. But mass production technology can turn a simple mistake into a catastrophe. In 1985, the failure of one large dairy plant to pasteurize its milk properly led to more than 190 thousand cases of salmonellosis in Illinois. In 1994, an outbreak of SE that affected approximately 224 thousand people in forty-eight states was linked to consumption of a gourmet ice cream produced at a single plant (Hennessy, Hedberg, Slutsker, et al. 1996). In that outbreak the investigators found that tanker trucks used to transport a pasteurized premix to the ice cream plant were also used to carry unpasteurized liquid eggs. The premix was not pasteurized again after delivery to the plant. There were rules about washing out the tankers after delivery of the liquid eggs, but to save time drivers often chose to bypass that procedure.

Burritos with a Difference

Children who complain about the meals served in their school cafeterias had something new to whine about when a food-borne disease of unknown cause emerged in sixteen separate outbreaks beginning in October 1997. In all but one of the outbreaks, children at school suddenly became ill with nausea, vomiting, and abdominal cramps shortly after eating at their school lunchrooms. In all, the outbreaks affected more than seventeen hundred people in seven states. Investigators quickly linked the new illness to eating mass-produced burritos made by either of two unrelated food companies (Centers for Disease Control and Prevention 1999c). More than two million pounds of the implicated burritos were then recalled or held from distribution, but the causative agent of the illness has not been easy to identify.

Because the fillings in the burritos differed in each outbreak, investigations have centered on the wheat flour tortillas in which the fillings were wrapped. But tests on the tortillas have ruled out every plausible infectious agent and known chemical toxin. Outbreaks of a similar illness were reported in China since the 1960s, and again in India in 1987. In those outbreaks the disease was linked to eating foods made from grains contaminated with various fungi. These fungi can produce powerful toxins known to induce vomiting in humans and animals. But none of these fungal toxins has yet turned up in any of the suspect burritos. While laboratory investigations continue, the elusive agent remains at large. For now, it goes by the name "burrito associated regurgitation factor," or B.A.R.F. for short.

Preserving Food, Promoting Pathogens

Sometimes new ways to package or store food can have unexpected effects on its safety. When plastic wrapping of fresh mushrooms was first introduced in 1967 to preserve freshness, the rapid absorption of oxygen by the mushrooms created an oxygen-free environment suitable for the growth of *Clostridium botulinum*, the bacteria that cause botulism. It became necessary to punch holes in the plastic wrap around mushrooms to allow oxygen transfer without sacrificing freshness. Plastic bags also brought botulism to Alaskan natives, who had traditionally fermented their foods in porous containers placed in holes dug into the cold permafrost. *C. botulinum* grew when they began to ferment foods above ground in the airtight environment of the plastic bags.

Listeria moncytogenes is another food contaminant that is able to prosper in the modern kitchen. Most microbes found in food cease to grow when placed in a cool refrigerator, but *Listeria* continues to multiply without difficulty at refrigerator temperatures. It is particularly common in soft cheeses, unpasteurized milk, stored salads and coleslaw, and in chilled, precooked deli meats. Healthy people rarely develop serious disease from *Listeria*, but in pregnant women an infection can cause a flu-like illness and lead to miscarriage or stillbirth. Other groups at high risk are newborn babies, frail elderly people, and those with compromised immunity. For these people, the disease can cause meningitis or blood poisoning, leading to death.

Listeriosis made headline news in 1985 when an outbreak affecting pregnant women in Los Angeles resulted in thirty deaths among their unborn and newly born babies. The disease was linked to a particular brand of soft cheese that is a staple in the diet of the city's large Hispanic population. In 1998 and early 1999, another large outbreak of listeriosis occurred, this one affecting at least 101 people in 22 states. In all there were fifteen adult deaths and six miscarriages. In this episode, transmission occurred by way of hot dogs sold under many brand names but produced by a single manufacturer in Michigan. Investigators surmised that a major construction project at the hot dog factory had contaminated the plant's processing equipment (Dunne 1999). The epidemic ended when thirty-five million pounds of hot dogs and deli meats were recalled.

In the future we can expect microbes to play an increasing role as biologic control agents, "environmentally friendly" tools to improve crop production and control plant diseases that affect the foods we eat. One agent recently put forward for this purpose is *Burkholderia cepacia*, a bacterium first described as a cause of onion rot in 1949. Ironically, *B. cepacia* is now being extolled for a number of beneficial agricultural uses, including the control of fungal diseases in crops and the degradation of potent herbicides and pesticides for the bioremediation of contaminated soils. The potential economic and ecological benefits of *B. cepacia* seem enormous. But *B. cepacia* is already recognized as a human pathogen, especially among cystic fibrosis patients. It is inherently resistant to many antibiotics, and it has an unusually large genetic endowment, suggesting that it is suited for rapid genetic adaptations and potentially radical changes in its virulence to humans. Researchers in Europe and America have called for a moratorium on the widespread use of *B. cepacia* in agriculture until more is known about its risks to human health (Holmes, Govan, and Goldstein 1998).

Infections from Medical Technology

Like cathedrals in medieval Europe, hospitals today are more than buildings. They are symbols of our faith in science, they are temples of technology inside which we experience birth, sickness, healing, and death. They are shrines in which we invest our capital and place our hopes for a better life. Without question, new medical technologies have delivered immeasurable benefits to millions of people. Today's health consumers expect, and increasingly receive, the latest and most sophisticated diagnostic tests, surgical procedures, and medical therapies. "The impact of technology on the practice of medicine is among the most salutary changes that has occurred during the twentieth century," writes Robert Breiman (1996) of the CDC. But hospitals and other medical settings are also hot zones for infections. Approximately 2.1 million Americans acquire new infections every year while receiving treatment in acute care hospitals. This amounts to about one new infection for every twenty patients admitted. In developing countries, this rate may be five to ten times higher. Hospital-acquired infections lead directly to more than sixty thousand deaths per year in the United States, making them one of the leading causes of mortality today. They also add about $4.5 billion to the annual cost of medical care, mostly through prolonged hospital stays. For infections that end up in the bloodstream, hospital stays are often extended by ten to fourteen days. With costs reaching $1,500 per day, such infections can increase hospital expenditures by $15 thousand to $21 thousand per patient. Bloodstream infections also increase the risk of dying in the hospital by a factor of twenty (Pittet and Wenzel 1995).

Infections acquired in health care settings—sometimes called "nosocomial infections"—are all too common today because of a constellation of factors inherent in modern medicine. First, hospitals are where people with serious infections come for treatment. If these infections are not well contained they can be easily spread within the hospital environment—on surfaces such as floors, on improperly disinfected instruments, or on the hands of health care workers. Secondly, hospitals treat large numbers of people with suppressed immunity, people who are more susceptible to infections than the general population. Such patients include the elderly, premature babies, those with HIV infection, those recovering from severe trauma or burns, those receiving chemotherapy for cancer or autoimmune diseases, those undergoing radiation treatment, and those receiving immunosuppressive drugs for organ transplantation. Thirdly, the vast quantity of antibiotics used in hospitals exerts selective pressure on the organisms found there, favoring the survival of resistant strains. Nearly a third of hospitalized patients receive antibiotics during their stay. Because of antibiotic resistance, infections picked up in hospitals are often the hardest kinds to treat. Finally, many of the procedures carried out in hospitals—operations, transfusions, and insertions of innumerable tubes—are highly invasive. The potential of hospital treatments to introduce infections into normally sterile compartments of the body is tremendous.

Opportunities from Invasive Procedures

In 1997, Britain's Public Health Laboratory Service reported that the risk of hospital-acquired infection is seven times higher when an invasive device is used (Swafford 1997). Among the nineteen hospitals studied for the report, the incidence of infections varied in relation to the use of invasive procedures. The overall rate of nosocomial infection was three per one hundred admissions. But for intensive care patients, on whom invasive devices are used more frequently, the rate was one in five admissions. The most common nosocomial infections are those of the urinary tract. Most of these infections are caused by bacteria that normally reside without harm on the surface of the body. In hospitals, these bacteria gain entry to the bladder through the everyday practice of inserting a catheter to drain away a patient's urine.

Risk of Catheter Use

Urinary catheters are not the only medical devices that invite infections. Patients placed on mechanical ventilators are likewise predisposed to infections, this time in the respiratory tract. The tubing inserted in these patients' upper airways interferes with the normal cough reflex and other physical mechanisms by which the lungs are kept free of pathogens. At least sixty-nine mechanically ventilated patients developed pneumonia from *Burkholderia cepacia* at two Arizona hospitals over a two-year period beginning in 1996. This organism, the same one proposed for bioremediation of contaminated soils, was growing in bottles of mouthwash used to provide routine oral care for patients who were unable to breathe on their own (Centers for Disease Control and Prevention 1998b). Intravenous catheters—the lines doctors use routinely to administer fluids and drugs directly into the bloodstream—also provide easy access for accidental infections. It is estimated that at least four hundred thousand infections due to IV catheters occur each year in the United States. Most of these infections originate either from microbes on the skin where the catheter is inserted into a vein, or from the unclean hands of medical personnel who handle the catheter while it is in place.

Inadequate Disinfection

Occasionally, outbreaks of serious disease can arise from the contamination of medical devices used on multiple patients. Recently two separate outbreaks of tuberculosis have been linked to bronchoscopes that had not been adequately disinfected between patients. Bronchoscopes are flexible, fiber-optic tubes used by doctors to examine the airways of the lungs. About 497 thousand patients undergo the procedure in the United States each year. In the first outbreak, a patient underwent bronchoscopy seventeen days after the procedure was performed on a patient with multidrug-resistant TB at a hospital in South Carolina (Agerton, Valway, Gore, et al. 1997). The second patient then developed active TB infection due to a strain identical to that of the first patient. Another patient exposed to the bronchoscope twelve days after the first patient was also infected but did not become ill. The three patients had no other contact that could explain the outbreak. In the second episode, a patient with lung cancer underwent bronchoscopy with the same instrument that had been used two days earlier on a patient with active TB (Michele, Cronin, Graham, et al. 1997). Again, the second patient developed tuberculosis, and the organism involved had a DNA fingerprint identical to the first case.

In each instance the bronchoscopes were not disinfected between patients in the manner specified in published guidelines.

"We observed numerous opportunities for bronchoscope contamination," the investigators of the South Carolina outbreak wrote (Agerton, Valway, Gore, et al. 1997). Bacteria hiding in a bronchoscope could bypass the lung's normal defenses against infection by penetrating small abrasions in the lining of the airways caused by the procedure. If only 1 percent of bronchoscopies were performed on patients with TB, and only 10 percent were not properly disinfected, there would be four hundred to five hundred people in the United States exposed to TB each year through bronchoscopy, according to Richard Wenzel and Michael Edmond (1997) at the University Medical College of Virginia. If TB can be transmitted this way, so can other virulent organisms. Increasingly, hospitals are using automated reprocessing machines to disinfect bronchoscopes instead of manual cleaning. This saves time, but individual bronchoscopes are not always compatible with the machines used to clean them. "Hospitals and clinics cannot afford to trivialize the importance of routine and thorough cleaning of reusable parts of the bronchoscope," Wenzel and Edmond wrote in an editorial (1997).

Unsanitary Reuse of Supplies

Medical procedures that spread serious infections need not be sophisticated. For example, during 1996, two separate outbreaks of hepatitis B were linked to reusable fingerstick blood sampling devices. One outbreak was in a nursing home in Ohio, and the other was in a New York hospital (Centers for Disease Control and Prevention 1997b). Spring-loaded fingerstick devices are widely used for blood-sugar monitoring of patients with diabetes. The device is stabilized on the finger of a patient with a small plastic platform. This platform contains a hole through which a sharp lancet punctures the skin, creating a drop of blood for analysis. Lancets are routinely changed between patients to control the spread of blood-borne infections; but in these outbreaks, blood contaminated with hepatitis B virus spilled onto the platform. Because the platform was not replaced between patients, it transmitted hepatitis B to many of the patients subsequently tested. Hepatitis B has also been transmitted by a jet gun injector used to deliver drugs for weight reduction without the jabbing pain of needles. In 1985, at least thirty-one patients at a weight-loss clinic in Long Beach, California, were infected with hepatitis B after blood from a highly infectious carrier contaminated the nozzle tip of the clinic's jet injector (Centers for Disease Control 1986).

Open Surgery Environments

Nothing done in hospitals is more invasive than open surgery. Most hospitals go to great lengths to ensure the safety of operating room procedures with regard to infection. But infections related to surgical wounds are the third most common hospital-acquired infections. On rare occasions surgeons can spread their own infections to their patients; this was the case when a Los Angeles surgeon infected with hepatitis B transmitted the virus to nineteen of his patients before hospital authorities caught on and prevented him from operating (Harpaz, Von Seidlein, Averhoff, et al. 1996). Pathogens on surfaces in operating suites, or on surgical instruments, have also found their way deep into the bodies of patients having surgery. Recently, a study showed that viruses can sometimes seep through the latex gloves worn by surgeons as a barrier against spreading infections (Medical Device Technologies 1997). The porous quality of latex, together with the inescapable fact that gloves can be torn or punctured, mean that microbes on the hands of surgical staff can sometimes end up inside patients on the operating table.

That was probably how eight surgical patients at a hospital in California were infected with *Serratia marcescens*, including one who died (Passaro, Waring, Armstrong, et al. 1997). *S. marcescens* is an opportunistic pathogen that settles in the blood, lungs, bone, heart valves, or skin of hospitalized patients who are already weakened by other illnesses. The only factor the California patients had in common was a particular scrub nurse during their operations in 1994. Bacterial cultures of her hands were negative. But when investigators went to the nurse's home they found a jar of exfoliative cream in the shower that had a heavy growth of *S. marcescens* bacteria. The cream, made from crushed olive pits and almond shells, provided an ideal environment for bacterial growth. The nurse tended to use the cream on Sundays, which explained why most of the cases occurred after operations early in the week. How the organism was transmitted from the nurse's hands to the patients was never established, but the fact that she wore artificial nails may have played a part. Artificial nails are known to increase the carriage of bacteria on the hands, and the nurse recalled tearing her gloves during the time of the outbreak.

Bloodthirsty Pathogens

Sometimes the infections patients pick up in hospitals originate from biological products they receive as part of their treatment. About four million Americans receive transfusions of blood or blood products as part of their medical care each year. These transfusions, made possible by donations of blood from eight million volunteers, are safer from the risk of infection today than at any time in the past. But the stakes are high, as more than twenty-five different infectious agents are known already to spread through transfusions, and new threats to the blood supply in the future cannot be ruled out. We have seen how at least one million Americans may have been exposed to hepatitis C through blood transfusions they received before 1992. Tainted blood has also infected up to forty-five thousand Canadians with hepatitis C. Class-action lawsuits brought on their behalf forced the Canadian Red Cross Society to file for bankruptcy protection in 1998. In developing countries, the risks from transfusion are much greater, and so is the array of pathogens transmitted this way. We have already mentioned how Chagas disease is starting to spread to blood recipients in Latin America, as the disease has moved into urban populations (see chapter 4).

Certain viruses, bacteria, and parasites are able to survive for days or weeks in stored blood, and can be passed unknowingly to transfusion recipients. For example, *Yersinia enterocolitica*, an emerging cause of food-borne diarrhea, is able to proliferate in blood packets that can now be stored in hospital refrigerators due to recent technological breakthroughs. Blood collected from a donor with a mild or inapparent case of yersiniosis can cause overwhelming sepsis and death in a recipient. In the United States, about two cases of *Yersinia* blood poisoning are reported after transfusions each year, but this number probably underestimates the true incidence.

Fractionated blood products, which are made from plasma that is pooled from multiple donors, present a special risk. Without adequate disinfection, the effects of a pathogen introduced by a single donor can be amplified through the manufacture and distribution of vast quantities of the final product. A major health care crisis erupted in Ireland in 1994 when it was discovered that batches of Rh_oD immune globulin (RhIG) given to pregnant women during 1977 and 1978 had been contaminated with hepatitis C virus from a single donor. RhIG is a concentrated blood product made from the pooled plasma of donors who are immunized to produce high levels of a particular antibody. It is routinely given to pregnant women whose Rh blood type may be incompatible with that of her fetus. The 1994 discovery prompted an international effort to locate and screen all Irish women who had received RhIG since the early 1970s. So far more than sixty-five thousand women have been screened for hepatitis C, of whom at least 390 were found to have chronic infections.

Hepatitis C has also been transmitted in the United States through a commonly used antibody concentrate. During 1994, at least 113 people who received a particular brand of intravenous immune globulin became infected with hepatitis C. Like RhIG, immune globulin is derived from pooled human plasma, but it contains a much wider range of antibodies. It is commonly administered to treat immune deficiencies and to prevent certain infections after a known exposure, particularly hepatitis A. Another outbreak, in 1996, required a worldwide recall of more than 115 thousand vials of Albuminar, a brand of human albumin. In this instance, patients who received the product developed bloodstream infections with *Enterobacter cloacae* bacteria. Albumin is a protein in plasma that doctors give in concentrated form to treat severe bleeding and sometimes liver disease.

Fortunately, infections acquired from blood and fractionated blood products are becoming rare in developed countries. Thirty years ago the risk of hepatitis following a blood transfusion was one in three, but today the odds are less than one in one hundred thousand. Before 1985 more than eight thousand people in the United States were infected with HIV through transfusions of blood or blood products. This included hundreds of hemophiliacs whose repeated injections with blood clotting factors, derived from pooled plasma donations, contained the virus. Now that the blood supply is carefully screened, fewer than two units in a million are thought to be contaminated with HIV in the United States. But the picture is not so rosy everywhere. In regions of Africa, where AIDS is common and little testing for HIV is performed, the virus contaminates as much as 13 percent of the blood supply. In these countries, inadequately screened blood represents a major ongoing source of new infections.

While medical science searches for a safe artificial blood substitute, blood collection centers in most developed countries are taking prudent steps to protect the blood supply from infections. The first of these steps is to make blood donation voluntary, to eliminate people who would give blood primarily for monetary gain. Secondly, all prospective donors answer detailed questions about their lifestyles and medical history. Those who report IV drug use or other risk factors for common blood-borne infections are deterred from donating. Thirdly, units of donated blood are laboratory-tested for the agents that cause syphilis, hepatitis, and AIDS. Finally, donors are given permission to advise the blood bank later that their blood may not be suitable if they have second thoughts about their risk.

Despite this, no safeguards are completely foolproof. A study of more than thirty-four thousand blood donors by the American Red

Cross showed that nearly 2 percent were at risk of HIV and other blood-borne infections but did not report this at the screening interview (Williams, Thomson, Schreiber, et al. 1997). Laboratory testing inevitably misses at least a few cases among the millions of donations screened. Viral infections like HIV typically have a "window period" early in the infection when transmissible virus is present in the blood but the antibody response is not yet detectable by the laboratory. New tests under trial by the American Red Cross since 1999 promise to cut down on false-negative results by picking up viruses in blood before the donor's own immune system knows they are there, but such measures will not eliminate all transmission risks. Finally, there is always the possibility that a pathogen unknown today will contaminate the blood supply, as HIV did in the early 1980s. In view of these hazards, it is not surprising that doctors are becoming more conservative about ordering transfusions. Patients having elective surgery today may be advised to furnish units of their own blood prior to their operations if transfusions are considered likely.

British Blood Need Not Apply

Since August 1999, would-be blood donors who say they have spent six months or more in Britain since 1980 have been politely refused at American and Canadian blood banks. The reason is the theoretical risk that they are infected with the new variant form Creutzfeldt-Jacob Disease (CJD), and the even more speculative notion that the disease could be passed to others through their blood. In what was a controversial decision in both the United States and Canada, health authorities felt it was better to err on the side of caution and impose the ban. "The day you find out there is human transmission, you're too late to protect the blood supply," said Linda Detwiler (1999), a member of the expert panel advising the federal Food and Drug Administration on the issue.

As far as anyone knows, classic CJD has never been transmitted through blood. Given the sheer number of people exposed to blood, it seems likely that transfusion-related cases would have appeared by now if the disease could be spread that way. In one study, none of fifteen hundred patients who received blood products from a donor who later died of CJD were found to develop the disease themselves (Rahman 1999). But variant CJD (VCJD) may behave differently. It has already shown it can spread in ways that no one thought possible ten years ago.

The added layer of safety won't come without a cost. The American Red Cross predicts the new ban will deprive blood banks of 2.2 percent of their regular donors. In Canada, and in certain large cities of the Northeast, the percentage will be even higher. That's bad news at a time when blood shortages are an increasing problem. "It's very unsafe not to have enough blood," notes Richard Davey (1999), a Red Cross spokesman. As if the hypothetical dangers of vCJD weren't enough, a mysterious new virus has started turning up in blood supplies around the world. The newly found microbe, known simply as "TT virus," can be detected in 8 to 10 percent of American blood donors. As yet, no one knows whether the TT virus poses a threat to health. Let's hope not.

Transplanting Infections

Organ transplantation has moved from the realm of science fiction to everyday medical practice for patients with end-phase organ failure, especially since the introduction of improved drugs for immune suppression during the 1980s. These drugs help prevent rejection of the foreign organ, but they also diminish the recipient's ability to fight infection. For this reason, patients receiving transplanted tissue are at special risk of developing life-threatening infections. These infections might arise from organisms circulating in the hospital environment, or they may result from some of the pathogens already present in the body at low levels that are allowed to awaken because of the body's weakened immunity. Infections can also be spread from person to person by the transplanted tissues themselves.

Potential donors are usually tested extensively for pathogens known to be transmissible in donated organs, including HIV and hepatitis viruses. The agent most likely to be transmitted from donor kidneys, hearts, livers, and bone marrow is cytomegalovirus (CMV), a member of the herpes family. CMV infection is extremely common, although symptomatic disease is relatively rare. CMV is a latent virus, so infection is lifelong. In most situations doctors are reluctant to refuse an organ from someone infected with CMV, as otherwise viable donor organs can be in short supply. Usually, CMV in a donated organ causes no problems, but serious disease can result in about 25 percent of cases when an infected organ is transplanted into a CMV-negative recipient.

Tissues contaminated with the prions that cause CJD also create transplant risks. In 1974, a woman who received a cornea contaminated with CJD became the first person infected nosocomially with this disease. Since then, two other cases have been reported in recipients of corneal transplants. Since 1979, at least sixty-one patients have developed CJD after receiving surgical implants made from processed dura mater. Dura mater is the thickest layer of the meninges, the tissues that line the brain and spinal cord. Most of the contaminated implants were manufactured by a single company in Germany, which harvested them from cadavers. About forty of the infected implants ended up in patients in Japan, but they have also been linked to CJD in the United States, Canada, the United Kingdom, Germany, Italy, Spain, Australia, and New Zealand.

Hormones extracted from the pituitary glands of cadavers have also transmitted CJD. In the 1960s doctors began treating growth deficiency in children with human growth hormone obtained in tiny amounts from pituitary glands deep in the heads of cadavers. This practice ceased in most countries in 1985 after a series of case reports in the United States showed that some children receiving the hormones were developing CJD (Centers for Disease Control 1985). To date, at least seven cases of CJD have been transmitted this way in the United States. Cases have also been reported from Britain, France, Brazil, and New Zealand. In France, where fifty young people have developed CJD from growth hormone treatments, the problem has erupted into a major political scandal. Pituitary hormones given to induce ovulation in women have also transmitted CJD from cadavers to otherwise healthy people.

With demand for donor organs today far outstripping supply, there is growing interest in xenotransplantation, using animal sources for human organs. In 1984, a newborn infant was kept alive for twenty days with a heart transplanted from a baboon. There have also been attempts to transplant the hearts of chimpanzees, pigs, and sheep into human recipients. Nonhuman primates are often preferred for xenotransplantation because of their genetic similarity to humans; chimpanzees are in short supply, but baboons, which are not endangered, could provide a suitable donor pool. For many transplanted tissues, barnyard pigs would be perfectly acceptable alternates. Commercial farming of pig donors might someday provide an almost limitless supply of needed organs.

Cultural and ethical issues over xenotransplantation remain unresolved. Many people ask if it is appropriate to use animals for this purpose. There are even greater concerns about the potential of introducing unwanted infectious agents—both known and unknown—from animals into the human population. Known agents would include simian viruses that resemble HIV, Ebola virus, the monkeypox virus, and various herpes viruses. Such infections could be devastating for the recipients, whose immunity would be suppressed as part of their treatment. There is even the possibility that latent viruses embedded in the genetic code of an animal tissue graft could be awakened in the body of a new human host, causing disease and allowing new infections to disseminate to the general human population. Already two suspect viruses with potential to infect humans have been found woven into the DNA of pigs. In 1999, the parliamentary assembly of the Council of Europe called for a Europe-wide moratorium on trials of animal transplants into humans, out of fear that xenotransplantation might trigger an uncontrollable epidemic. Jean-Francois Mattei (1999), a French geneticist who pressed for the moratorium, said, "We do not intend to stop research on xenotransplantation permanently, but the risks are currently too high to be acceptable."

Contemporary technological changes are having far-reaching effects beyond the areas of food production and medical care that we have examined in this chapter. Around the world human activity is having profound effects on natural ecosystems, opening the door for new infectious diseases to emerge. The next chapter will discuss the infectious disease impact of environmental changes resulting from economic development and evolving global land use patterns.

What You Can Do to Prevent Blood-Borne Diseases

In the United States today, the blood transfused from one patient to another is more carefully screened for infectious agents than ever before. Still, no blood bank can promise there is no risk that infections will spread this way. To bring the risk essentially to zero, patients who are likely to need blood in an upcoming operation can donate their own blood in advance. These *autologous* donations are recommended by the FDA and the American Association of Blood Banks wherever possible for elective surgery, and they now account for nearly 5 percent of all donated blood. Those considering this option should be aware of the following:

- A unit of blood (just under a pint) can be donated as often as every three to four days, and donations can continue until seventy-two hours before surgery.

- Collecting blood before surgery may actually speed up recovery afterwards, as it stimulates the bone marrow to make new blood cells.

- Using autologous blood costs more, due to special handling and separate storage requirements.

- Autologous blood donation may be inadvisable for some patients, such as those with severe heart disease or blood vessel disease.

- Decisions about autologous blood should be made together with your physician.

Chapter 7

Ecological Changes: Land Use and Climate

We suffer for we have not taken better care of the Earth.

—Reflections of a Navajo Indian chief
during the epidemic of hantavirus
disease in Arizona, 1993

Runaway environmental change represents the greatest challenge facing human society today. Relentless pollution, deforestation, loss of biological diversity, and greenhouse warming of the atmosphere have combined to cause what ecologists are now calling "environmental distress syndrome." Irreversible damage to natural ecosystems has encouraged selection of opportunistic pests and has exposed increasingly stressed human populations to new and resurgent pathogens. To no one's surprise, we are finding that the health of the planet and its people are inextricably linked.

The scale of ecological change today is staggering. Unregulated logging and agricultural development are decimating ancient primary forests in South America, Africa, Southeast Asia, and the islands of the South Pacific. Nearly ten million acres of Amazon forest are cleared for pasture each year, an area roughly the size of Switzerland. Sumatra, an Indonesian island that is larger than California, has lost virtually all its lowland forests in the past twenty-five years. Such massive change in the character of tropical forests has exerted profound effects on the complex biological web that supports all living things, including humans. Of the ten to twenty million species of plants, animals, and other life forms believed to exist on Earth, half face extinction by the middle of the twenty-first century. With them will go countless natural sources for new medicines, such as antibiotics and painkillers. At the same time, the loss of natural controls on species abundance has allowed some species to flourish, amplifying the spread of dangerous pathogens to humans.

Ecological calamities on land are closely tied to profound changes occurring in the lower atmosphere. Worldwide carbon emissions resulting from combustion of fossil fuels now exceed six billion tons per year. The amount of carbon dioxide accumulating in the troposphere is now at least 20 percent greater than in preindustrial times. Like a greenhouse, CO_2 in the troposphere traps much of the sun's radiant heat that would normally reflect off the surface of the Earth. As forest fires, industrial pollution, automobile fumes, and other human undertakings have pumped more CO_2, methane, ozone and other so-called greenhouse gases into the air, average global temperatures have progressively increased. There is only one chance in forty that the global warming documented in the past three decades is due to a natural variation (Merritt 1998).

Models that attempt to predict the effects of a warmer global climate involve considerable guesswork. But they suggest that higher temperatures will cause an increase in the world's total precipitation, accelerated melting of the polar ice caps, a rise in global mean sea level, and marked changes in the present distributions of many living things. Instabilities in global climate are already leading to turmoil in various natural ecological communities. Recent anomalies in weather, including those brought on by the El Niño phenomenon, have had serious implications for the occurrence of infectious diseases.

This chapter will examine infectious disease threats emerging because of today's unprecedented ecological changes, particularly recent shifts in land use and extraordinary disturbances in weather. The tropical rainforest of Africa is a good place to begin. Here the recent appearance of human monkeypox offers a clear-cut example of how people can precipitate disease emergence when they impose their designs on a landscape and disturb the natural balance of the biosphere.

Deforestation and Monkeypox

In late July 1996 health officials in Zaire began receiving reports from the Katako-Kombe region that villagers there were becoming ill with a serious new disease. Since mid-February at least seventy-one people in this remote jungle district had developed the disease, six of whom had died. More than half the cases, including three of the deaths, had occurred in a single village with only 346 residents. The disease began with a fever, followed a few days later by a rash. The rash, typified by large, pus-filled blisters, was concentrated on the face and limbs. Such a clinical picture reminded older doctors of smallpox, that great scourge of humanity that once swept through continents killing many millions over the centuries. But smallpox had not been seen in Central Africa since the 1960s, and the smallpox virus had been eradicated from the entire world by 1977 through a heroic public health campaign. What then could this be?

The disease turned out to be human monkeypox, an affliction caused by a close relative of the smallpox virus. Monkeypox virus primarily infects subhuman primates and other mammals inhabiting the tropical rainforests of Central and West Africa. The virus was first discovered in 1958, when it turned up in some laboratory monkeys in Copenhagen. The first human infection was reported in 1970, in northern Zaire. Since then it has been sporadically reported in humans along an equatorial band of rainforest villages stretching from Sierra Leone in the west to the eastern frontier of Zaire. There had been no large-scale outbreaks until the Katako-Kombe outbreak began in 1996. That outbreak, which spread into the neighboring Lodja region, grew to include more than five hundred cases by October 1997. "I hate to be accused of pushing the alarmist button, but for practical purposes, smallpox is back," Peter Jahrling (1997) told the journal *Science* at the peak of the epidemic. Jahrling is a virologist and the chief scientist at the United States Army Medical Research Institute of Infectious Diseases.

Most cases of human monkeypox have resulted from the direct handling of an infected animal. Children living in small villages are at greatest risk, especially during the months of the year when they are active outside the home, tilling crops or hunting for game. A person infected with the monkeypox virus is able to transmit the disease to others, but monkeypox was always thought to be less contagious among humans than smallpox was. However, in the Katako-Kombe outbreak, about three-quarters of those who became ill believed they were infected by other people. If true, this would represent the highest rate of person-to-person transmission ever reported.

Sustained outbreaks of monkeypox transmission among human contacts might be the result of declining immunity to smallpox following the cessation of vaccinations in 1980. Smallpox vaccine used to confer partial immunity to monkeypox as an incidental benefit. Ironically, the successful eradication of smallpox may have created a large pool of individuals susceptible to full-blown monkeypox,

epidemics within human communities wherever the virus is
:ed. Extensive transmission of monkeypox among humans
has some experts worried: "This is not just an outbreak of some rare,
exotic disease in the middle of nowhere. I'm personally concerned
about what would happen if this disease showed up in a major city,"
said Ali Khan (1997), an epidemiologist with the CDC. Khan spent
five days visiting twelve villages at the center of the outbreak in
mid-1996, until civil unrest cut short his investigation.

Before humans can transmit monkeypox among themselves, the
virus has to be passed from its usual animal hosts. That requires
human contact with the wild mammals that circulate the virus naturally. Expansion of human populations into previously uninhabited
jungle regions of Africa throughout the 1990s has certainly increased
the chances of an accidental exposure to monkeys and other normal
mammalian hosts of the virus. At the time of the Katako-Kombe outbreak, Zaire was experiencing a civil war. Displacements of villagers
during the war undoubtedly forced many people into uncharted rainforest to eke out an existence hunting wild animals for food, including some animals that carry the virus.

But the mere encroachment of human hunters into the traditional habitats of the monkeypox virus is not sufficient to explain the
emergence of the disease today. To account fully for the eruption of
monkeypox we must consider the unprecedented environmental
changes that have come with recent human intrusions into primordial African woodlands. Conversion of vast areas of rainforest into
more open terrain has forever altered the delicate ecosystems in
which the monkeypox virus lives. At least half of the first-growth
rainforests of Zaire have in recent years been degraded by human
occupation into what ecologists call "secondary" forests, where space
has been opened up between trees to allow the grazing of domestic
animals and the planting of some crops. Many trees remain, but these
altered environments are unable to support most of the larger wild
animals that once inhabited the original, dense rainforests.

With the top predators removed, the meek have inherited the
Earth. In Africa, newly created secondary forests have opened up a
niche for enormous populations of rodents and other small animals,
particularly squirrels of the *Funisciurus* type. Unfortunately, these
squirrels are prime hosts for the monkeypox virus. In some areas of
Zaire, nearly half of captured *Funisciurus* squirrels have antibodies
indicating infection with monkeypox (Khodakevich, Jezek, and Messinger 1988). The squirrels thrive on the nuts of oil palm trees that
grow widely in the secondary forests that surround small human settlements. The squirrels can number in the hundreds per square mile,

and they are a favorite source of meat, especially for young children making their first forays as hunters.

So the emergence of human monkeypox is not surprising when seen in the context of the profound changes occurring in the ecosystems of the virus' natural hosts. Prolonged deforestation, and its unforeseen effects on squirrel populations, has created conditions that favor the propagation of a potent virus among animal hosts that are in close contact with humans. This ecological disturbance has occurred at the same time that the human population is losing its collective immunity to the virus, following the end of smallpox vaccination. Ironically, control of human monkeypox may ultimately depend on a progressively worsening degradation of the natural environment, eliminating the habitats of infected squirrels. Human monkeypox is uncommon in areas of Central Africa where agricultural development is more advanced and wild animals are no longer available as a source of animal protein. Sadly, the threat of monkeypox may only disappear when there is an even more severe destruction of Africa's dwindling rainforests.

Accidental Epidemics of the Green Revolution

Monkeypox is but one of several new diseases emerging from an almost limitless pool of animal viruses, most of which are still unknown to science. The vast majority of infectious agents that are spread among animals are poorly adapted for transmission to humans. But there are key exceptions, most notably HIV. Increasingly, some of the rare animal pathogens that can cause diseases in *Homo sapiens* are finding their way into human populations today, thanks to our profound perturbations of the natural environment.

Perhaps no human activity has had a more conspicuous impact on natural ecosystems than agricultural development. The world's growing demand for a secure supply of food has resulted in huge tracts of undeveloped land being put into cultivation in recent years, permanently altering the original ecosystems. Not all the effects of these changes have been helpful. Harmful effects include the emergence of viral hemorrhagic fevers in South America and the persistence of river blindness in Africa, all of which have occurred with the clearing of land and the spread of agriculture into new territories.

The Junin Virus

Until the mid-twentieth century the Argentine pampas was a fertile, temperate grassland that supported a wide variety of wildlife. The predominant rodent was the South American field mouse, *Akodon azarae*. During World War II, both sides in the conflict turned to Argentina for grain, and much of the pampas was plowed for the production of maize. Initial harvests lagged behind expectations because the pampas' prolific grasses competed with the maize for sunlight, and the grasses had to be removed by hand.

After the war, new herbicides suppressed these grasses and transformed the pampas overnight: Then, maize could grow unimpeded to its full height. This change favored a new, shade-tolerant understory of grasses. The altered ecology displaced the South American field mouse, *Akodon azarae*, with a new dominant species, the vesper mouse. This mouse, also known as *Calomys musculinus*, feeds off the seeds of the shade-tolerant grasses. *Calomys* mice had always been present in the pampas, but in low numbers. Now the land supported twenty times as many *Calomys* per acre.

It turns out that the vesper mouse, *C. musculinus*, is the natural host for the Junin virus, a member of the *Arenaviridae* family. The Junin virus causes no symptoms in the mice, but it can infect them for life, and it is shed profusely in their urine and feces. Farm workers and other people who inhale aerosolized particles given off by infected mouse excretions, or eat food contaminated with the excretions, began to develop a bleeding disease now called Argentine hemorrhagic fever. Since it was first recognized in 1953, between two hundred and two thousand people have been reported with the disease each year. Death results in 10 to 20 percent of cases. With the ongoing spread of maize production the geographic range of the virus continues to grow.

The Machupo Virus

Further north, in the tropical savanna (grasslands) of eastern Bolivia, another virus of the *Arenaviridae* family has emerged since 1960: The Machupo virus. Its natural host is the small mouse *Calomys callosus*, a cousin of the Argentine *Calomys*. This mouse has traditionally lived in small numbers along the forest-grassland margins of the region. With the forced break-up of large, foreign-owned rancheros since the 1950s, many rural Bolivians have returned to subsistence farming. The most fertile lands available are those areas of prairie that border forested outcrops, the very zones where *C. callosus* mice prefer to live.

Hemorrhagic Fever

The mice have flourished in the ramshackle dwellings and gardens of the new settlers. With so much close contact they have had little difficulty sharing the Machupo virus with their human neighbors. The result has been the emergence of Bolivian hemorrhagic fever, a bleeding disease resembling the Argentine variety. Household rodent control was successful in eliminating human cases of the disease for several years after 1973, but, since 1994, the Machupo virus has returned. Guanarito virus, yet another member of the *Arenaviridae* family, turned up among settlers clearing native forests for food production in the Portuguese state of central Venezuela during 1989. It causes Venezuelan hemorrhagic fever, and is spread by two local rodents that are also well adapted to the rough-and-tumble environments of farmhouses and gardens.

The Lassa Fever Virus

The most notorious member of the *Arenaviridae* family is the Lassa fever virus, found in West Africa. Lassa fever produces a prolonged illness characterized by fever, sore throat, chest pain, bleeding, and shock. Death occurs in as many as a quarter of hospitalized cases, and deafness is a common complication. Lassa fever virus is spread by contact with the excretions of various species of *Mastomys* rodents, or "multimammate" rats. These fast-breeding rats have a fondness for human houses, where they scavenge on poorly stored foods and deposit infected droppings on floors and beds, and in food or water. Unlike most *Arenaviridae* diseases in South America, Lassa fever can also be spread from person to person. It was first recognized in 1969 when three nurses successively developed the disease at a missionary hospital in Nigeria.

Today, Lassa fever has become a major public health problem in parts of Guinea, Liberia, Sierra Leone, and Nigeria. The disease causes about five thousand deaths per year and leaves many thousands of others with permanent hearing loss. In some areas of Liberia and Sierra Leone, the disease accounts for more than 10 percent of all hospital admissions. Eastern Sierra Leone has become a hotbed for Lassa fever in recent years following an influx of workers to the region's burgeoning diamond mines. This impoverished rural area had previously offered little promise to *Mastomys* rats seeking to extend their range from coastal cities. But the new diamond fields have created a chaotic boomtown environment in the region. *Mastomys* rats have found plenty of food in the refuse of the mining towns, and they are now well-established local hosts of Lassa fever.

River Blindness

Another particularly vicious disease affecting rural people is onchocerciasis, better known as river blindness. Onchocerciasis is caused by a parasitic worm, *Onchocerca volvulus*, which lives up to fourteen years in the human body. The female worm, which grows up to twenty inches in length, brings forth millions of tiny offspring called microfilariae that migrate everywhere in the body. In the skin, these miniature worms can cause intense itching and depigmentation. They also attack the optic nerve and retina, leading to blindness. Onchocerciasis has caused blindness in 270 thousand people who are alive today, and it has left half a million others with serious visual impairment. The disease has been a major impediment to socioeconomic development in the thirty-four tropical countries where it is found, but especially in Africa. Until recently, large tracts of fertile lands in the Volta River basin and other areas of West Africa were simply abandoned out of fear of the disease.

Microfilariae are transmitted through the bites of the black fly, *Simulium damnosum*. The fly breeds in the fast-flowing water of mountainous streams and seeks blood meals from people who live and work nearby. Strains of *Onchocerca* worms that are most associated with blindness have always been more common among subgroups of black flies inhabiting the sparsely wooded riverbanks of the savanna. Strains that predominantly cause skin disease have generally been passed by subgroups of flies that prefer dense forests. Now, deforestation threatens to redistribute the flies, giving the most blinding strains of the worm access to new turf (Brown 1992). A quarter-century of aerial spraying has dramatically reduced the numbers of black flies in savanna and forest alike in eleven West African countries. Where efforts to control the flies have been successful, the scourge of onchocerciasis is disappearing. But the relentless clearing of primary rainforests in Liberia, Ghana, and Côte d'Ivoire has seen advances of the savanna varieties of black flies into new territories, and this raises fears that recent progress in reducing river blindness will be reversed.

The Weeds Choking Africa's Great Lakes

Introduced plant species can have dramatic effects on local environments. Ask residents of the state of Georgia about kudzu, the Japanese vine that blankets much of the countryside. Such introductions can sometimes have unforeseen consequences on infectious disease emergence. In the 1980s, South American water hyacinths (*Eichhornia crassipes*) were imported to Africa as an ornamental plant. This broad-leafed plant floats on top of garden ponds and brings forth numerous showy blue flowers. But hyacinths accidentally released into Lake Victoria and East Africa's other Great Lakes have flourished, with disastrous results for lakeside communities (Epstein 1998). This has occurred in the absence of any natural enemies for the plant and with the help of unregulated industrial and agricultural run-off into the rivers and streams feeding the lakes. In many areas, the hyacinths have proliferated into an endless mat that blocks much of the shoreline and depletes the water of oxygen. With boats trapped and spawning grounds choked by the plants, communities dependent on the fishing industry have suffered. At the same time, the tangled web of hyacinths is supporting numerous gastrointestinal pathogens, some of which are ending up in the local drinking water. The hyacinths also aid the breeding of mosquitoes, including those that transmit malaria and other diseases.

Diseases Helped along by Dams

At the same time that large tracts of forest and grassland have been placed under cultivation, millions of acres have been flooded to create new artificial lakes. Throughout the world, governments have been constructing massive new hydro projects to control floods, to generate electric power, and to provide a reliable supply of water for agricultural and urban uses. Today there are some thirty-five thousand large dams in the world, and more so-called mega-dams are under construction every year. By radically altering the natural environment, these enormous projects sometimes have unintentional effects on disease emergence.

Rift Valley Fever

Like dengue fever, Rift Valley fever is an emerging viral disease characterized by fever, inflammation of the brain, and bleeding. First described in 1931 in East Africa, it is transmitted by certain *Aedes* mosquitoes. Initially, Rift Valley fever was largely confined to sheep and cattle, and, before 1977, it was never seen outside sub-Saharan

Africa. But that year approximately two hundred thousand people in Egypt developed the disease, including 598 who died. In retrospect, the Egyptian epidemic can now be traced to the construction of the Aswan Dam, completed in 1970. This enormous dam flooded two million acres for Lake Nasser and elevated ground water levels in the Nile Valley. This allowed standing water to puddle, offering new breeding sites for *Aedes* mosquitoes. With the concurrent migration of infected people and livestock into the area, there were favorable circumstances for an epidemic of Rift Valley fever among Egypt's large, nonimmune population. In 1987, this scenario was repeated in the African country of Mauritania, following the completion of the Diama Dam on the Senegal River during the previous year (Jouan, LeGuenno, Digoutte, et al. 1988).

Parasitic Disease—Schistosomiasis

These same dams, among others, have also been implicated in the emergence of schistosomiasis in parts of Africa recently. Schistosomiasis is caused by five species of water-borne flukes (flatworms) called schistosomes. With more than two hundred million people now infected in seventy-four developing countries, schistosomiasis is a parasitic disease second only to malaria in its public health importance. People become infected with larval forms of schistosomes when they are working, swimming, or fishing in fresh water inhabited by particular snails. Unique species of snails act as intermediate hosts for each species of schistosome, and determine its range. Once attached to a human host, schistosome larvae penetrate the skin and migrate to the liver, where they mature and reproduce. From there they relocate to the veins of the intestines or bladder, and pass their eggs back to the environment in feces or in urine. With chronic infection a heavy load of worms will retard growth in children. It will also cause weakness and lethargy, so that adults are unable to work. Ultimately, schistosomiasis can severely damage the liver and the urinary tract, and sometimes it leads to cancer.

Drowned vegetation under the surface of artificial lakes is rich in nutrients, able to support large numbers of snails involved in the life cycle of schistosomiasis. Before construction of the Taabo and Kossou dams in Côte d'Ivoire during the 1970s, schistosomiasis was rarely detected in children living along the Bandama River. A pre-dam survey of 120 children living in villages around the proposed Taabo Dam found only four with evidence of schistosomiasis. When researchers went back in 1992, the prevalence of urinary schistosomiasis in the 258 children they surveyed had risen to 73 percent (N'Goran, Diabate, Utzinger, et al. 1997). Similar increases were found in most villages around the Kossou Dam.

New dams can even have effects on schistosomiasis incidence hundreds of miles downstream. The altered environment downstream from African hydro projects has repeatedly favored populations of some snails at the expense of others, exposing humans nearby to new forms of the disease. Urinary schistosomiasis, caused by *Schistoma haematobium*, had been common in Egypt since the time of the pharaohs. But since the construction of the Aswan Dam, the types of snails that carry *Schistoma mansoni*, the major cause of intestinal schistosomiasis, have come to dominate the lower Nile (Mott, Nuttall, Desjeux, et al. 1995). Similar shifts in snail populations have followed complex ecological changes downstream from new dams on the Senegal and Volta Rivers, resulting in recent epidemics of intestinal schistosomiasis in West Africa.

At present, public health officials in China are attempting to predict the impact of the Three Gorges mega-dam on transmission of schistosomiasis in the Yangtze River Basin. Begun in 1994, this epic, $24 billion project will create a lake covering twenty thousand square miles when completed in 2009. It is possible that the lake, which will displace 1.4 million people, will promote breeding of the *Oncomelania* snails that act as intermediate hosts of *Schistoma japonicum* (Zheng, Xu, Hotez, et al. 1997). Schistosomiasis is already well established in villages just twenty-five miles downstream from the dam site. If the disease expands into the area around the giant new reservoir, this would occur at a time when countless new migrants who are susceptible to schistosomiasis are predicted to arrive in the region to exploit new work opportunities in aquaculture.

Ecological Changes in Developed Countries

Developing countries are not the only ones where environmental changes are hastening the emergence of infectious diseases. Countries that enjoy a relatively high standard of living are also experiencing ecological shifts, with consequent impacts on human infections. Oppressive pollution of the air and water around urban centers is an obvious outcome of expanding industrial and commercial land uses. Suburban sprawl is obliterating productive farmlands in the United States at an alarming rate. Around Atlanta alone, five hundred acres

---

Emerging Infections on the Most Remote Continent

If there is one place on Earth that is free of dangerous pathogens, surely it must be Antarctica. Here, at the bottom of world, where international treaties protect a vast, frozen wilderness from mining and other commercial exploitation, one does not expect to find problems with epidemic diseases. But there is mounting evidence that some of the icy continent's unique wild inhabitants are becoming ill from the impact of human visitors. Sewage left behind by the growing number of scientists and tourists who visit Antarctica and its subantarctic islands may be infecting local birds and marine mammals with human diseases. Feces collected from fur seals, penguins, albatrosses, and other unique wildlife have now been shown to contain *Salmonella* and *Campylobacter* bacteria. *Salmonella* was one of the organisms found when more than fourteen hundred New Zealand sea lions died mysteriously in early 1998 in the subantarctic Auckland Islands.

Human foods also present a threat, particularly poultry. Even after processing, poultry can carry pathogens that are harmful to other birds. Discarded chicken bones have been spotted in the nests of skuas, large sea birds with a habit for snatching from their neighbors. Now antibodies to a virus usually found in chickens have turned up in Emperor penguin chicks and adult Adélie penguins living near scientific stations (Gardner, Kerry, Riddle, et al. 1997). The virus suppresses the birds' immune systems, leaving them susceptible to other infections. With tourist numbers expected to reach fourteen thousand by the summer of 2000-2001—double the level of 1992-1993—improved standards for food preparation and sewage treatment must be adopted to protect Antarctica's delicate ecosystem.

---

of field and farmland are swallowed up every week. Such unbridled growth is increasing our reliance on cars, and adding to the toxins that cars release into the air. Children who endure prolonged exposure to urban smog are at greater risk of developing respiratory infections and middle ear infections. The problem is compounded by uncontrolled forest fires, like those that raged in Indonesia and neighboring countries in 1997. Heavy smoke from those fires blanketed many of Southeast Asia's booming cities, shrouding the glass and steel skyscrapers of downtown Singapore, Kuala Lumpur, and beyond. The stifling pollution, when added to the usual urban haze, caused increased respiratory ailments of all kinds, including infections.

Illness from shoreline pollution remains a problem for beach-goers in even the wealthiest nations. Sewage outflows mean that certain beaches are off-limits, while others can become risky for bathers when currents shift. One recent study showed that swimming in the early morning hours is especially hazardous (Pearce 1999). Fecal bacteria are five times more common in the morning than in the afternoon, after the sun's ultraviolet rays have disinfected the water. In Los Angeles, even rainwater flowing into the sea from storm drains has been making surfers and other ocean bathers sick. About fifty to sixty million people visit the beaches of Santa Monica Bay every year. Now it appears that people who swim near storm drain outfalls are 50 percent more likely to suffer from bacterial and viral infections than those who swim at least fifty yards away (Haile, Witte, Gold, et al. 1999). Swimming in a tidal soup of infectious agents increases the risk of many adverse health outcomes, including diarrhea, fever, ear infections, skin rashes, wound infections, and respiratory disease.

Expensive new projects to pump sewage sludge further out to sea from major American cities aim to improve water quality on our coastlines. But no one really knows what becomes of microbes dumped in the ocean abyss. Some scientists fear that pathogens can maintain themselves at sea for months or years, only to return to shore in an upwelling current. Human pathogens were recovered in the 1980s from sewage sludge dumped in the ocean off New York City more than two years after such dumping ceased. "We don't know the consequences of adding sewage to the sea," notes Paul R. Epstein (1999), an environmental health expert at Harvard University. "We're just beginning to look at how climate change can affect ocean circulation and bring these bugs back to haunt us."

Diarrhea is also on the increase where seafood is harvested from waters that are polluted by sewage and industrial waste. Untreated sewage was a key factor in the resurgence of epidemic cholera in Hong Kong during 1994 (Lee, Lai, Lai, et al. 1996). Coastal waters around Hong Kong Island have become heavily polluted from tons of untreated sewage and industrial wastewater that are discharged every day. Restaurants there customarily keep fish and shellfish alive in tanks before they are cooked and served in meals. Water for those tanks is typically drawn straight from Hong Kong's filthy harbor.

Polluted water is also behind the rising incidence of harmful algal blooms around Hong Kong, Japan, the Atlantic seaboard of North America, the North Sea, the Baltic Sea, and elsewhere. During August 1997, thousands of fish died suddenly in the Pocomoke River and adjacent waters of Chesapeake Bay. During the previous year, many fish had been seen with open, bleeding sores. The outbreak, which devastated the region's fishing industry, was linked to the explosive growth of *Pfiesteria piscicida*, toxin-producing dinoflagellates that environmental scientists have recently been tracking in coastal waters from Delaware to Alabama's Gulf Coast. These tiny algae-like creatures thrive in warm, brackish waters polluted by excess nutrients. Such nutrients have been finding their way into coastal estuaries from many sources: the run-off of sewage treatment plants and septic tanks; nitrogen-rich fertilizers flushed from suburban gardens and market farms; manure produced by large poultry operations and cattle feedlots; and air pollutants that settle on the land and water. In the Chesapeake Bay outbreak, commercial fishermen and others having prolonged exposure to affected waters suffered from headaches, a burning sensation of the skin, and disturbances of memory and higher cognitive functions (Grattan, Oldach, Perl, et al. 1998).

The emergence of Lyme disease in the northeastern United States can be traced to a different sort of change in land use patterns. In the early 1800s the native oak and hickory forests of the region were cleared to open lands for cultivation and to supply the wood needed to fuel America's growing industries. Deforestation greatly reduced the native deer population. This deprived adult *Ixodes* ticks of a ready source of blood meals, a requirement for their reproduction, and their numbers declined. But by the early twentieth century, many farms were abandoned as the rural population of the region drifted into cities. Gradually the land was reoccupied with forest.

In the absence of natural predators, deer populations rebounded as their woodland habitat grew. By the 1980s, the region supported more deer than when Columbus sailed for America in 1492. As deer herds have grown, the *Ixodes* ticks that feed on them have thrived. For people visiting forested areas, that has meant an increased risk of bites from ticks, including those infected with *Borellia burgdorferi*, the curly bacterium that causes Lyme disease. Deer apparently suffer no ill effects from *Borellia*. Neither do the smaller mammals and birds on which immature *Ixodes* ticks feed and from which the ticks acquire the infection before they are ready to go after larger animals like deer. But for accidental hosts, like humans, tick bites present a real danger of unpleasant disease. In highly endemic areas of Connecticut and elsewhere, up to 80 percent of *Ixodes* ticks are now infected with *Borellia* bacteria.

Reforestation in the northeastern states has occurred at the same time that increasing numbers of city dwellers have returned to the region's woodlands for recreation, and, increasingly, to live. Like many semirural areas now plagued with a high incidence of Lyme disease, the area of eastern Connecticut that hosted the first epidemic of the disease is popular with urban refugees fleeing New York or Boston in search of a country lifestyle. Sadly, the debilitating effects of Lyme disease have shattered many dreams of rustic bliss. Since World War II, reforestation and the proliferation of deer have also led to the emergence of Lyme disease in Central Europe. As in North America, the recovery of deer populations has fostered a multitude of *Ixodes* ticks that occasionally snatch a meal from passing humans. Surveys in endemic areas of Sweden have found antibodies to *B. burgdorferi* in more than a quarter of local residents (Gustafson, Svenungsson, Forsgren, et al. 1992).

Dust in the Wind

Although most environmental changes that trigger disease emergence can be linked to human activities, sometimes diseases appear through an "act of God." On the morning of January 17, 1994, a magnitude 6.7 earthquake shook Southern California. The earthquake, centered on the suburb of Northridge, killed seventy-two people and caused damage estimated at $23.8 billion. Strong ground-shaking from the main quake and subsequent aftershocks caused innumerable landslides in the nearby Santa Susana Mountains, sending dense clouds of dust into the air. Brisk Santa Ana winds then blew the dust westward into Ventura County, particularly into the suburban city of Simi Valley. During the next several weeks 203 cases of coccidioidomycosis were reported in Ventura County, including 114 cases among residents of Simi Valley. Three people died. Coccidioidomycosis, commonly known as valley fever, is caused by the *Coccidioides immitus* fungus that grows in the topsoil of semiarid regions of the southwestern United States. Infection results from inhalation of air-borne spores, which can be dispersed when the soil is disturbed. Although most infections go unnoticed, many infected people experience a prolonged flu-like illness with fever, chills, and a cough. Investigators concluded that the Ventura County outbreak was caused by dissemination of *Coccidioides* spores released during the earthquake (Schneider, Hajjeh, Spiegel, et al. 1997).

Blame It on the Weather

Eccentric weather patterns can bring additional pressure to overburdened ecosystems, upping the ante for human epidemics. A recent epidemic of Rift Valley fever in northeastern Kenya and southern Somalia was linked to rainfall that was sixty to one hundred times heavier than normal during late 1997 and early 1998 (World Health Organization 1998b). More than eighty-nine thousand people were infected during the epidemic, including about 250 who died. The floodwaters that covered much of the normally arid region permitted innumerable virus-infected mosquito eggs to hatch. In a similar manner, fifty-five people in North America's Great Plains were infected with western equine encephalitis in 1975 after a disastrous flood of the Red River led to the proliferation of *Culex* mosquitoes. This viral disease, which causes acute inflammation of the brain and spinal cord, also affected hundreds of horses and other domestic animals during the outbreak.

The 1993 outbreak of hantavirus infection on the Indian reservations around the Four Corners was probably the outcome of weather-associated changes in the local density of deer mice, *Peromyscus maniculatus*. That year, heavy winter rains after six years of drought brought forth a plentiful supply of pine nuts and grasshoppers, staples in the diets of deer mice. With abundant food and insufficient numbers of predators, the population of mice soared. Scientists who study rodents call these dramatic and temporary population surges "irruptions." In all likelihood, the hantavirus that we now call "Sin Nombre" (see Chapter 2) had long been present at low levels in local *Peromyscus*. However, the ten-fold increase in mouse numbers that year escalated their interaction and helped to propagate the infection. As the rodent irruption started to overwhelm the carrying capacity of the local ecosystem, competition for food and water increased rodent-to-rodent contact even more, especially when precipitation plummeted during late spring and summer. The decline in natural food sources then drove many of the infected mice from their underground burrows into human dwellings and other structures nearby. There the virus spread accidentally to people who inhaled some of the dried excretions the mice left behind, and the epidemic began (Engelthaler, Mosley, Cheek, et al. 1999).

Hantavirus pulmonary syndrome made an unwelcome comeback in the Four Corners in 1998 and 1999, after heavy rains and mild winter temperatures again created ideal conditions for another rodent irruption. Environmental factors have also played a major role recently in several large hantavirus epidemics in South America. In a pattern remarkably similar to that seen in the Four Corners, abnormally high rainfall followed by a drought sparked an outbreak in western Paraguay in 1995 and 1996. In the Río Negro and Chubut provinces of southern Argentina, fires and mild winters in 1994 and 1996 increased local numbers of the long-tailed rice rat (*Oligoryzomys longicaudatus*). This grain-loving rodent is the favored host of the

Argentine hantavirus, known as the Andes virus, which spread quickly from infected rodents to humans living close by. In 1997, the same virus caused an outbreak in southern Chile when the flowering and fruiting of a local species of bamboo caused another rodent irruption. The bamboo, which provided abundant food for *Oligoryzomys* rats, bursts forth this way only once every ten to thirty years.

In a similar way, the rise and fall of Lyme disease incidence in the northeastern states may reflect fluctuations in woodland deer and mouse populations. If the weather is favorable, the region's oak trees will produce a bumper crop of acorns during the autumn months every two to five years. Scientists call this process masting. When masting occurs, more deer are drawn into the forests where adult *Ixodes* ticks live. Ticks that can feed on deer at that critical time of year are able to mate and lay eggs the following year. Abundant autumn acorns also improve winter survival rates for white-footed mice and other small animals of the forest that maintain the core reservoir for the curly bacteria *Borellia burgdorferi*. In the year after masting, these small animals provide ready meals for larval ticks, infecting the larvae in the process. These ticks then spend another year on the forest floor as they grow into adolescent "nymphs," ready to bite humans and other innocent passersby. If this scenario holds true, peaks in the local incidence of Lyme disease among humans will follow masting by about two years (Jones, Ostfeld, Richard, et al. 1998).

The Various Moods of El Niño

Many of the world's recent weather anomalies, including the heavy rains that sparked the hantavirus epidemics around the Four Corners, have been linked to a volatile pattern of global climate variation known as the El Niño Southern Oscillation (ENSO). El Niño, meaning "Christ child," refers to a change in sea surface temperatures that begins at Christmastime every three to five years off the west coast of South America. We now know this seemingly local event has profound effects on weather patterns around the world. El Niño arises from shifts in atmospheric pressure over the equatorial Pacific, known as the Southern Oscillation. As an El Niño episode begins, trade winds that normally blow to the west from the eastern Pacific start to weaken, causing intense tropical storms to drift eastward from Indonesia. These changes stimulate swarms of very long ocean waves that displace cold currents on the sea surface with much warmer waters as they head east. As these warmer waters collect on the South American seaboard, evaporation increases over the eastern

...ic causing severe storms. In turn, these atmospheric changes disturb the normal course of the world's high-altitude jet streams, setting in motion unusual weather in many distant places.

Predicting the global effects of El Niño events is fraught with uncertainty. But usually El Niño years will bring droughts to India, Southeast Asia, parts of Africa, and Australia; heavy rainfall and flooding to California and certain arid regions of Latin America; and mild winters to much of North America and Europe. In years when the Southern Oscillation is reversed, and cold surface waters are restored in the eastern Pacific, opposite sorts of weather prevail worldwide. Not surprisingly, climatologists call this phase of the cycle La Niña, which literally means "little girl." An especially intense El Niño event during late 1997 and early 1998 caused severe drought and dry winds in much of Southeast Asia and the Western Pacific. These tinderbox conditions fanned uncontrollable fires across one million acres of Indonesian forests and brought a disastrous famine to Papua New Guinea. Elsewhere, that winter's El Niño delivered typhoons to Japan, flash floods and mudslides to California, tornadoes to Florida, freak snowstorms to Mexico, and catastrophic ice storms to Canada. As far away as Kenya and Somalia, the worst floods in forty years unleashed the epidemic of Rift Valley Fever we discussed earlier. Cholera also emerged because of the floods.

Evidence is growing that extremes in weather brought about by ENSO can have profound effects on other infectious diseases too. The transmission potential of malaria seems especially sensitive to ENSO weather disturbances. In the Punjab region of northeast Pakistan, malaria incidence can increase five-fold during the year following an El Niño event (Bouma and van der Kaay 1996). The above-average monsoon rainfall that follows the Punjab's dry El Niño years boosts the abundance and longevity of local *Anopheles* mosquito populations. Malaria cases also increase in Venezuela during the year after El Niño, for similar reasons (Bouma and Dye 1997). Here too, El Niño is associated with lower than usual rainfall, and the adage that "fever years follow famine years" holds well. In both regions it seems likely that the reduction of malaria transmission during dry El Niño years reduces population immunity, resulting in a rebound of cases when more normal rains return. Dry conditions may also diminish the predators of larval *Anopheles* mosquitoes, and the recovery of predator numbers in the first months after an especially dry year may lag behind that of their larval prey.

Human cases of Murray Valley encephalitis in southeast Australia can be predicted when the Southern Oscillation ushers in a La Niña episode (Nicholls 1993).

Infection with the Murray Valley virus, a relative of the dengue fever agent belonging to the flavivirus family, can cause a severe inflammation of the brain. Death results in one-third of patients, while an equal number suffer from permanent neurological deficits. During La Niña conditions, the states of Victoria, New South Wales, and South Australia that surround the Murray River can be subject to extended periods of heavy summer rainfall and flooding. These conditions favor the *Culex* mosquitoes that transmit the disease to humans.

La Niña's heavy summer rains also benefit the *Culex* and *Aedes* mosquitoes that pass on Ross River virus in temperate Australia. After high summer rainfall during 1992 and 1993, more than eight hundred cases of arthritis, fever, and rash due to the virus were reported in the state of South Australia, up from the usual thirty or fewer cases per year (Seldon and Cameron 1996). Since 1970, dengue fever outbreaks in the island nations of the South Pacific have also correlated with fluctuations in the Southern Oscillation (Hales, Weinstein, and Woodward 1996). At the El Niño part of the cycle, rainfall increases in the central and eastern islands, boosting *Aedes* mosquito numbers and increasing dengue transmission. During the La Niña phase, rainy conditions are seen further west, heightening the dengue fever risk there.

Diarrhea outbreaks have likewise been noted where El Niño has increased local temperatures and reduced essential rainfall. During Southeast Asia's severe drought in late 1997, water rationing was imposed in Manila to cope with an acute shortage. This made hygiene more difficult in the city's many impoverished districts, which led to an increased incidence of diarrhea, especially among infants and other young children. The situation was worsened when thirsty residents began siphoning off water from underground supply lines. This water inevitably became contaminated, and it helped to spread diarrheal infections far and wide (Easton 1997). Since then, the torrential rains associated with La Niña conditions have also plagued Manila's shantytowns. Floodwaters that funnel down city streets have been badly contaminated with infectious rat urine, leading to an epidemic of leptospirosis (Easton 1999).

El Niño Southern Oscillation-related increases in sea temperatures off Peru may have also played a role in starting Latin America's cholera epidemic in 1991. As in Chesapeake Bay, nitrogen-rich runoff had been accumulating in Peru's coastal waters for years. The sudden warming of surface seawater stimulated new algal blooms, significantly increasing the local biomass of free-floating plankton. Direct algal toxicity was not a problem, but it soon became evident that these marine organisms could harbor immense populations of

Vibrio cholerae bacteria. From the refuge of the algal blooms, the bacteria eventually found their way into the human food chain (Colwell 1996). Increases in sea surface temperature in the Bay of Bengal have also been linked to human cholera outbreaks in Bangladesh. Not surprisingly, the return of El Niño conditions to Peru at the end of 1997 coincided with an upturn in cholera cases there. During the first three months of 1998 more than sixteen thousand cholera cases were reported in Peru, including 146 deaths. Increases were also noted in Bolivia, Honduras, and Nicaragua.

Ominous Long-Term Weather Predictions

Climatic instability attributed to ENSO may be only a foretaste of what is in store in the years ahead, due to greenhouse warming. Average global temperatures have risen by approximately one degree Fahrenheit during the past century, and are likely to climb between two and six degrees Fahrenheit by the year 2100. These changes may seem small, but a decrease of only about nine degrees Fahrenheit is sufficient to trigger an ice age. The first nine months of 1998 were among the warmest on record throughout most of the Northern Hemisphere. Unseasonably hot temperatures returned to North America and elsewhere during the summer of 1999. Judging from studies of tree rings and glacial ice cores, summers haven't been this hot since at least the Middle Ages. Greenhouse gases in the atmosphere today may be at their highest levels in 420 thousand years. Once released in the atmosphere, many of these gases take a very long time to dissipate. Without determined efforts to stop deforestation and reduce our dependence on fossil fuels, the heat-trapping blanket that covers the earth will only get thicker. Our planet is overheating and there is no relief in sight.

Just as no one can say for sure how warming of the lower atmosphere will alter global climate, no one can be certain how such changes will affect disease emergence. It does seem likely, however, that higher temperatures and consequent increases in heavy rainfall will permit certain disease vectors to expand their usual ranges. Already, various mosquito vectors appear to be enlarging their distributions at rates correlated with the retreat of mountain glaciers. In Mexico, *Aedes aegypti* mosquitoes, the principal vectors of dengue fever, have been found at elevations as high as fifty-five hundred feet (Herrera-Basto, Prevots, Zarate, et al. 1992). Transmission of dengue had not been seen above four thousand feet before 1986, but since then it has returned there every summer. Since the 1980s, epidemic malaria has moved into highland populations in Rwanda, Zambia, Ethiopia, and Madagascar in tandem with increases in temperature and rainfall. By 2050, an additional one hundred to seven hundred million people may be at risk of malaria infection because of human influences on climate.

Besides malaria, other major diseases of the tropics, including schistosomiasis and visceral leishmaniasis, may extend their distributions into more temperate areas if global warming continues unabated. African trypanosomiasis, also known as sleeping sickness, is a parasitic disease spread by infected tsetse flies. The disease produces severe lethargy and other neurological disturbances in about twenty-five thousand people each year. Without expensive medical treatment, African trypanosomiasis is almost invariably fatal. At present, the disease is limited to localized areas of tropical Africa by the temperature preferences of tsetse flies. When researchers examined the effects of a five degree Fahrenheit increase in average temperature across Kenya and Tanzania, the potential range of tsetse flies expanded markedly (Rogers and Packer 1993).

Global warming may not only enlarge the territories of important disease vectors; it may make those vectors more efficient in transmitting disease. For example, when daily temperatures rise from eighty-six degrees Fahrenheit to more than ninety degrees Fahrenheit, the time required for an *Aedes* mosquito to become infectious after its first exposure to the dengue fever virus drops from twelve days to seven days (Sehgal 1997). A warmer ambient temperature also reduces the size of mosquito larvae, which results in smaller adults. Smaller adult females must bite more frequently to nourish their eggs. This too increases the risk of dengue transmission to humans. Warmer temperatures also shorten the time for malaria parasites to mature in the stomachs of *Anopheles* mosquitoes, making them infectious sooner.

In the eastern United States, computer models for climate change are predicting more warm, wet winters and hot, dry summers. If this forecast is correct, epidemics of St. Louis encephalitis (SLE) seem likely (Patz, Epstein, Burke, et al. 1996). The SLE virus is a close relative of the West Nile virus that struck New York City in 1999 (see preface and chapter 3). Epidemics of SLE are highly correlated with dry spells in summer that exceed eighty-five degrees Fahrenheit for days on end, especially in years where the winters had been mild and rainy. Like the West Nile virus and Australia's Murray River virus, certain *Culex* mosquitoes spread the SLE virus, and it too can cause an inflammatory disease of the brain. When New York's encephalitis epidemic erupted during a prolonged heat wave after the second-worst summer drought on record, epidemiologists could be forgiven for initially thinking the disease was SLE. Other diseases likely to increase with greenhouse warming are the traditional hot-weather infections associated with food, such as *Salmonella* and *Campylobacter*. Diseases transmitted by ticks may become less common in southern states, where ticks may not tolerate higher temperatures. But further north, tick-borne diseases may increase because of a longer transmission season.

Thus far we have focused on many of the common ways that modern human activities have precipitated emergence. Factors related to changes in the host-agent environment are undoubtedly of greatest importance for explaining most cases of emergence. But as Richard Krause (1994) points out, "Microbes are not idle bystanders, waiting for new opportunities offered by human mobility, ignorance, or neglect." Krause, a researcher with the National Institutes of Health, notes that sometimes "microbes possess remarkable genetic versatility that enables them to develop new pathogenic vigor." Clearly, some organisms that infect humans are becoming more vicious today, while others are simply becoming harder to kill. The next chapter will consider how rapid evolution in the microbial world occasionally turns relatively tame organisms into dangerous pathogens.

What You Can Do To Prevent Rodent-Borne Diseases

Hantaviruses and other pathogens spread by rodents can be avoided by making the environments in and around our homes as unattractive to mice and rats as possible. It will never be possible to eliminate rodents altogether, but the CDC recommends a few simple measures that will reduce the likelihood of contact with these animals and the diseases they transmit:

- Keep your home clean, especially the kitchen. Keep food covered in rodent-proof containers, and keep a tight-fitting lid on garbage.

- Set spring-loaded traps near baseboards, as rodents tend to run along walls. If you use EPA-approved rodenticides, follow instructions carefully.

- Seal holes and cracks around your house where rodents might gain entry.

- Clear all brush, grass, and junk away from the foundation of your house.

- If you discover a rodent-infested area in or around your home, do not stir up any dust by sweeping or vacuuming. Instead, thoroughly wet the area and mop or sponge it with a disinfectant. For heavy infestations, consider calling a professional exterminator.

- When outdoors, don't disturb rodent burrows, and never feed or handle rodents in the wild.

Chapter 8

Microbial Adaptation and Change

Mutants of contemporary viruses are created every minute. They are part of the heterogeneous population of virus particles produced in every case of viral infection.

—Edwin D. Kilbourne,
New York Medical College

Infectious organisms, like all living things, evolve over generations to adapt to new circumstances and to compete effectively with other organisms vying to occupy the same niche. Due to their immense numbers and exponential rates of reproduction, bacteria and viruses can run the evolutionary race at breakneck speed. Among the countless varieties of micro-organisms that inhabit this planet, pathogenic organisms encounter especially powerful pressures on their survival, for they are constantly besieged by the immune defenses of their human or animal hosts. They must be quick in the face of adversity, or they face extinction.

To endure in this dangerous world, many microbes have developed an ingenious capacity to reinvent themselves via manipulation of their genetic makeup. Through random point mutations and various techniques of genetic reshuffling they manage to stay one step ahead of their hosts in the battle for life. Sometimes such evolutionary tactics give pathogens access to new kinds of cells in their usual hosts, or even allow them to break through "the species barrier" from one animal host to another, including humans. Genetically remodeled pathogens might be able to evade antibiotics or other drugs designed to kill them, as we will explore in the next chapter. They might also be able to release new toxins into the cells they infect, or simply acquire the means to bypass the normal workings of the human immune system.

Occasionally the result of such genetic reconstruction is the emergence of an apparently "new" disease. From our perspective, a previously unknown or seemingly harmless microbe has suddenly turned vicious, triggering a deadly epidemic of human disease. From the viewpoint of the microbe, the human misery of the epidemic is just an accident that comes with the territory of maintaining its fitness for survival. Fortunately, the spontaneous emergence of strikingly new microbial variants is a relatively rare cause of massive human epidemics. More often, the mechanisms of emergence related to social and environmental change—like those we have examined in previous chapters—are responsible. But a few organisms, particularly certain viruses, do have a penchant for sudden variations in their innate virulence. The results can be devastating for their unsuspecting hosts. Sometimes a common but innocuous viral ailment, familiar to humans throughout their history, can put on a new face and shake us from complacency. Such was the case in 1918.

The Epidemic of the Twentieth Century

Early in the morning of March 4, 1918, Albert Gitchell, a cook serving in the United States Army at Fort Riley, Kansas, reported to sick bay with a fever, sore throat, cough, and muscle aches. The cook had all the classic symptoms of an influenza infection, better known as "the flu." He was advised to stay off his feet, drink plenty of fluids, and rest. But by noon that day, doctors at Fort Riley saw 107 men with the same complaints. By the end of the week 522 cases had occurred. Over the next month another 605 personnel at the fort would succumb to the disease. In all there were forty-six deaths.

That spring, no one could have imagined that the Fort Riley flu outbreak would presage the most devastating pandemic the world has known since the Black Death swept Europe in the fourteenth century. No one would have believed that by the end of the year more than twenty million people, from almost every country, would be dead from the flu. World War I, which was drawing to a close in November that year, had cost more lives than any previous war. But the flu would kill more men, women, and children in just 120 days than the global military conflict had killed in four years.

The first wave of the flu, which followed American soldiers to Europe for the closing offensives of the war, spread quickly across the globe but caused relatively few deaths. With the world's attention on the war, the initial outburst of the epidemic provoked little alarm. By summer it had dissipated, as would be expected for a disease that has a striking preference for the colder months. But the hiatus that summer was brief. By late August the flu was back, this time with a vengeance.

Doctors quickly recognized that the strain of the new flu virus was similar to that of the first wave, as those who had fallen ill with flu earlier in the year were immune this time around. But somehow over the summer the virus had become more deadly. Now, within hours of becoming ill patients could be overcome by the infection. Many would simply collapse, unable to breathe because of the fluid filling their lungs. Jeffery Taubenberger (1997), a pathologist who has recently examined lung tissue from victims of the 1918 epidemic says, "These people were drowning. There was so much liquid in the air spaces of their lungs that patients would have bloody fluid coming out of their noses. When they died, it would often drench the bed sheets."

The second wave of the flu epidemic surfaced almost simultaneously in France, North America, and West Africa. It swept across Europe, tracing the movement of soldiers and supplies involved in the war. Suffering was particularly relentless in Spain, and probably for this reason the pestilence came to be known as the "Spanish flu" in most of the world. Outbreaks among German soldiers undoubtedly contributed to Germany's defeat in the war. A 1918 dispatch in *The New York Times* noted that among captured German soldiers, "the new fever is said to strike down the men so quickly that they drop in their tracks while on duty." Kaiser Wilhelm himself was forced to return home from the front in France because of the malady.

Away from the battlefields, the mortality in the second wave was staggering. On just the first day of October there were 202 deaths from the flu in Boston. On October 23, there were 851 deaths in New York City. During two weeks in the middle of October more than seventy-six hundred people died in Philadelphia. The Catholic Charities of Philadelphia organized six horse-drawn wagons to search the streets for the discarded bodies of flu victims. They found more than two hundred. Cadavers in the city morgue were stacked up three and four deep as embalmers refused to come to work. Coffins grew scarce, and a black market developed to meet the demand.

Normal life ceased as the flu descended. Factories and offices shut their doors. Homeless children wandered the streets. Alfred Jay

Bollet, a Yale University medical historian, has likened American cities during October 1918 to London during plague outbreaks in the late Middle Ages: "All places of public assembly were closed, including schools and churches. Liberty Loan drives, parades, and even football games were canceled. Ordinances were passed requiring everyone to wear gauze face masks in public, and stiff fines were imposed on people who sneezed or coughed in public without a handkerchief," wrote Bollet (1997).

Perhaps the most disturbing aspect of the 1918 pandemic was its terrible toll on young adults. Death from influenza is usually confined to the elderly and those with underlying medical problems. For reasons still not fully understood, the 1918 virus selectively struck down robust individuals in the prime of life. Mortality rates during the pandemic were highest for those between the ages of twenty-five and twenty-nine years. As Malcolm Gladwell noted in a 1997 article for *The New Yorker*, "This wasn't just a deadly infectious disease. It was a deadly infectious disease with the singular and terrifying quality of being better at killing the young and healthy than the old and infirm."

Overall, the 1918 epidemic claimed more than six hundred thousand American lives, of whom 99 percent were under the age of sixty-five. Smaller waves of influenza would return in the winter of 1919, and again in 1920, but the pandemic strain would soon fade to oblivion, vanishing from the human species as mysteriously as it had first appeared. To date, the world has not witnessed another outburst of mortality from any cause like that seen in the latter months of 1918. The means to capture influenza viruses in the laboratory and study them was not available until 1933. By then, all that remained of the Spanish flu was the imprint of the deadly virus on the immune systems of those who had survived it. For more than eighty years the legacy of the Spanish flu has resided only in the antibodies of those who endured it, and in the fading memories of a grieving generation.

How Flu Viruses Remake Themselves

Viruses that cause flu are relatively primitive life forms, but they possess a genetic versatility unequalled in nature. Their genetic code is written in a single strand of RNA. As a group, RNA viruses cause a disproportionate share of emerging diseases in humans and animals, in part because they mutate one hundred thousand times more easily than DNA viruses do. During viral replication, mistakes are inevitably made in copying the genetic code from a parent virus to its many millions of progeny. Those mistakes can then be passed on to succeeding generations, creating a new virus variant. Although DNA viruses also make mistakes, they possess "proofreading" enzymes that correct such errors, so fewer mutations are passed on. Most mutations offer no advantage to the virus, and many are downright suicidal. But every so often a mutation, or an accidental cluster of mutations, bestows new powers on a virus that promote its survival.

Flu viruses are particularly adept at accumulating point mutations that work to their advantage. They need to be adept. Every winter they unleash themselves on a global human population that possesses powerful antibodies against flu, acquired from previous infections. They survive among such unfriendly hosts and escape the neutralizing effects of the antibodies they encounter in the course of infection by taking advantage of slight mutations that arise from year to year. As such mutations accumulate, flu viruses can rearrange the three-dimensional structure of their surface proteins, called antigens, and thus disguise themselves from detection by the hosts' defenses. This annual subterfuge is called "antigenic drift," and it explains why people infected one year with the flu are not completely immune the next time the disease comes around. Flu vaccines are updated annually to take account of these gradual revisions in the viral contours.

But flu viruses have another evolutionary trick up their sleeves. Every so often they emerge suddenly with an entirely new look, displaying a radically different protein coat to the immune systems of their prospective hosts. When this happens no one on Earth is immune, and a life-threatening andemic is born. Flu experts call this dramatic, unforeseeable change an "antigenic shift." One way these shifts arise is from a process called genetic reassortment. Reassortment occurs when pieces of genetic material from one strain are mixed with those of another, like ingredients in a tossed salad. Flu viruses partition their RNA into eight neat segments, each segment comprising one or two genes. When the cells of a single host are dually infected by two viral strains certain segments of one virus can be exchanged with corresponding segments of another. The result of this swapping can be a potent hybrid strain never encountered before by human populations.

Influenza Type A

There are two main varieties of influenza virus, unimaginatively named A and B. A third group, type C, is not a serious pathogen.

Influenza A is by far the most mutable, and because it is the only type that undergoes antigenic shift, it alone causes human pandemics like the one in 1918. For that reason we will concentrate here on influenza A. The surface of the virus carries two key proteins, the hemagglutinin (called H) and the neuraminidase (called N). The H protein plays a major part in binding the virus to the host cells it invades. Once bound by its H protein, the virus induces the cell to swallow it. There the virus hijacks the cell's normal metabolic machinery, forcing it to produce countless new viral offspring. Eventually the infected cell explodes, releasing a hoard of new viruses that are ready to repeat the process in other cells. There are least fifteen subtypes of H and nine subtypes of N, each with a characteristic chemical composition and shape. Strains of influenza A virus are classified by the numbers given to their H and N proteins. For example, most flu viruses in circulation among humans in recent years are of the H3N2 variety.

The viruses of the H3N2 family undergo antigenic drift each year, so although a certain Wuhan strain dominated global flu incidence in 1997, the "Australian flu" (so named because it was first isolated in Sydney) chalked up the most victims in 1998 and 1999. Today's H3N2 strains are all descendants of the last major antigenic shift, the sudden viral makeover that provoked the "Hong Kong flu" pandemic of 1968. A second variety of influenza A making the rounds today is of the H1N1 type. We know from antibody studies of elderly people that the 1918 pandemic was also due to an H1N1 strain, one that supplanted another type that had been prevalent for at least eighteen years. But the viral descendants of the Spanish flu strain found themselves displaced by an antigenic shift to H2N2 in 1957, a shift that prompted the "Asian flu" pandemic that year. The current batch of H1N1 viruses stems from the appearance of the "Russian flu" in 1977, an outbreak that actually began in the Anchan province of China. This strain has coexisted with H3N2 for more than twenty years without displacing it.

The Recipe for Disaster: How Reassortment Occurs

Most strains of influenza A cannot easily infect humans because our cells lack suitable receptors to which most viral H proteins can bind. Until recently it was thought that only three hemagglutinin subtypes (H1, H2, and H3) can readily infect humans. In contrast, aquatic birds possess the needed receptors to play host to the entire range of influenza subtypes. Wild ducks, geese, seagulls, and other migratory birds turn out to be the definitive hosts for influenza viruses, the natural "reservoir" for the flu. Humans and the few other mammals that end up with flu infections are by comparison mere bystanders in a highly evolved bird-virus interaction. Typically, waterfowl that carry flu viruses suffer no disease as a result. Avian flu viruses replicate silently in the cells lining the birds' digestive tracts and are excreted in high concentrations in fecal droppings. Young birds acquire the virus as it is shed by adults into the waters where the young birds are raised. The migratory behavior of many waterfowl allows flu viruses to spread in a rapid but benign fashion among wild birds over vast areas.

Although the panoply of avian flu viruses cannot generally infect humans, they can infect pigs. Since 1918, veterinarians have reported seeing the classic symptoms of flu in pigs during and between human flu epidemics. When the Hong Kong flu struck in 1968, H3N2 viruses like those afflicting humans were recovered from pigs around the world. Researchers wondered whether pigs have a role in the evolution of influenza among humans. It turns out that pig cells uniquely possess receptors for both avian and human flu viruses. It is plausible that a pig could be infected simultaneously with flu viruses from birds and humans. In China—where most new strains of influenza emerge—pigs, ducks, and humans often share the same living quarters. A pig infected with an avian flu virus might pick up a human flu virus from a farmer and become an ideal "mixing vessel" for genetic reassortment. According to this hypothesis, gene segments from an avian virus might intermingle with segments from a human virus in the pig, yielding a hybrid virus with the virulent features of both. The unwitting pig, whose coughs and sneezes recycle the recombinant virus back to humans, becomes the bridge to a new pandemic.

From Where Did the Spanish Flu Virus Come?

It now seems certain that genetic reassortment caused the pandemics of 1957 and 1968, presumably with the help of Chinese pigs. Unfortunately, the origins of the 1918 pandemic are much less clear. One theory holds that it too arose from a reassortment event, possibly in Kansas, where the first human cases were reported, but probably in China. According to this scenario, flu-carrying ducks dropped infected feces into ponds and pastures along their migrations, infecting local waterfowl. The bird virus then passed into a pig, probably from swallowing water contaminated with infected feces. The unknown pig, which also acquired a human flu virus, then cradled a genetic reassortment that resulted in an entirely new H1N1 strain, infectious to humans.

But recent genetic sequencing of the 1918 virus has called this theory into question. No one was able to grow the Spanish flu virus in a laboratory in 1918, but in the last few years it has become possible to recover minute fragments of the viral RNA from preserved human specimens. Careful analysis of these "fossil" fragments has shown that the 1918 virus was closely related to swine flu viruses still circulating among pigs during the 1930s (Reid, Fanning, Hultin, et al. 1999). This supports the idea that pigs were involved in conveying the new virus to humans. But investigators have found no evidence for genetic reassortment in the virus, no sign that human and bird viruses had been knitted together into an entirely new pathogen. Perhaps infected pigs acted as intermediate hosts, helping to adapt an avian virus for infection in humans over a period of years. If so, it now seems they did this without mixing and matching bird and human segments of the viral genome.

Alternatively, pigs may have had nothing to do with the entry of the lethal new virus into the human population. This view asserts that the Spanish flu virus was entirely the result of bird-to-human gene transfers, in which humans themselves were the mixing vessels. Maybe the pigs that developed a flu-like disease in 1918 were actually infected by nearby humans. For now, the jury is still out on the cause of the antigenic shift behind the 1918 epidemic. Whatever the exact mechanism of interspecies transfer, a mild wave of human flu emerged that March at Fort Riley, where crowded living conditions facilitated its spread. The new virus was not particularly lethal until August, when, after one or more further mutations, it turned deadly.

Why Was the Spanish Flu So Deadly?

As yet, the genetic basis for the Spanish flu's sudden virulence in August 1918 is unsolved, but a 1983 flu epidemic among chickens might provide some clues. That year, a mild outbreak of H5N2 flu at several huge commercial chicken farms in Pennsylvania suddenly became deadly. Normally, flu viruses infecting birds can only commandeer the cells that line the animals' intestines. After binding, successful invasion depends on cleavage of the virus' H protein, which is done by an enzyme found only in the digestive tract of birds. Similarly, human flu viruses must stage their attack in our respiratory tract, as the enzyme needed for cleavage is only found there in humans. But the transformed chicken virus in Pennsylvania attacked every tissue in the body of the birds in a frightening display of carnage. Ultimately, seventeen million chickens had to be slaughtered to control the outbreak. Researchers later found that it was a single point mutation in the gene for the H protein that had made the virus so virulent (Webster, Kawaoka, and Bean 1986). That tiny change enabled the virus to use a more common enzyme to cleave the H protein, an enzyme found in cells throughout the bodies of the infected chickens.

Perhaps then the 1918 pandemic became so deadly because the Spanish flu virus also carried a modified H protein, one that gave it unlimited access to virtually every cell of its unfortunate human hosts. Maybe this was how the disease cut down so many young and otherwise robust people with such fury. This explanation for the pandemic's extreme virulence is tempting, but a mutation like the one observed in the chicken epidemic has not yet been found at the analogous site of the Spanish flu virus. Investigations are continuing to find other pernicious aberrations in still unexplored regions of the viral genome. It may turn out that multiple genes working in concert caused the exceptional virulence of the 1918 virus.

Such work is only possible because of recent attempts to recover trace amounts of viral RNA from the preserved body parts of 1918 flu victims. The first breakthrough came in 1995 when the pathologist Taubenberger (1997) and his colleagues obtained preserved lung tissue from a twenty-one-year-old Army private who died from the flu on September 26, 1918, at Fort Jackson, South Carolina. For nearly eighty years his lungs, fixed in formalin and embedded in paraffin, had been preserved, stored at the Armed Forces Institute of Pathology in Washington, D.C. Since then the same team has salvaged the 1918 virus from the stored lungs of a thirty-year-old soldier stationed at Camp Upton, New York. He had died the same day as the first case, seven hundred miles away. A third specimen was found in August 1997, when a retired pathologist retrieved the lungs of an Inuit woman whose body he had exhumed from a mass grave in the hard-frozen permafrost at Brevig Mission, Alaska. Like approximately 85 percent of the residents in this tiny arctic settlement, she had perished from the disease after an infected mail carrier delivered the virus to her village by dogsled. The more these specimens and others containing the virus are studied, the better the chances will be of unlocking the cause of the Spanish flu's lethality.

Although secrets regarding the origins and deadliness of the 1918 pandemic remain, there is no mystery about why a variant virus appearing at that moment in history spread as extensively as it did. When the new virus surfaced on the plains of Kansas, the world was engaged in what was being called "the war to end all wars." Vast demographic shifts were occurring at an unprecedented level. Diseases like the flu, spread by respiratory contact, thrive when people are forced into crowded living situations, such as military camps, trenches, and battlefield hospitals. The intercontinental movement of troops and equipment during the final months of the war carried the virus very efficiently into large, susceptible populations. Finally, there was little public health knowledge at that time about how to control influenza, and public resources in most countries were diverted primarily to the war effort anyway. In retrospect, a malignant new virus could not have appeared at a worse time. Once it began, the pandemic of 1918 was virtually unstoppable.

Fowl Play in Hong Kong

Fears of another unstoppable flu epidemic shook the world in 1997. In late March that year outbreaks of influenza A broke out at three chicken farms in Hong Kong's New Territories. By early May, poultry deaths exceeded forty-five hundred, representing about 70 percent of the birds in the flocks. Tests revealed that an H5N1 virus had caused the outbreaks. This strain, first identified in South Africa during the 1960s, has become a recognized source of deadly epidemics among poultry. But an H5 virus had never caused disease in humans. Then, on May 21, just as the chicken epidemic was subsiding, a three-year-old boy died in a Hong Kong hospital from acute respiratory distress secondary to influenza pneumonia. His death followed a twelve-day illness that began with a fever, sore throat, and a cough. Routine tests on various respiratory specimens could not identify which strain of influenza A was involved. Finally, with the help of international experts, a startling answer emerged by early August: The boy had died from infection with an H5N1 virus. Subsequent genetic sequencing showed that this virus was virtually identical to the one implicated in the chicken farm outbreaks.

As the discovery of "bird flu" in a human host electrified the world's news media, the international flu experts who converged on Hong Kong sought to assure the public that the tragic death of the little boy was probably an isolated incident. But, by early December, three more cases occurred, including another fatality. "Everybody is wondering whether this is the beginning of another pandemic," admitted Keiji Fukuda (1997), a Centers for Disease Control and Prevention (CDC) epidemiologist interviewed in Hong Kong on December 11. Within two days another three cases were diagnosed, and Hong Kong hospitals went on alert for a full-blown epidemic. As Christmas approached, emergency supplies of drugs to treat the flu were flown to Hong Kong, and efforts to produce a vaccine against the new strain intensified. On December 23, Hong Kong authorities suspended chicken importation from mainland China, and six days later they ordered that all live chickens in the former British colony be destroyed. Within three days more than 1.3 million chickens collected from 1,000 markets and 160 farms were gassed, sealed in plastic bags, and buried in landfill sites.

The slaughter of Hong Kong's chickens was an unpopular decision at the time, but it may have prevented the twentieth century's fourth flu pandemic. The eighteenth and final human case of H5N1 flu was diagnosed on December 28, the day before the slaughter began. In most of the human cases, transmission of the virus could be explained by direct exposure to live chickens. There was little evidence that the new virus was very efficient at person-to-person spread, which could have triggered a pandemic. But to flu experts it was only a matter of time before the "bird flu" virus acquired the ability to pass easily from one human to another. This change might have arisen by a spontaneous mutation, or via the coinfection of human hosts with conventional human flu viruses, allowing the kind of genetic reassortment well-known to occur in pigs. By removing people's exposure to chickens, authorities may have averted such a doomsday scenario just in time.

Even without the dramatic risks presented by the 1997 "bird flu" outbreak, there is no doubt that influenza is one of humanity's most formidable enemies. During an ordinary flu season the disease still claims about twenty thousand lives in the United States. Fatal outbreaks of ordinary flu strains erupt throughout the world every year, especially during the winter months. In 1999 alone, major flu epidemics were reported in Afghanistan, Nepal, Japan, and several countries in Europe. In the Afghan outbreak the disease was especially fierce because of poor hygiene, inadequate nutrition, and crowded living conditions. Within days, mortality rates in parts of the Badakhshan province reached 1 to 2 percent of the total population. Summertime travelers to Alaska and the Yukon Territory have also been victims of recent flu outbreaks. In 1998 about forty thousand travelers and tourism workers there developed the disease. Epidemics involving Alaskan land and sea tours returned during the summer of 1999. Earlier in the year Hong Kong braced itself for a rerun of the "bird flu" incident, as two young girls were found to be infected with another novel avian flu virus, H9N2. Five additional cases in mainland China were also suspected. So far this strain seems relatively mild in humans, but it bears watching. We have not seen the last of bird viruses crossing directly into humans.

Could a 1918-Style Pandemic Happen Again?

In a word, yes. It is a safe bet that another major flu pandemic will occur some time, but it is impossible to predict when the current "interpandemic period" will end. Certainly, living conditions on this crowded planet, compounded by high-speed transport systems, are well suited for a novel flu virus to disseminate globally, once an antigenic shift takes place. Treatment of the flu has recently improved, and new medicines able to halt viral replication in cells are on the horizon. But for the time being the potential for a 1918-style catastrophe is high.

Influenza pandemics have been documented at least thirty-one times since 1580. With twentieth century pandemics erupting in 1918, 1957, and 1968, it is plain that antigenic shifts do not occur with any predictable regularity. Some say that with no major antigenic shift in more than thirty years the world is overdue for one now. To most flu experts, Hong Kong's 1997 "bird flu" outbreak was an extremely close call. "Next time, humankind may not be so fortunate," write W. Graeme Laver, Norbert Bischofberger, and Robert Webster (1999). "If a virus as deadly as the Hong Kong strain tore through the world's crowded communities today, 30 percent of the world's population could conceivably be dead (from the virus itself or from secondary bacterial infections) before a vaccine became available."

Newly published projections of the impact of the next pandemic on the United States make sober reading. Martin Meltzer and colleagues (1999) predict there will be 89 thousand to 207 thousand deaths in this country alone. The pandemic will also cause 314 thousand to 734 thousand hospitalizations and require 18 to 42 million outpatient visits to doctors. Without large-scale immunization, the United States economy will lose up to $166 billion fighting the disease. Serious disruptions to commerce and social institutions also seem likely. For example, if many long-distance truck drivers are kept from working because of the flu, deliveries of fresh foods may be curtailed to some communities. If too many schoolteachers are stricken, classes will have to be suspended. Staffing shortages at health care facilities would be especially troublesome.

Robert Webster, one of the virologists who discovered the mutation that caused the great chicken flu catastrophe of 1983, notes that all the genes of past influenza pandemics are alive and well in the aquatic bird reservoir. Like most flu experts, Webster urges constant vigilance. He compares the vulnerability of humans today to that of the boiler-house chickens who perished in the 1983 epidemic: "The chicken population in Pennsylvania is like the world is at the moment—hundreds of thousands, even millions of chickens just waiting to be infected" (1993).

Other Shifty Viruses

Flu viruses are not the only microbes that actively redesign themselves. HIV-1, the principal AIDS virus, can also undergo brisk genetic changes. It does this through point mutations in its RNA, and by genetic recombinations assembled from distinct viral subtypes within the same host. Molecular geneticists have been amazed at HIV's capacity for genetic divergence during the few short years since it was first isolated. It is not unusual for a patient infected only once with HIV to carry a complex mixture of viral subtypes when examined years later. The remarkable mutability of HIV has made it difficult to develop a vaccine against AIDS, as the virus presents researchers with a moving target. Similar problems confront the control of hepatitis C, another innately unstable RNA virus. As with HIV, people infected with hepatitis C play host to a multitude of viral "quasispecies," a throng of genetically diverse mutants whose many faces baffle the body's normal immune defenses. This genetic diversity is probably why hepatitis C infections so often become chronic.

Enteroviruses

Another group of RNA viruses that undergo a high rate of mutation within their human hosts are the enteroviruses, including those which cause hand, foot, and mouth disease (HFMD). This common illness of childhood is characterized by a mild fever, sores in the mouth, and a blister-like rash seen on the hands and soles of the feet. Hand, foot, and mouth disease is most often due to infection with coxsackievirus A16, and its clinical course is almost always benign. A less common cause of HFMD is enterovirus 71 (EV71). Since its discovery in 1974, EV71 has occasionally been linked to serious neurological disease, including meningitis and polio-like paralysis.

Enterovirus 71 infection has also been responsible for encephalitis, leading to death. But its clinical features have varied greatly in each place the virus has turned up.

In 1998 the EV71 virus turned up in Taiwan. During the spring and summer months that year an outbreak of HFMD struck the southern portion of the island, affecting as many as three hundred thousand young children. Most recovered with little difficulty, but at least 320 children were hospitalized and 55 died (Centers for Disease Control and Prevention 1998c). In each fatal case the child's condition suddenly deteriorated about three days after the onset of illness, prompting immediate hospitalization. Clinical signs of neurological involvement were common, especially signs pointing to inflammatory disease around critical life-support areas of the brainstem. Death typically followed within twenty-four hours, despite mechanical ventilation and repeated attempts at cardiovascular resuscitation. In ninety-seven cases where the viral cause was sought, EV71 was found.

The savage course of the Taiwan epidemic had only been seen with EV71 outbreaks twice before. The first time was in 1975, when forty-four young children died in Bulgaria during an outbreak that did not feature HFMD (Melnick 1984). The other occasion was during the spring months of 1997, when twenty-eight children died in Malaysia following the eruption of HFMD in Sarawak province on the island of Borneo. A few of the Malaysian deaths may have been due to other viruses, but an EV71 strain genetically distinct from the Taiwan strain was isolated from at least two children. In 1999, still another EV71 virus appeared in Perth, Western Australia, during a large epidemic of HFMD. This time the virus was linked to six cases of polio-like paralysis and twelve cases of meningitis, but it did not appear to attack the brainstem of its victims (McMinn, Stratov, and Dowse 1999). Why different strains of EV71 appear when they do—and how they cause such a variety of highly pathogenic syndromes—remains a mystery. We can only hope that molecular biology will provide some answers about this eccentric virus before it surfaces again.

O'nyong-Nyong Virus

Occasionally, a spontaneous genetic change in a known viral pathogen can alter the way it is transmitted and lead to new cases of disease. This accounts for the brief appearance of the O'nyong-nyong virus in East Africa, starting in 1959. The new virus turned out be a close relative of the Chikungunya virus, an RNA virus still commonly encountered in Africa and South Asia. Chikungunya virus takes its name from the Swahili expression for "that which bends up," referring to the severe pain and swelling in the joints that this febrile infection can cause. Like the dengue fever virus, the Chikungunya virus is transmitted by the bite of an infected *Aedes* mosquito. In many urban centers of the tropics its incidence has increased as *Aedes aegypti* mosquitoes have proliferated, and there is concern that the disease may spread soon to vulnerable new populations in the Western Hemisphere.

But during the early 1960s, it was the O'nyong-nyong virus that was on the move (Monath 1993). In only a few years it had infected at least two million Africans across an area stretching from Uganda to Malawi. O'nyong-nyong means "swelling." The new disease had many clinical similarities to Chikungunya fever, but it was spread among human hosts by *Anopheles* mosquitoes, the ever-present vectors of malaria, instead of *Aedes* mosquitoes. Today it seems likely that O'nyong-nyong virus arose from acute alterations in the genetic makeup of the Chikungunya virus, changes that allowed it to switch insect vectors. The O'nyong-nyong virus persisted for only a short time, but it illustrates how new viral variants with epidemic potential can arise abruptly from suitably volatile precursors like the Chikungunya virus.

Rocio Virus

Sometimes an entirely novel virus develops through the mingling of genetic material from two viral species circulating in the same region. This is the most likely explanation for a mysterious outbreak of encephalitis in the Santista lowlands of the São Paulo state of Brazil during 1975 and 1976 (De Souza Lopes, de Abreu Sacchetta, Francy, et al. 1981). In that epidemic, about one thousand people came down with the disease, ninety-five of whom died. More men were affected than women or children, and infection was associated with a high frequency of mosquito bites. Eventually, virologists isolated a previously unknown RNA virus from some of the victims.

The new pathogen, dubbed the Rocio virus, turned out to be related to the virus of St. Louis encephalitis (SLE), the infamous mosquito-borne agent first thought to be the cause of New York's West Nile virus epidemic in 1999. At the time of the Rocio outbreak SLE was a well-known menace in southern Brazil. But the newly found pathogen also bore some resemblance to the Ilheus virus that inhabits the area, a virus that only rarely causes human disease. Both of the SLE and Ilheus viruses used the same species of local birds as their primary reservoirs, and both could be transmitted by the same local mosquitoes. It is now presumed that the Rocio virus resulted from a genetic exchange between the two precursor viruses. Humans were accidental or "dead-end" hosts, as it seemed they could not actively participate in the reproductive cycle of the virus; but they could develop serious disease from infectious mosquito bites. Fortunately the Rocio virus has vanished, but other such mosaic viruses seem likely to emerge somewhere in the world again.

Bacteria: Traders of Virulence

Bacteria are far more complex than viruses, but they have the same need to adapt quickly to new environments, to resist host defenses, and to overcome competition from other micro-organisms. To gain access to a host, and then to grow and multiply within the host, pathogenic bacteria possess "virulence factors," functional proteins derived from virulence genes. Products of virulence genes include: adhesins that help bacteria stick to host tissues; hemolysins that disintegrate host blood cells; hyaluronidases that perforate host tissues for bacterial invasion; enzymes that coagulate the blood of hosts or dissolve coagulated blood; proteases that disarm local antibodies and other immune responses; drug resistance factors; and an array of toxins.

Because toxins are behind much of the harm that bacteria cause, we tend to dismiss their utility to the microbes that release them. But if we take a bacterial perspective we can see that toxins can be helpful in disrupting the normal physiology of the host, knocking down defenses and enabling a successful invasion, all while suppressing competing microbes. They also aid in spreading the organism from one host to the next, such as when a toxin from an intestinal pathogen induces diarrhea in the host.

New genes for bacterial virulence factors must arise slowly through complex evolutionary processes. How is it then that bacteria sometimes emerge out of nowhere with new invincibility? This occurs most often because bacteria have clever ways of passing around ready-made virulence genes. Two of the key "mobile genetic elements" by which bacteria share genes among themselves are plasmids and bacteriophages.

Plasmids

Plasmids are loops of DNA that exist outside bacterial chromo-
somes and replicate autonomously. They can be transferred between
bacteria that come into close contact by a process called conjugation.
The bacteria involved in conjugation need not be of the same species,
so the virulence factors inherited from plasmids can be spread among
a range of different bacterial pathogens that simply find themselves
residing in the same neighborhood. Such indiscriminate sharing has
given plasmids a major role in the transfer of antibiotic resistance (see
chapter 9). Plasmids also have direct effects on bacterial virulence.
For example, it is plasmids that encode for the neurotoxin of tetanus,
for the invasive capacities of *Shigella* bacteria in the intestine, for the
edema factor that triggers swelling around the skin lesions of
anthrax, and for the toxin that loosens the bowels in traveler's
diarrhea.

Bacteriophages

Bacteriophages are viruses that prey on bacteria. They insert
their own genes into the bacterial genome, including genes that code
for toxins. Other bacteriophages simply "turn on" toxin genes
already present in the bacterial DNA. The bacteria that cause botulism and diphtheria probably acquired their toxic potential from bacteriophages. The toxin produced by *Staphylococcus aureus* in toxic
shock syndrome is the product of a viral hijacker, as are the shiga-like
toxins of *Escherichia coli* O157:H7.

Recently the lethality of *Vibrio cholerae* was linked to a viral
predator (Waldor and Mekalanos 1996). It turns out that a thread-like
virus is able to infiltrate cells of *V. cholerae* through their pili, the
same external fibers the bacteria use to latch onto the human digestive tract. Inside the bacterium, the virus, named CTX, inserts its own
DNA into the bacterial genome. It now seems likely that it is the
gate-crasher's DNA that provides the genetic recipe for the powerful
toxin of cholera. Once released into the human gut, the cholera toxin
activates enzymes in the intestinal lining that pump salt ions into the
bowels. Massive quantities of water follow the salt into the gut
because of osmosis, leading to "rice water" diarrhea of up to fifteen
liters a day. Without immediate fluid replacement, the result is profound dehydration, shock, and death.

It is possible that each of the world's cholera pandemics since
1817 arose from insertion of toxin-coding genes by a virus like CTX
into otherwise innocuous strains of *V. cholerae*, using their pili as

receptors. This is worrisome, not only because it means that other toxic strains of cholera may yet emerge in the future. John Mekalanos (1996), one of the discoverers of CTX virus, has noted that other bacteria—including some species commonly found in the human gut—possess pili like those of *V. cholerae.* Might the CTX virus some day find the pili of such bacteria suitable as receptors, rendering a normally mild-mannered strain of *Escherichia coli* into another killer like cholera? "A virus is not going to be limited to the bacterium it lives on if the receptor is not limited to that bacterium," Mekalanos says.

Virulence in Bacteria: Lessons from Brazil

A startling case of enhanced bacterial virulence came to light in the town of Promissão in southern Brazil during 1984. There, some young children who acquired conjunctivitis, a mild infection of the eye commonly known as "pink eye," later developed high fevers with vomiting and abdominal pain. These symptoms rapidly progressed to a blotchy, purple rash and shock due to vascular collapse. Ten children died in the outbreak, all within forty-eight hours of the onset of fever. Similar cases were reported in nine nearby towns and from a city in a neighboring state in 1986. During 1990, the disease surfaced again, in the Mato Grosso state of central Brazil. This time it claimed six young lives.

The new disease, which came to be called Brazilian purpuric fever (BPF), was caused by a deadly variant of *Haemophilus influenzae* biogroup aegyptius, a common bacterium known to cause pink eye in various regions of the world, including Brazil. How this minor pathogen changed into a ruthless killer is still unknown. One investigation has shown that the rogue organisms in the Promissão outbreak all possessed a specific plasmid that is not usually found in other Brazilian strains of *H. influenzae* biogroup aegyptius (Brazilian Purpuric Fever Study Group 1987). But it is not clear where this plasmid came from or whether it codes for virulence factors that made the bacteria so noxious. In the meantime, regions of the world where *H. influenzae* biotype aegyptus commonly causes pink eye await outbreaks of BPF. One such area, the Australian outback, has already had at least one case presumed to be BPF, reported in a three-year-old boy from Alice Springs in the Northern Territory. The child survived, but he required amputation of gangrenous limbs.

Fortunately, new bacterial diseases like BPF are rare. More often, microbial adaptation and change underpins the re-emergence of all-too-familiar agents of disease: organisms that have developed resistance to the drugs which humans have devised to kill them. The next chapter will examine some of the key pathogens that are re-emerging as serious threats because of antimicrobial resistance.

What You Can Do To Prevent Influenza

Every winter, as new breeds of the influenza virus travel the globe, needless deaths occur among people who could have been protected by annual flu shots. About one-third of Americans over age sixty-five years still don't bother with influenza vaccines, even though their age group accounts for the largest share of the twenty thousand flu deaths that occur each year in the United States. While a sudden antigenic shift in the future might leave too little time to produce enough vaccine to protect the population, in ordinary years scientists are usually well equipped to predict the annual antigenic drift and update the vaccine accordingly. In those years, vaccines given to the elderly in time for the flu season can reduce the risk of hospitalization by up to 70 percent, according to the CDC. In addition to those aged sixty-five years or older, the CDC recommends annual flu vaccination for the following groups:

- Residents of nursing homes and other chronic-care facilities.

- People of any age with chronic diseases of the heart, lung, or kidneys; people with diabetes, immunosuppression, or severe forms of anemia.

- Health care workers and others in contact with people at high risk.

- Anyone who wishes to reduce the likelihood of becoming of ill, particularly those who provide essential community services.

Chapter 9

Antimicrobial Resistance

If we do not make serious attempts to address this issue, it won't matter that we have antibiotics in twenty years' time. They simply won't work. We are running out of time and need to act now.

—Einar Krag,
chief medical officer of Denmark

The resistance of disease-causing organisms to antimicrobial drugs has recently taken center stage as a major public health concern. For the first time in half a century, doctors are voicing genuine fears that soon they may be powerless to stop bacteria and other pathogens that were once treatable with safe and effective antibiotics. Increasingly the "wonder drugs" that we have taken for granted in the battle against life-threatening infections are unable to work their wonders. In today's combat with microbial foes our "magic bullets," as drugs like penicillin were once described, have lost much of their magic. Some doctors even speculate that a "post-antibiotic era" waits in the wings, when humanity is laid waste by a host of invincible bacterial adversaries, as it was in centuries past.

The modern antibiotic era began in 1928 when the Scottish physician Alexander Fleming observed that a substance released by the common fungus *Penicillium notatum* inhibited the growth of bacteria on agar plates. Mass production of that fungal by-product, penicillin, began during World War II. For the first time, military doctors could cure most wound infections, and war-related deaths and amputations declined significantly. As new classes of antibiotics became available after the war, the burden of incurable bacterial disease hastily departed, at least from industrialized countries. But almost as soon as penicillin appeared, occasional reports in the medical literature told of inexplicable treatment failures. In those cases, the targeted bacteria were digging in and somehow circumventing the antibiotic's lethal force. Such cases raised little alarm at the time, as a cure was usually achieved with one of the many new drugs arriving on the scene. Sadly, the development of new compounds today has slowed to a trickle, as the costs of bringing new drugs to market have exploded. This has happened at a time when a growing number of pugnacious bacterial strains have devised ingenious ways to circumvent most, if not all, of the one hundred or so antibiotics left in our armory.

Antibiotics come from natural substances produced by various living things to inhibit microbial competitors in their environments. They work by disrupting bacterial cell wall synthesis, or by tampering with the vital machinery inside microbial cells involved in growth and reproduction. Bacteria spontaneously develop resistance to antibiotics in the same ways that microbes develop other inheritable characteristics that confer survival advantage. We saw in the chapter 8 how the immune systems of natural hosts exert pressure on pathogens to adapt to hostile surroundings or die. In the same way, antibiotics present populations of bacteria with the threat of imminent extinction. In the face of such intimidation, any variant organisms that can withstand a drug's deadly effects enjoy a substantial advantage over other individuals in the pool. Such variants are able to pass on their drug-rebuffing traits to future generations, giving rise to resistant strains. The more that antibiotics are used, whether they are needed or not, the more selective pressure they will exert on the bacteria they are designed to kill. Nowadays, the magnitude of the selective pressure applied by our antibiotics far exceeds the pressures from any natural sources. The result has been the rapid evolution of bacteria possessing the genetic apparatus to resist any insult that our drugs can dish out.

The scale of antibiotic use today is staggering. The annual consumption of antibiotics in the United States alone is more than fifty million pounds, up from about two million pounds in 1954. Approximately half of all antibiotics produced worldwide are fed to farm animals to promote growth, a highly questionable practice. Of the portion destined for human consumption, at least one-third is wasted on patients with viral infections and other ailments that antibiotics cannot cure. In many developing countries antibiotics are readily available without a prescription and are devoured like vitamins. The result of this recklessness is that antibiotics can now be found everywhere, in the foods we eat, in the water we drink, and even in the soil beneath our feet.

Within the average person there are approximately one hundred trillion cells, of which only 10 percent are actually human. The remaining cells belong to the bacteria, fungi, protozoa, worms, and other primitive organisms that exist along with us in a symbiotic fashion. Many of these organisms are vital for our health, and they often protect us from the few renegade germs that cause disease by limiting their proliferation. Antibiotics that are intended to kill infecting pathogens, real or imagined, can have unexpected harmful effects on these indigenous bystanders. When these benign organisms are repeatedly exposed to antibiotics they too are pressured over time to obtain the means to repel the threats. Such resistance may arise spontaneously through random mutations of the bacterial genome, or it may be acquired externally in the form of ready-made resistance genes encoded in mobile bits of DNA, such as plasmids. Careless use of antibiotics thus enables a reservoir of resistance genes to develop in close association with human hosts, genes that might accidentally fall into the hands of a pathogen.

Resistant bacteria fend off antibiotics in a variety of ways. Some produce enzymes that inactivate the drug. Others block the uptake of the drug or alter its target molecules in the bacterial cells. They might even devise ways to bypass the metabolic pathways the drugs are designed to disrupt. Strains resistant to one antibiotic can often stand up against any drugs in the same class. Doctors confronting pathogens resistant to conventional antibiotics are forced to rely on "second-line" drugs to treat sick patients. These drugs often have more toxic side effects and may be more difficult to administer. Beyond this, they are invariably more expensive than first-line drugs. Antibiotic resistance adds between $100 and $200 million a year to America's health care costs; that is a price that poor patients in developing countries are unable to pay.

Now even the second-line agents are no longer beneficial against certain pathogens. The stockpile of useful antibiotics is becoming leaner, even in the richest countries. The likeliest place in any community to encounter drug-resistant pathogens is the local hospital. Today about 70 percent of hospital-acquired infections in the United States are resistant to at least one antibiotic. No hospital-based pathogen has rebuffed the panoply of modern medical weaponry more proficiently than *Staphylococcus aureus*, the tenacious bacterium that some recent news headlines have christened the "super bug."

Is the "Super Bug" Germ Unstoppable?

When the report first appeared at the end of May 1997, infectious disease experts around the world shook their heads and heaved a collective sigh. The day they had long been dreading had arrived. A four-month-old boy in Japan had developed an infection with a strain of *S. aureus* that was partially resistant to the antibiotic vancomycin. "The emergence of vancomycin-resistant *S. aureus* is a public health emergency," declared William Jarvis (1997a), the top hospital infection specialist at the Centers for Disease Control and Prevention (CDC).

S. aureus is one of humanity's most formidable bacterial enemies. Worldwide it accounts for 2.5 million cases of pneumonia and 7 million cases of ear infection each year. It is a leading cause of fatal meningitis and it is the most common serious infection acquired in hospitals. Before the advent of antibiotics, 80 percent of bloodstream infections with *S. aureus* ended in death, most often in young adults. At any one time, 20 to 30 percent of the population carries the organism silently in their noses, spreading it to susceptible people via unwashed hands. In recent years, *S. aureus* has been acquiring resistance to one potent antibiotic after another. But doctors always had vancomycin in their armamentarium to fall back on. Even at times when every other drug failed, doctors could steadfastly depend on vancomycin to overcome *S. aureus* and save the patient. So the doctors in Tokyo caring for this four-month-old boy were stunned to find that vancomycin therapy did not work.

The boy had picked up *S. aureus* in Juntendo University Hospital while he was recovering from a heart operation performed to correct a birth defect (Hiramatsu, Hanaki, Ino, et al. 1997). As we know from chapter 6, nosocomial infections following invasive procedures are all too common nowadays. Nothing about the case looked unusual at first. The boy had a fever, and there was a milky white discharge oozing from his surgical wound. Bacterial cultures of the discharge grew *S. aureus,* and a routine check of antibiotic sensitivities showed it was a strain resistant to a broad range of drugs. Doctors refer to such troublesome strains as MRSA, for "methicillin-resistant *S. aureus.*" Methicillin is a semisynthetic derivative of penicillin that was developed in the 1950s when penicillin was rapidly becoming ineffective against *S. aureus* infections. At first, methicillin produced miraculous results, but by the mid-1970s about

2 percent of *S. aureus* strains showed they could defy methicillin treatment in the way their ancestors had stood up to penicillin. By the 1980s, methicillin resistance was becoming a common predicament in hospitals worldwide. Even worse, methicillin resistance increasingly signified invincibility to a bevy of other antibiotics as well. Today, MRSA accounts for about half of all *S. aureus* strains isolated in American hospitals. Half of these strains now resist every known drug except vancomycin. In Japan, MRSA takes an even larger share of *S. aureus* infections.

So there was nothing too usual about finding MRSA in the baby boy's surgical wound. The boy's infection just meant that he needed a course of intravenous vancomycin. This antibiotic, which belongs to a class of compounds called glycopeptides, kills bacteria by interfering with the synthesis of their cell walls. It was introduced in 1958, but it was used only infrequently at first because less toxic alternatives, like methicillin, were equally effective against *S. aureus*. At high doses vancomycin can damage the auditory nerves, resulting in permanent hearing loss. It can also disturb the normal function of the kidneys, so doctors were initially cautious about using it widely. But with the emergence of MRSA, vancomycin usage had surged by the 1980s. Doctors still worried about its toxic side-effects, and they knew that overuse of a single drug could invite disaster by selecting for bacterial genes that could resist the drug's lethal powers. But at the bedside they often had no choice, as vancomycin was their last line of defense against strains of MRSA that no other drug could kill.

Given this, it was hardly a surprise that resistance to vancomycin turned up by 1987 in some of the bacteria that reside benignly in the human intestine, the enterococci. Enterococci are among the most common bacteria lining the digestive tract. In hospitalized patients with compromised immunity they can cause serious infections, particularly if they escape to the urinary tract or the valves of the heart. But in general, the enterococci are not aggressive pathogens, preferring to live in peaceful coexistence with humans and their other animal hosts in the complex ecological matrix of the gut. What they lack in innate virulence the enterococci make up for with a remarkable intrinsic resistance to many common antibiotics. They have an even more striking ability to acquire new mechanisms of drug resistance as the need arises.

As vancomycin usage increased during the 1980s certain strains of enterococci were able to procure at least two transferable genes that produce high-level resistance to the drug. The origin of these genes, called *vanA* and *vanB*, is unknown, but bacteria that possess either of them can prevent vancomycin from binding to its usual target site on the cell wall. The efficient transfer of plasmids that encode for these resistance genes has allowed vancomycin resistance to enter susceptible strains of enterococci in both humans and animals around the world. The proportion of nosocomial infections caused by vancomycin-resistant enterococci (VRE) increased twenty-fold in the United States between 1989 and 1993. By 1997, VRE accounted for 17 percent of enterococcal infections of the bloodstream, some of which were invincible against any available drugs.

The emergence of potentially untreatable enterococci was bad news, but doctors had a bigger fear. What if the growing reservoir of VRE infections helped vancomycin resistance genes find their way into much more belligerent human pathogens, such as MRSA? They knew that enterococci have a penchant for sharing useful bits of genetic material with other bacteria in their neighborhood. Perhaps vancomycin resistance genes could be transferred between strains of VRE and MRSA within a patient infected with both organisms. These concerns were heightened in 1992 when a British research team observed the transfer of *vanA* from a species of enterococcus to *S. aureus* in the laboratory (Noble, Virani, and Cree 1992). The researchers promptly destroyed the new hybrid, but preventing such genetic trading in the real world outside the laboratory would not be as easy.

Then came the perplexing case of the baby boy in Japan. Despite twenty-nine days of vancomycin treatment at the usual doses, his infection showed no signs of improvement. Fortunately for him, when the laboratory analysis revealed "intermediate" levels of vancomycin resistance there was still hope that his strain of MRSA could be treated. A combination of other antibiotics, including a new agent for MRSA not licensed in the United States, eventually led to recovery, and the boy was discharged from the hospital. How the strain's reduced susceptibility to vancomycin arose could not be explained at the time, but doctors could take some comfort that in this case the transfer of resistance genes from enterococci was probably not involved. What they did know right away was that modern medicine had turned a new corner with MRSA. An emerging class of resistant bugs had arrived, and there was no looking back. As other cases started turning up in the United States and elsewhere, the tough new bacterial breed came to be called by a new name: "glycopeptide intermediate-resistant *S. aureus*," or GISA for short.

The Genie We Can't Put Back in the Bottle

It did not take long for GISA to surface again. Within months of the report from Japan, a case appeared in a fifty-nine-year-old Michigan man with end-stage kidney disease. The man had been on a type of home dialysis in which a solution is introduced into the abdomen to allow the peritoneum, the natural membrane that lines the abdominal cavity, to filter out waste products as the kidneys are meant to do. Such patients are prone to frequent infections of the peritoneum, and this patient had received repeated courses of vancomycin for MRSA-associated peritonitis. Weeks later, another case of GISA came to light, this time in a sixty-six-year-old man living in New Jersey. He too suffered from serious underlying illnesses and had numerous previous bouts with MRSA that required prolonged treatment with vancomycin. Then, in early 1998, a third case was reported, this time in a seventy-nine-year-old man from New York. Like the others, he had been infected with MRSA and had received vancomycin repeatedly for long periods. All three men died, but it is difficult to say whether their GISA infections or their other medical problems were responsible. In healthier patients these infections may have been successfully treated.

But multiple cases of GISA in the United States may be harbingers of an unknown future where serious infections become untreatable with all currently available drugs, even in otherwise healthy people. Theresa Smith and the other CDC researchers who examined the first two United States cases made no attempt to hide their concerns. "The emergence of *S. aureus* with intermediate glycopeptide resistance threatens to return us to the era before the development of antibiotics," they wrote in *The New England Journal of Medicine* (Smith, Pearson, Wilcox, et al. 1999). Jarvis was even more blunt (1997b): "The timer is going off. We were concerned it would emerge here, it has emerged here, and we are concerned we are going to see it popping up in more places." Since the New York case in 1998, GISA has popped up Hong Kong, where it has caused at least one death, and in two patients in Scotland. Moreover, clusters of vancomycin resistant organisms have been identified among susceptible organisms in nearly 10 percent of MRSA strains tested at university hospitals in Japan (Hiramatsu 1998).

Fortunately, no cases of GISA investigated thus far have arisen from the transfer of prefabricated resistance genes from VRE or any other source. Instead, it appears that prolonged exposure to vancomycin has selected for naturally occurring mutants from the pool of MRSA organisms infecting each host. The exact mechanism is not yet worked out, but in the New York case it appears that the organism developed a thickened cell-wall structure with which it could mop up any nearby vancomycin, diverting the drug from its usual target site. DNA fingerprinting of the MRSA strain that infected this patient before it expressed resistance to vancomycin showed it was closely related to a group of strains prevalent in eight different New York area hospitals at that time. All eight of the sibling strains could be induced in the laboratory to develop intermediate resistance to vancomycin by means of exposure to low levels of the antibiotic, selecting for subsets of mutant organisms that could withstand the killing power of the drug (Sieradzki, Roberts, Haber, et al. 1999). If intermediate resistance can evolve this way naturally under the drug's selection pressure, how long before fully resistant strains appear in our hospitals?

The most dire public health nightmare would see the strains of GISA arising in hospitalized patients spread to the wider community. This ominous possibility seemed unlikely until recently, as there had been relatively few instances of significant MRSA transmission outside of hospitals or long-term health care facilities. The scant reports of MRSA acquired in community settings had been largely confined to individuals with identifiable risk factors, such as injecting drug use or frequent contact with health care facilities. But a report by Betsy Herold and colleagues in 1998 showed that community-acquired infections with MRSA may now be on the rise. In their study of inner-city children in Chicago, nearly three-quarters of children with MRSA infections had no predisposing risk factors for the disease. Community-acquired MRSA has also emerged recently in Minnesota and North Dakota (Centers for Disease Control and Prevention 1999d). Fortunately, community-acquired infections in the United States are still susceptible to a number of drugs besides vancomycin, and they can usually be treated successfully if proper drugs are started early. But the sudden emergence of MRSA outside of hospital walls raises the ante for limiting the spread of vancomycin resistance now before the problem of GISA spins out of control.

For the moment, staphylococcal vancomycin resistance remains rare, even in hospitals. But the surprise emergence of GISA is unmistakable proof that no antibiotic is completely trustworthy in this dangerous world. Francis Waldvogel (1999), a Swiss expert on MRSA, has likened the world's reaction to GISA to the final outcry of Julius Caesar, who realized only at the moment of death that his adopted son Brutus had betrayed him. "*Et tu* vancomycin?" many doctors have asked. But like the death of Caesar, the emergence of GISA surely could have been foretold. "The adaptive potential of the microbial world is such that for each new antibiotic that is introduced, several escape mechanisms are soon devised," Waldvogel says. "The action of antibiotics and resistance to these drugs are linked like light and shadow: One does not exist without the other. It was naïve to believe for forty years that vancomycin could remain an exception to this law."

Making a Bad Thing Worse

The evolution of antibiotic resistance may well be unavoidable, as Waldvogel asserts. Through natural selection of resistant strains, each new antibiotic gradually sows the seeds of its own undoing. But society's abuses of these powerful weapons have greatly accelerated their decline in recent years. Our misguided impulses to treat the first signs of any infection with the most potent antibacterial drugs, and our willingness to fatten farm animals by lacing their food with excessive amounts of antibiotics, are two key ways that human actions have promoted the emergence of resistant pathogens. Both factors require a closer look, because with better stewardship of the priceless resource that antibiotics represent, fewer drugs would become insensitive to common bacterial pathogens

Excessive Human Consumption

There is no question that human consumption of antibiotics has been rising in all industrialized countries. The annual number of prescriptions in the United States for sinusitis (inflammation of the sinuses around the nose) more than doubled to nearly thirteen million between 1985 and 1992. During the same period, the number of prescriptions for middle-ear infections rose from about fifteen million to more than twenty-three million per year. By 1999, ear infections accounted for thirty million antibiotic prescriptions. It is not unusual for American children today to spend three months on oral antibiotics for the treatment of ear infections during their first two years of life. Similar trends have been documented in Europe, Canada, Japan, and New Zealand. Part of the increase may reflect a growing burden of infection arising from changing social conditions. With more children attending early childhood education, there are more opportunities for them to transmit bacterial pathogens. Homelessness also increases a community's rate of bacterial infection, as does the improved survival of elderly and chronically ill people kept alive by medical advances. But increased transmission of bacterial disease does not begin to explain the ongoing surge in human antibiotic use.

Understanding the scope of modern antibiotic consumption requires an appreciation of human psychology and the doctor-patient relationship. Today two-thirds of consultations with family doctors end with the issuing of a prescription. Many patients have come to believe that antibiotics will cure whatever ails them, and they often demand prescriptions even when antibiotics are clearly not the answer. Doctors frequently acquiesce to such pressure because they want to seem helpful. They also fear that they may lose the patient's business, and they want to cover themselves "just in case" there is a hidden bacterial infection after all. Professional anxieties about legal liability can also influence treatment decisions; the dispensing of antibiotics in questionable cases has become part of practicing "defensive medicine" today. Similarly, in situations when there is just cause to offer an antibiotic a doctor may prescribe a "broad spectrum" drug, able to annihilate a wide range of organisms, when a more narrowly acting agent would almost definitely produce a cure.

In this country alone, as many as fifty million antibiotic prescriptions given out every year are of dubious value. The CDC estimates that up to 63 percent of the vancomycin that patients receive is not really necessary, and only adds to the selective pressure creating resistance. A study by Gonzales and others in 1997 showed that more than half of American adults presenting to family doctors with colds and other viral infections of the respiratory tract were needlessly prescribed antibiotics. The authors estimated that such infections accounted for more than one-fifth of all adult antibiotic prescriptions. Similar results have been reported in studies of pediatric office visits (Nyquist, Gonzales, Steiner, et al. 1998). Pressures on doctors to prescribe can be overwhelming. Half of the pediatricians surveyed recently for the American Academy of Pediatrics reported that parents of sick children always or often pressure them to prescribe antibiotics in situations when the drugs are not indicated (Bauchner, Pelton, Klein, et al. 1999). One-third said they sometimes or usually give in to such requests and prescribe antibiotics against their better judgment. Franz Kafka may have been right when he said, "To write prescriptions is easy, but to come to an understanding with people is hard."

At the same time that doctors are feeling compelled to prescribe unnecessary antibiotics, many patients are failing to complete the full course of treatment. For uncomplicated infections doctors might direct patients to take an antibiotic for a week or ten days. But often patients will stop the medication early if they are feeling better. They may even hoard the remaining pills to medicate themselves or family members the next time an illness strikes. In either instance, such improper dosing exposes bacteria to subtherapeutic levels of the drug. It allows surviving pathogens to persist, and supports the emergence of drug-resistant strains. The risks are even greater in most developing countries, where sales of antibiotics are completely unrestricted. In some of these countries counterfeit drugs compound the problem. These medications contain deliberately reduced quantities of the active ingredients, and add to resistance pressures through failed treatments.

Killing Germs Wherever We Find Them

In keeping with the popular view that "the only good germ is a dead germ," makers of household products have started to cash in on a wide range of new antibacterial goods. This marketing fad carries frightening implications for the evolution of antibiotic resistance. Until recently, chemical disinfectants and antiseptics were confined to hospital use, or to the homes of patients with extra susceptibility to infection because of impaired immunity. Now these compounds are turning up in soaps, lotions, and dishwashing detergents intended for ordinary domestic buyers. They have even been impregnated into cutting boards, toilet seats, mattress pads, ballpoint pens, tooth pastes, plastic toys, and car steering wheels. It's a worrisome trend that threatens to spawn a new generation of recalcitrant bugs. A recent study showed that mutations in a single gene from a laboratory strain of *E. coli* could produce resistance to triclosan, one of the most common antibacterial compounds added to consumer products (McMurry, Oethinger, Levy, et al. 1998).

"Germ resistant" products have become especially popular in Japan, where the big 1996 outbreak of *E. coli* O157:H7 made a lasting impression. A spokesman for the maker of Zeomic, the antibacterial powder that is used in most of Japan's "clean" products, anticipates even bigger sales in the future. "We are now working on construction materials so that whole buildings can be antibacterialized," the spokesman said in an interview with Jon Watts in 1997. The problem with the cleanliness craze is that indiscriminate use of disinfectants in the household environment puts pressure on harmless bacteria to develop genetic resistance that can be passed to dangerous pathogens. The same cellular mechanisms that allow bacteria to resist chemical disinfectants may enable pathogens to repel life-saving drugs. Far from protecting us from disease, these unregulated household chemicals may ultimately accelerate the emergence of untreatable human infections. The quest for a sterile home environment is foolish and is doomed to failure.

Antibiotics down on the Farm

The other major factor facilitating antibiotic emergence is the recklessly extravagant use of these compounds in agriculture. Some antibiotics are used justifiably in veterinary medicine to treat and prevent infections in farm animals. But globally about 90 percent of the antibiotics these animals receive has been added to their food and water at subtherapeutic levels with the aim of enhancing growth. This practice began almost by accident in the 1940s, when high-quality chicken feed was in short supply because of World War II. Feed makers turned to soybean meal, but found it was deficient as a source of vitamin B12. To supply the missing vitamin they spiked the feed with byproducts left over from the manufacture of a new antibiotic, chlortetracycline. These byproducts prevented vitamin deficiencies in the chickens, but to everyone's amazement the animals receiving the additive gained substantially more weight than those which had not. By the 1950s feed makers applied to the United States Food and Drug Administration (FDA) to add chlortetracycline itself to a variety of animal feeds. Approval was granted, and other antibiotics quickly followed. The reasons for the growth-promoting effects of antibiotics are still not completely understood, but the results, in terms of improved meat output, were indisputable from the start.

Soon the growth-enhancing uses of antibiotics surpassed all other uses throughout the world. In the United States, at least 40 percent of antibiotics by weight are now deployed in agriculture, predominantly to fatten up livestock. In Australia, 56 percent of the antibiotic supply ends up in feed supplements. Antibiotics are also sprayed liberally on fruit trees and other food crops as pesticides. In aquaculture, 110 to 130 pounds of antimicrobial agents may be dumped annually on each acre of a salmon farm. These practices have enormous economic benefits for food producers, but ultimately they may promote the emergence of resistant organisms that can pass directly into the human food chain. When the organisms in the chickens, pigs, or cattle that we grow for food develop resistance to an antibiotic added to animal feeds, the organisms typically show cross-resistance to all other antibiotics having the same mode of action. Resistance to one agent confers resistance to an entire class of drugs, including those used in human medicine.

Unfortunately, many antibiotics used in animal husbandry today are closely related to the drugs doctors use to cure human infections. Squandering these precious agents on growth enhancement of farm animals may ultimately threaten the effectiveness of vital human medicines. Some agents used in livestock feed belong to classes of antibiotics that are only beginning to find uses in human medical care. Doctors will be counting on antibiotics from these classes in the future to replace existing agents that have become ineffective through overuse. How tragic it would be if tomorrow's new drugs are already obsolete because animal consumption of similar agents has already selected for resistant bacteria. It is not surprising that the World Health Organization has joined concerned medical and citizens' groups around the world in calling for reductions in antibiotic usage outside of human medicine.

The full effects of agricultural antibiotics are unknown, but there are hints that they are already putting human health at risk. We have seen how the overuse of vancomycin in hospitals has led to the emergence of vancomycin-resistant enterococci (VRE) in the United States. In Europe and elsewhere, VRE has also emerged as a major public health problem, but for different reasons. In these countries, VRE has turned up most often outside of hospitals, typically in people who develop diarrhea in the community or in symptomless-carriers. Curiously, neither of these groups would have had exposure to vancomycin or to other people who received the drug in hospitals. The source of their infections had to be somewhere else in the community, but where? Eventually investigators realized that people were becoming infected with VRE from the foods they were eating, particularly meats derived from animals that had been fed avoparcin.

Avoparcin is a glycopeptide similar to vancomycin. It was approved as a growth promoter in most European countries in 1974. Numerous investigations have now shown that use of this compound in livestock feeds created a major reservoir of drug-resistant enterococci in animals raised for food (Wegener, Aarestrup, Jensen, et al. 1999). This reservoir then put humans at risk of acquiring VRE. The reasoning goes like this: As avoparcin use increased, enterococci residing in the intestines of many farm animals found themselves bathed in a constant stream of the drug at low doses. Over countless generations these bacteria acquired resistance, in part from passing around off-the-rack genes, such as *vanA*. Humans who ate undercooked meats or other foods contaminated by raw meats from these animals then picked up the resistant bugs themselves. Avoparcin was never licensed in the United States because of its potentially carcinogenic effects. So VRE didn't enter the human food chain here. Similarly, food-borne transmission of VRE has not been a problem in Sweden. Avoparcin was taken out of use there in 1986 when Sweden banned all agricultural growth promoters.

But wherever avoparcin has been widely used, human VRE infections have inevitably followed. Denmark was hit especially hard.

Danish farmers were once among the heaviest users of avoparcin. In 1994, they used more than fifty thousand pounds of the drug in animal feeds, at a time when Danish doctors were using just fifty pounds of vancomycin each year to treat human infections. The discovery that agricultural use of avoparcin might cause VRE in humans led the Danish government to ban the drug as a growth promoter in 1995. Germany imposed a similar measure in 1996, and in 1997 avoparcin was banned in all member states of the European Union (EU). The EU outlawed four additional antibiotics as animal feed additives in 1999, including virginiamycin. This growth promoter, which is still widely used in poultry production in the United States, is closely related to a new human medicine called Synercid. Ironically, Synercid is the first antibiotic proven to be effective against human VRE infections when all other drugs fail. Continued use of virginiamycin in animal feeds could render Synercid useless, but so far the FDA has not followed Europe's lead. Instead, American food producers and drug companies claim that reducing antibiotic supplements to livestock foods will jeopardize animal health and drive up food costs.

Treating Animals, Promoting Resistance

Although most concerns about agricultural antibiotic use have focused on growth promotion, questions recently have been raised about the inappropriate use of antibiotics in treating and preventing disease in farm animals. Like their counterparts in human medicine, veterinarians are finding themselves under increasing pressure to dispense powerful antibiotics to treat sick animals that may not always benefit from such medicines. When a single infection appears among a herd of intensively reared animals, veterinarians may even feel obliged to treat the entire herd to prevent further cases and minimize a farmer's economic losses. Indiscriminate use of animal antibiotics can have disastrous effects on bacterial resistance to their human analogues. This truth came home to American consumers in 1999, when researchers in Minnesota showed that the *Campylobacter* bacteria that commonly contaminate poultry products are becoming resistant to fluoroquinolones.

Fluroquinolones are a major class of antibiotics at the front line of humanity's defenses against a wide array of bacterial pathogens. When drug makers asked the FDA to license fluroquinolones for use in American poultry, an expert panel recommended caution because of the potential consequences for human medicine. After all, when fluroquinolones were licensed for use in poultry in the Netherlands in 1987 there was soon a sharp increase in fluroquinolone-resistant *Campylobacter* recovered from Dutch chickens. The same trend appeared in Spain after fluroquinolones were licensed for veterinary use there in 1990. No one wanted that to happen in the United States, but in 1995 the FDA went ahead and licensed the drugs for use in poultry production.

Now, the report from Minnesota has revealed an eight-fold increase since 1992 in human infections due to fluroquinolone-resistant *Campylobacter* (K.E. Smith, Besser, Hedberg, et al. 1999). Many of the resistant infections had been acquired in developing countries, where agricultural fluroquinolone abuse is rampant. But the incidence of resistant infections acquired at home in America increased significantly after 1996. As part of the study, the investigators went shopping for chickens at eleven retail markets. Poultry sold at the markets had been procured from producers in five states, as far away as Florida. Of the ninety-one chickens they purchased, 88 percent were contaminated with *Campylobacter*. Nothing surprising there. The shock came when they found that 20 percent of the chickens harbored *Campylobacter* that was resistant to fluoroquinolones. The DNA fingerprint of the supermarket strains was identical to that of organisms recovered from people who had acquired their infections domestically. It's getting harder than ever to deny the connection between animal antibiotics and risks to human health.

Four More Militant Bugs

Since resistance to penicillin was first reported in the 1940s, nearly every bacterial pathogen has developed at least a measure of diminished sensitivity to first-line antibiotics. The exceptions include *Streptococcus pyogenes*, *Chlamydia trachomatis*, and *Treponema pallidum*. *Streptococcus pyogenes*, the cause of strep throat, remains sensitive to penicillin, although the drug concentrations needed to kill the organism have been increasing steadily. Fortunately, *Chlamydia trachomatis* also remains sensitive to the tetracyclines, a class of drugs introduced in 1948. It was always thought that *Treponema pallidum*, the cause of syphilis, was universally sensitive to penicillin, but resistance has recently started to emerge in Africa (Hart 1998). Resistance has also arisen against new antiviral agents, such as those used to treat genital herpes, influenza A, and HIV infections. It is not possible here to examine all the pathogens that are mounting serious challenges to humanity's antimicrobial arsenal. But before we leave this topic, one hardy parasite and three additional bacterial agents deserve special mention in view of their immediate risks to public health.

Malaria

As we saw in chapter 2, malaria is one of the most pernicious diseases in the world today, affecting up to three hundred million people each year. Endemic in more than ninety countries, malaria kills more people than any infectious disease, except tuberculosis and AIDS. It is caused by four different species of *Plasmodium* protozoa, the most lethal being *P. falciparum*. A big reason for malaria's recent comeback is this parasite's frightening ability to develop resistance to antimalarial drugs. Malaria has been treated for centuries with quinine, a substance that Amazon Indians extracted from the bark of cinchona trees. They introduced quinine to Jesuit missionaries, who took the drug back to Europe during the seventeenth century. Quinine is still used to treat *P. falciparum* infections today, whenever more modern drugs fail. But doctors avoid quinine whenever possible because of its many unpleasant side effects, which include headaches, ringing in the ears, and blurred vision.

Given these problems, the development of chloroquine during the 1940s was met with much rejoicing. Here was an agent that could kill malaria parasites like *P. falciparum*, but with few of quinine's toxic effects. It was inexpensive to produce, easy to administer, and it was safe, even during pregnancy. In fact, chloroquine was so well tolerated that it could be given to prevent malarial infections, not merely to treat them once they had started. With the best of intentions, the United Nations made massive amounts of chloroquine available to malaria control programs throughout the tropics. The drug was even added to table salt in Southeast Asia, South America, and sub-Saharan Africa. In hindsight it is obvious that the mass distribution of a single agent to millions of people exerted powerful selection pressure on *P. falciparum*, allowing the emergence of drug-resistant strains possessing genetic traits that would have been extremely unlikely to arise on their own. The problem was worsened when patients using chloroquine for treatment of active disease took suboptimal doses in order to economize. As patients shared their pills with children and other family members at home, the parasites were exposed repeatedly to subtherapeutic drug levels, encouraging the rapid evolution of resistance.

By the early 1960s, chloroquine-resistant *P. falciparum* was appearing simultaneously in South America and Southeast Asia. By 1978, it arrived in sub-Saharan Africa, brought by Asian laborers building a railway from Mozambique to Zaire. Today, chloroquine remains a useful drug against *P. falciparum* in only a handful of malarial regions. The other major malarial parasite, *P. vivax*, is also beginning to resist the drug. The disturbing loss of chloroquine in the battle against malaria has forced other, more toxic drugs to the forefront. Chief among these is mefloquine, a derivative of chloroquine that has been linked to an alarming number of neuropsychiatric side effects. Mefloquine is not safe in pregnancy, and by the dose it costs up to eighteen times as much as chloroquine.

But now doctors worry that even mefloquine is biting the dust. Foci of mefloquine-resistant *P. falciparum* have appeared in Thailand, both on the border with Myanmar to the west and on the border with Cambodia to the east. In some of the densely forested areas along the Cambodian border there are strains of *P. falciparum* that respond to no known drugs. Increasingly, these multidrug-resistant strains are turning up in other areas of Southeast Asia. The emergence of highly resistant *P. falciparum* along Thailand's border with Cambodia probably arose from the parasite's erratic exposure to antimalarial drugs consumed by the itinerant gem miners working in the region during the past decade (Shell 1997). Unlike the poor refugees who flooded the area to escape the Khmer Rouge, these miners had enough money to buy mefloquine and other drugs to keep them going in the jungle as they sought their fortunes. Popping one pill after another, they eventually cultivated resistant strains of *P. falciparum* that spread readily to nearby refugees and other susceptible hosts.

Gonorrhea

Gonorrhea is a sexually transmitted disease affecting sixty-two million people each year. Worldwide, it is the leading cause of pelvic inflammatory disease, female infertility, and ectopic pregnancy. One in three infected mothers will pass gonorrheal infection to their babies at birth; this can cause blindness if there is no treatment. In sub-Saharan Africa up to 4 percent of babies are born with gonorrheal eye infections. In the United States, gonorrhea is second only to *Chlamydia* infection as the most common bacterial sexually transmitted disease. About eight hundred thousand new cases of gonorrhea occur in this country each year, incurring medical costs of $1.98 billion.

Gonorrhea was once easily treated with penicillin. By the early 1970s low-level resistance began to appear in developed countries, so the recommended dosage of penicillin was increased. This resistance was thought to be related to a mutation in the bacterial chromosome. In 1976, high-level resistance to penicillin emerged almost simultaneously in Africa, Asia, Europe, and North America. This resistance arose from a plasmid that encoded a bacterial enzyme called penicillinase; this enzyme could protect the bacteria from penicillin by inactivating any of the drug lurking in its vicinity. Soon penicillinase-producing *Neisseria gonorrhoeae* (PPNG) strains surpassed penicillinase-negative strains in much of Africa and Asia. In the United States, rates of PPNG rose abruptly after 1984, so that by 1988 PPNG accounted for one-third of cases in certain regions. At about the same time, chromosomally mediated resistance to penicillin became more intense, and resistance to tetracyclines and other antibiotics appeared. By 1989, half of *N. gonorrhoeae* infections in the United States had one form of antibiotic resistance or another.

In response to these events, gonorrhea treatment guidelines in the United States and elsewhere moved away from penicillin, in favor of other, more costly antibiotics that were still effective. These included agents from the fluoroquinolone group and certain members of a class called cephalosporins. Because fluoroquinolones can usually be given in a single dose by mouth they have often become the preferred choice. Not surprisingly, strains resistant to these drugs are starting to appear. One study has shown that 10 percent of gonorrhea strains in Hong Kong and the Philippines are now resistant to fluoroquinolones, and as many as half of the strains in other East Asian countries are at least partially resistant (Knapp, Fox, Trees, et al. 1997). The easy availability of fluoroquinolones without a prescription in the Philippines has undoubtedly helped to promote resistance there. Sporadic case reports of treatment failures with fluoroquinolones have also appeared recently in Europe, Australia, Canada, and the United States.

Salmonella

Salmonella infections with antibiotic resistance are likewise becoming a public health problem worldwide. Some countries, especially in Europe, have witnessed a ten- to twenty-fold increase in human disease from *Salmonella* since 1980. Uncomplicated episodes of *Salmonella* diarrhea are best treated with rest and rehydration. Antibiotics in such instances actually increase the chance of developing persistent infection, and may lead to resistance. But in serious cases where organisms invade the bloodstream, antibiotic treatment can be lifesaving. Unfortunately, the proportion of antibiotic-resistant infections has also been steadily increasing. Today, at least one-third of *Salmonella* infections in the United States are resistant to one or more of the traditional mainstays of antibiotic therapy. Patients infected with these strains are more likely to require hospitalization and they tend to have longer recovery times.

Of the more than twenty-three hundred known serotypes of *Salmonella*, by far the two most prevalent varieties causing human disease are *S. enteritidis*, which was discussed in chapter 6, and *S. typhimurium*. Both are common intestinal pathogens for a menagerie of wild and domestic animals, and human disease is usually contracted through ingestion of contaminated foods of animal origin. In the late 1980s a resistant strain of *S. typhimurium* called "definitive type 104" (DT 104) emerged among cattle in the United Kingdom. The strain then appeared in poultry, sheep, pigs, horses, and humans. By 1995, DT 104 was the second most common cause of human *Salmonella* infections in England and Wales. More than 90 percent of DT 104 infections have involved a variant called R-type ACSSuT, which is resistant to five antibiotic classes that can usually eradicate *Salmonella*. Approximately 10 percent of people who acquire this multidrug-resistant variant require hospitalization, and 3 percent die. DT 104 organisms with this highly resistant R-type did not trigger human outbreaks in the United States until the mid-1990s. But recently they have made significant inroads among both cattle and human hosts, and may now be causing about 9 percent of all human *Salmonella* infections in this country (Glynn, Bopp, DeWitt, et al. 1998).

As antibiotic-resistant strains have grabbed an ever-larger share of *Salmonella* infections in both humans and animals, there has been greater reliance on the two principal drugs that generally remain effective. But antibiotic overuse in any species inevitably leads to resistance. In England and Wales, resistance to the drug trimethoprim among human DT 104 cases increased from 1 percent to 27 percent between 1993 and 1995. It is likely that this rapid change resulted from overzealous attempts to combat multidrug-resistant DT 104 in British cattle. By 1997, resistance to trimethoprim there had declined to 17 percent. But resistance to ciprofloxacin, a type of fluoroquinolone, has continued to increase, rising from 0 percent in 1993 to 6 percent in 1995 to 12 percent in 1997. This trend might be explained by overuse of ciprofloxacin in human medicine, or it could reflect excessive dependence on fluroquinolones in British agriculture. As we saw with drug-resistant *Campylobacter*, the growing veterinary use of fluoroquinolones throughout the world is raising alarm. It would be even more disastrous to lose this class of drugs in the fight against human *Salmonella* infections, as they generally cause more serious disease than infections with *Campylobacter*.

Streptococcus Pneumoniae

Streptococcus pneumoniae is a leading cause of sickness and death worldwide. In the United States alone *S. pneumoniae* accounts for forty thousand deaths each year. It causes three thousand cases of meningitis, five hundred thousand cases of pneumonia, and more than seven million middle-ear infections. It is the foremost cause of bacterial blood infections, of which nearly 30 percent are fatal. *S. pneumoniae* (also called the "pneumococcus") is spread by respiratory secretions, and it thrives in crowded settings, such as institutions and child care centers.

Mutants of *S. pneumoniae* resistant to penicillin could be induced in laboratory experiments as early as 1945, but clinical pneumococcal infections remained uniformly susceptible to penicillin until 1967. That year a resistant strain was isolated from the sputum (a thick mucus coughed up from deep in the respiratory tract) of a patient in Australia. Subsequently, other penicillin-resistant strains were identified in Australia and Papua New Guinea. By the mid-1970s, resistance was cropping up in Israel, Poland, Spain, South Africa, and the United States. In Spain, the proportion of penicillin-resistant *S. pneumoniae* (PRSP) increased from 6 percent in 1979 to 44 percent by 1989. By 1992, more than half of pneumococcal infections in Hungary were due to PRSP strains. Two-thirds of *S. pneumoniae* organisms recovered from South Korean patients were resistant to penicillin by 1997.

Today at least 25 percent of the *S. pneumoniae* specimens routinely analyzed in the United States are not completely susceptible to penicillin. One specimen in seven is now considered "highly resistant." Penicillin resistance has been steadily increasing since 1992, when fewer than 10 percent of specimens showed any degree of resistance. Within the United States the geographical variation in resistance patterns is striking. Benjamin Schwartz and colleagues reported in 1998 that pneumococcal resistance is most common in United States counties with the highest rates of antibiotic use. Compared to people from counties in the lowest quartile of antibiotic use, people living in the highest quartile counties have roughly twice the risk of infection from a resistant strain. As penicillin resistance has emerged among pneumococci, so has resistance to other major antibiotics. Multidrug-resistant *S. pneumoniae* was first observed in South Africa during the late 1970s. Such strains then surfaced in Spain, from where they traveled to the United States, the United Kingdom, and elsewhere. Now some cases of pneumococcal meningitis in the United States can only be treated with vancomycin. Unrestricted use of this agent raises the dismaying prospect of vancomycin-resistant *S. pneumoniae* in the future. "Pneumococcal disease remains almost as great a challenge as it did one hundred years ago," notes Stephen Ostroff (1999) of the CDC.

For doctors whose treatment options are shrinking, each new report of drug resistance is met with a sense of déjà vu. They know that the answer to the antibiotic crisis is not new drugs, although more research and development for at least a few new antimicrobial agents are desperately needed. The solutions lie in reducing the inappropriate use of these powerful weapons, and this can only be achieved by waking up an apathetic public to the dangers of resistance. As Lord Soulsby noted in 1998, what is needed most is a change in attitudes. That year his Select Committee on Science and Technology tabled a report in Britain's House of Lords on antibiotic resistance. "Misuse and overuse of antibiotics are now threatening to undo all their early promises and success in curing disease. But the greatest threat is complacency, from [government] ministers, the medical professions, the veterinary service, the farming community, and the public at large," he said. Complacency and a lack of forward thinking have given rise to a number of other emerging pathogens, a few of which will be examined in the next chapter.

What You Can Do to Prevent the Spread of Antibiotic Resistance

We have seen how antibiotic overuse is steadily exhausting the ability of once mighty antibiotics to cure infections. Taking antibiotics when they are not needed does no good, and may suppress some naturally occurring bacteria that the body depends on to keep out harmful agents. Beyond this, taking these drugs needlessly exposes you to possible side effects, and adds to the selective pressure on microbes to develop resistance. To reign in the medical overuse of antibiotics, the FDA and the Alliance for the Prudent Use of Antibiotics at Tufts University make these recommendations:

- Don't pressure your doctor to prescribe antibiotics when he or she determines they would not be appropriate.

- Antibiotics should only be used when prescribed by your doctor. Never take antibiotics given to you by someone else or prescribed for a previous illness.

- Take antibiotics at the prescribed dose. Reducing the dose may make the treatment ineffective and could promote resistance.

- Take antibiotics for the full amount of time prescribed by your doctor. After your symptoms have disappeared small numbers of bacteria can remain.

- Don't use soaps or other products with antibacterial chemicals, unless caring for a person with weakened immunity. Accept that germs are a normal part of the home environment and practice good hygiene to keep well.

Chapter 10

Breakdown of the Public Health Infrastructure

The city can have as much reduction of preventable disease as it wishes to pay for. Public health is purchasable; within natural limitations a city can determine its own death rate.

—Annual report of the New York City
Board of Health, 1915

Public health is society's collective response to threats against the people's health. It is both a science and an art, organized around preventing disease and creating conditions that promote well-being and fulfillment. Public health is not merely the provision of health care services at taxpayers' expense, although in practice it works closely with providers of therapeutic medical care to control disease and build healthy communities. Perhaps public health is best seen as a movement, a social institution informed by science, shaped by societal values, and served by a cadre of professionals in every community who quietly go about the job of protecting us from disease. In its 150 years of existence the movement can claim many successes, such as the control of deadly epidemics, provision of safe food and drinking water, improved safety in the workplace, and reductions in maternal and child mortality.

Despite this proud history, public health in most Western countries today is in the doldrums. Many countries have lost sight of the importance of public health. Such apathy has allowed cash-strapped governments to back away from fundamental public health activities, including those aimed at keeping infectious diseases under control. North Americans today are all too familiar with dwindling public sector expenditures, but the downsizing of key public health functions has been a global phenomenon. Even though the world's economy has grown by a factor of six since 1950, deaths from curable or preventable infectious diseases still occur at a rate of seventeen million per year. The money the world spends each year on military needs—about $800 billion—is more than thirty times what would be required to meet basic health needs for everyone, according to the United Nations. Today, poor countries are forced to suffer from infectious diseases that could be eradicated for the cost of "a couple of fighter planes," says Gro Harlem Brundtland (1997), director-general of the World Health Organization. Global public sector spending on malaria control is now a paltry $85 million, barely 25 cents for every reported case of the disease. Even wealthy countries seem unable to invest adequately in disease control programs. In 1995, the budget allocated for the United States strategy to prevent emerging infections barely exceeded what the actor Dustin Hoffman was paid for his performance in the movie *Outbreak* that year. Somehow our priorities have gone awry.

Given all the underlying factors promoting emergence today, an effective and organized system of public health may be society's best defense. In a world increasingly vulnerable to devastating new infections, public health may prove it is "the thin blue line" protecting humanity against the ravages of epidemic disease. A breakdown of this system courts disaster, as infections will inevitably emerge and reemerge whenever society lets down its guard. The rapid spread of cholera in Latin America and the resurgence of diphtheria in Russia are two obvious examples of what can happen when routine public health activities fall into disarray. Erosion of basic public health services takes many forms. This chapter will emphasize the dangers arising from failures to provide safe drinking water, to immunize children, to treat tuberculosis, and to eliminate the insects and rodents that carry human diseases. Examples will highlight the problems of advanced, industrialized countries, as the effects of today's public health breakdown are by no means confined to the developing world.

The Water that Made Milwaukee Famous

Milwaukee, the largest city in Wisconsin, is a dynamic metropolis of 1.5 million people situated on the western shores of Lake Michigan. The city grew rapidly during the nineteenth century, attracting waves of immigrants, first from Germany and then from Poland. By the 1860s, Milwaukee had become an important railway hub, receiving much of the Midwest's agricultural produce. Soon meatpacking, tanning, and steel making established Milwaukee as a leading industrial center, and today the city remains a major manufacturer of industrial equipment and farm machinery. But Milwaukee's best-known enterprises are its breweries. Several of America's leading brewers proudly call Milwaukee home. Some say that people in Milwaukee are serious about two things: their football and their beer. They cheer one of America's most successful football teams, the Green Bay Packers, and, on average, they consume seven times as much beer as other Americans.

As spring settled on Milwaukee during March 1993, people in the city had something new to be serious about. Pharmacists and supermarket managers were among the first to notice that something unusual was going on. More people than ever were purchasing over-the-counter remedies for the relief of diarrhea and upset stomach. Soon their supplies of such favorite liquid cure-alls as Pepto-Bismol and Kaopectate were disappearing as quickly as they could be restocked. At the same time, schools were reporting unusually high levels of absenteeism among students and teachers. Employees at breweries and other industrial plants were not turning up for work, and doctors were getting more than the usual number of complaints about "stomach flu." At first, local public health authorities were baffled. The city's medical laboratories were not detecting an increase in any of the usual pathogens that cause diarrhea. And the mysterious illness was widespread, affecting a diverse range of people in different parts of city. Surely the cases were linked in some way, but how?

One factor the ill people had in common was their drinking water. Nearly everyone suffering from watery diarrhea that spring had been exposed to treated tap water supplied to their homes or workplaces by the Milwaukee Water Works (MWW). To some the idea that drinking water was behind the outbreak seemed ridiculous. It was taken for granted that modern water treatment technologies had virtually eliminated the risks of transmitting infections through tap water, at least in wealthy countries like the United States. Contaminated water may remain a leading cause of diarrheal disease in developing nations, but surely in a modern city like Milwaukee the safety of the municipal drinking water supply was beyond reproach. Still, with no other leads to go on, public health investigators took a closer look at Milwaukee's drinking water system.

They found that the MWW had two treatment plants, the Linnwood Avenue Plant on the north side of the city, and the Howard

Avenue Plant on the south side. Both plants could supply the entire system, but each predominantly served its own end of the city. Investigators found that purification operations were similar at each plant. Water obtained from Lake Michigan was first treated with polyaluminium chloride, a coagulant that binds suspended material to form larger particulates. These particulates were then aggregated into even larger "flocs" as the water was gently agitated. Next the flocs were given time to settle out, before the water was forced through sand filters designed to remove any finer particles that still remained. These procedures aimed to produce clear, colorless water, which would also be disinfected with chlorine before it was supplied to customers.

Clarity of treated water is important because it indicates how well a treatment plant is doing the job of removing suspended particles. The more turbid, or cloudy, a batch of treated water is, the more likely it is that pathogens have slipped through the plant's filters into the community's tap water. Municipal systems that monitor the turbidity of their finished water today aim to keep it below 0.1 nephelometric turbidity units (NTU). Investigators in Milwaukee were startled to find that by the last week in March the turbidity of water supplied by the Howard Avenue Plant had reached unprecedented levels. Although turbidity at the plant had never exceeded 0.4 NTU during the previous ten years, by March 28 it peaked at 1.7 NTU, a level seventeen times higher than the current industry standard. The turbidity of water from the Linnwood Avenue Plant rose only slightly to peak at 0.45 NTU. These increases in turbidity, coupled with laboratory confirmation of a particular parasitic disease in eight newly-diagnosed cases, led investigators to suspect strongly that drinking water was the source of the outbreak. On the evening of April 7 the mayor of Milwaukee advised the public to boil its water, and the Howard Avenue Plant was closed two days later.

Within two weeks the epidemic was over, but not before Milwaukee entered the record books with the largest documented outbreak of water-borne disease in United States history. A telephone survey of randomly selected households found that during the outbreak 26 percent of the city's population had experienced bouts of watery diarrhea (Mac Kenzie, Hoxie, Proctor, et al. 1994). Applying that rate to the population of the metropolitan area, the investigators estimated that 403 thousand people were stricken during the epidemic. Of those, forty-four hundred had to be hospitalized. Subsequent analysis of death records showed that at least fifty-four people died in connection with the outbreak. Not surprisingly, disease rates were highest among those living in areas closer to the Howard

Avenue Plant. More than half the people surveyed in the southern part of the city reported having watery diarrhea during the outbreak.

The Vexing Parasite behind the Outbreak

The parasite that turned up in the eight laboratory specimens just as investigators zeroed in on Milwaukee's drinking water was *Cryptosporidium*. Most infected people had not bothered to see a doctor, and those who did were rarely tested for this protozoan parasite, so there was a delay in determining the agent behind the epidemic by the usual methods of disease surveillance. But in the days that followed the advisory for citizens to boil their water, sightings of *Cryptosporidium* were reported from medical laboratories all over town. Most local doctors, who had little experience with this disease, were soon running to their textbooks for guidance. There they would have learned that besides watery diarrhea, most people infected with *Cryptosporidium* experience unpleasant bouts of abdominal cramping. Vomiting, fatigue, weakness, and a mild fever are also common. Among confirmed cases in the Milwaukee outbreak, the diarrhea lasted an average of nine days and resulted in an average ten-pound weight loss.

Although *Cryptosporidium* has been known as a cause of disease in animals since the start of the twentieth century, it was not recognized as a human pathogen until 1976. Case reports remained rare until the mid-1980s, but since then *Cryptosporidium* has emerged as a leading cause of watery diarrhea in more than sixty countries scattered across six continents. There is no specific treatment for *Cryptosporidium* infection, other than rest and fluid replacement while the body's normal immune defenses bring the pathogen under control. For people with compromised immune systems, especially AIDS patients, *Cryptosporidium* infection can be devastating. In such cases, diarrhea can become prolonged, resulting in severe dehydration and even death. Of those known to have died from drinking Milwaukee's contaminated water, 85 percent had AIDS.

One reason for the success of *Cryptosporidium* as a pathogen is its high level of infectiousness. It can establish itself in a new host with the ingestion of relatively few organisms. On average it takes a measly 132 organisms for healthy adult volunteers to acquire the disease. Some experts suggest that with no prior exposure to the parasite people can become ill from swallowing a single organism! Beyond this, *Cryptosporidium* can survive in moist environments outside the mammalian intestine for long periods in the oocyst stage of its life cycle. During the height of infection, billions of oocysts—encysted forms of the parasite that initiate infections—are shed in the feces of animal hosts. This is especially true for relatively immature hosts such as calves, lambs, and children. When released in such numbers, fecal oocysts can easily contaminate even the most pristine lakes and rivers that provide raw water for municipal supplies. One survey has detected *Cryptosporidium* oocysts in 87 percent of the raw surface water sources supplying sixty-six large North American treatment plants (LeChevallier, Norton, Lee, et al. 1991).

The ubiquitous oocysts of *Cryptosporidium* are a water engineer's worst nightmare. They have thick walls that enable them to resist common disinfectants, such as chlorine. They are only four to six micrometers in diameter, so they are much more difficult to trap in filters than other water-borne parasites such as *Giardia*. To make matters worse, they are not easily detected in drinking water, as there are no simple methods to find viable oocysts in water. Ordinary measures of water purity, such as fecal bacterial counts, are useless because *Cryptosporidium* may still be present after chlorination has killed every bacterial contaminant. Even turbidity is an unreliable measure, as turbid water is not always infectious, and transmission of *Cryptosporidium* has occurred where turbidity was well within the comfort range, under 0.1 NTU.

Faced with such a formidable enemy, no city water scheme that is dependent on surface water sources can afford even a minor treatment lapse; a more serious breach like that which occurred at Milwaukee's Howard Street Plant is out of the question. In retrospect, the failure of conventional coagulation and filtration systems to remove *Cryptosporidium* oocysts at the plant that March can be blamed on several factors. First, the plant's intake in Lake Michigan was too close to the outlets of polluted rivers. At the time of the outbreak these rivers were swollen by spring rains and melting snow. Such run-off was probably rich in infectious oocytes originating from upstream animal operations, such as slaughterhouses, as well as a human sewage treatment plant. The water intake for the Howard Street Plant has now been moved farther out into Lake Michigan so that it will not be directly impacted by river pollution.

Secondly, when the plant was overwhelmed with dirty source-water its staff was unable to adjust the levels of required coagulants quickly enough to maintain low turbidity. The plant has since been fitted with special monitors that help determine the appropriate level of coagulants, according to the temperature, pH, and suspended particle load of the source-water. A costly new system to kill

Cryptosporidium with ozone has also been installed. Finally, it had been the custom to clean the plant's sand filters periodically by back-washing them with treated water, which was then recycled through the plant. Although this practice was not unusual, it may have increased the chances that oocysts found their way through the filters into the treated water. Backwashed water is no longer recycled through either of Milwaukee's treatment plants.

Water, Water, Everywhere—but Dare We Drink It?

After the outbreak, Milwaukee officials were quick to point out that both of the city's treatment plants had met all existing state and federal quality standards (Kaminski 1994). All required equipment was properly installed and was operating within regulatory limits before and during the outbreak. United States drinking water quality standards have since been tightened, as they were clearly inadequate to prevent a catastrophe in Milwaukee. But standards by themselves do not prevent water-borne epidemics. At least nine other *Cryptosporidium* outbreaks linked to treated drinking water have been reported since 1984, including two since the Milwaukee outbreak. Recent outbreaks in North America have also been attributed to *Giardia* and to the parasite *Toxoplasma gondii*, to bacteria such as *E. coli* O157:H7, and to viruses, all of which turned up in community water systems. It has been estimated that 14 percent of mild intestinal disease in North America today can be ascribed to tap water (Payment, Siemiatycki, Richardson, et al. 1997).

"There is a crisis looming in the whole area of water-borne disease," says Timothy Ford of Harvard University's School of Public Health. In 1996, Ford co-authored a report for the American Academy of Microbiology that warned of worsening epidemics from contaminated drinking water, even in wealthy nations. A big part of the problem is the failure of public officials to face up to the threat, to purchase and maintain adequate water treatment equipment, and to spend the money required now to upgrade decrepit urban reticulation systems. Pathogens such as *Cryptosporidium* need not end up in treated drinking water, but keeping them out is an ever more expensive undertaking, and some moderate sized and smaller communities are failing to keep up. "The distribution of safe water to the home can no longer be taken for granted, not even in the United States or Western Europe," Ford's report said.

Perhaps it can no longer be taken for granted in Australia either. At the end of July 1998, more than three million residents of Sydney were instructed to boil their tap water when high concentrations of *Giardia* and *Cryptosporidium* were discovered in the city's supply. Four weeks later, record levels of the parasites were again detected at one of the city's major filtration plants, prompting a second boil-water appeal. An inquiry into the first contamination crisis, which was made public shortly after the second incident, highlighted mismanagement and confusion at Sydney Water, the recently privatized firm in charge of the city's drinking water. The source of the contamination was unclear, but it was probably the result of natural winter run-off from rural lands in the water system's catchment area. There were no reported increases in diarrheal illness in Sydney following either incident, but concerns about further water problems have hung over the city as it prepares to host the Olympic Games in 2000.

Water-borne *Cryptosporidium* has become a leading public health problem in the United Kingdom, where reported case numbers recently have far exceeded those of the United States. In a 1997 outbreak in the North Thames area of England there were 345 confirmed cases, and undoubtedly many others that were not reported. The outbreak was traced to a municipal system that treated water collected from eight deep wells. Investigators surmised that the system's filters were overwhelmed when heavy rains washed a massive load of oocysts into the groundwater aquifers around one of the wells after the worst dry spell in at least two hundred years (Willocks, Crampin, Milne, et al. 1998). At the height of the outbreak nearly 750 thousand consumers were asked to boil their drinking water. In 1999, a *Cryptosporidium* outbreak in northwest England was also linked to contaminated municipal water. This time 188 cases were reported in an area served by the water treatment works at Grasmere, in Cumbria.

Since the Milwaukee catastrophe, most large municipal water providers in the United States have invested heavily in filtration equipment and other apparatus to eliminate risks such as *Cryptosporidium*. But millions of Americans still drink untreated surface waters where oocysts and other pathogens are likely contaminants. Of the 171 thousand public water systems in the United States, fewer than eight thousand are operated by large or medium-sized water utilities that can realistically afford many of the newer water safety technologies. Fortunately, these systems supply water to more than 80 percent of American households, but even big city dwellers are exposed to water from much smaller systems when they travel to rural environments for work or vacations. Since the mid-1980s, an average of fifteen disease outbreaks associated with drinking water have been reported annually in the United States. These include outbreaks due to chemical contaminants or unknown causes, as well as confirmed microbial agents, such as *Cryptosporidium*. Nowadays very small systems that supply water to temporary visitors are often implicated as the sources of infection.

In one of the largest recent outbreaks of water-borne illness, nearly one thousand people who attended the Washington County Fair in upstate New York during late August 1999 became ill with diarrhea (Centers for Disease Control and Prevention 1999e). At least sixty-five people had to be hospitalized, and two died. Most infections were due to *E. coli* O157:H7, although some were caused by *Campylobacter*. The source of the outbreak was unchlorinated water from a shallow well that supplied one part of the fairgrounds. Several food vendors had used the water to make beverages and ice. This occurred after a torrential downpour had washed manure from a nearby dairy farm into an underground aquifer feeding the well. For many New Yorkers who had never thought much about the water they drink, the incident highlighted the dangers of using water from small, untreated systems. The New York State Health Department ordered all county fairgrounds that rely on wells to disinfect their water and monitor it daily when hosting public events.

As threatened as drinking water supplies have become in industrialized countries, the situation is still far worse in most developing nations. Today more than one billion people live in urban areas where water supplies are under constant danger from hepatitis A, typhoid fever, cholera, and a host of worms and other parasites. Water-borne diseases kill nearly four million people each year, most under five years of age. In the Philippines, where twelve million of the country's seventy million people do not have access to safe water, dehydration due to diarrhea is the fourth leading cause of death in young children. Circumstances are probably most appalling in sub-Saharan Africa. For example, in Abidjan, the capital of Côte d'Ivoire, more than one-third of the city's two million residents has no access to piped water. Fifteen percent lack toilet facilities and must defecate in the open. Providing safe water for everyone on Earth could cost as much as $68 billion during the next ten years. This sum, while huge, is less than what Western Europe and the United States now spend on pet food, perfumes, and cosmetics every two years.

Diseases from Recreational Water: Making a Splash

Having a drink of water isn't the only way to pick up a water-borne infection these days. Having a swim may also be risky. Swimming is the second most popular recreational activity in the United States, according to the Census Bureau. When people swim they can inadvertently swallow small amounts of water. If those waters are contaminated with pathogens, disease can result. We have already seen how polluted ocean waters have added to the hazards of family holidays at the beach. Swimming pools and lakes where large numbers of swimmers tend to congregate can also be breeding grounds for large epidemics. Fecal accidents and other inadvertent contamination of these waters can expose hoards of unsuspecting swimmers, who can recycle the infections to others. The dangers are particularly acute in large new water parks designed to accommodate many thousands of guests with a variety of water play activities such as water slides and wave pools. More than nine hundred such facilities now belong to the World Waterpark Association.

Water parks and other swimming pool operators generally try to protect their patrons by chlorinating and filtering pool waters. Unfortunately, the recommended levels of chlorine for swimming pools are not sufficient to kill *Cryptosporidium* oocysts. Higher chlorine levels aren't pleasant or even safe for swimmers. Beyond this, *Cryptosporidium* oocysts are small enough to pass through the sand filters installed in most public pools today. Filters able to remove smaller particles can be bought, but they are costly and may be more difficult to maintain. But even with an effective, well-maintained filter it would take many hours, even days, after a pool is contaminated to sift out the millions of oocysts released from a single dirty diaper. That gives the organism lots of time to infect other swimmers.

Since 1988, at least twenty-four *Cryptosporidium* outbreaks have been reported in swimming pools and water parks. The largest outbreak, in 1995, involved a water park in Georgia where more than five thousand people became ill after a fecal accident in the children's pool. The following year up to three thousand visitors at a California water park became ill after water from a jet ski was sprayed on an audience watching a show. Inadequately chlorinated swimming pool water can also transmit bacteria and viruses that cause disease, as can rivers and lakes when feces is introduced. Perhaps recreational waters play a bigger role in disease transmission than once was thought. According to Charles Gerba (1997), a microbiologist who studies pathogens in recreational water, the average bather releases about ten teaspoons of urine and about a quart of sweat per hour of active swimming. He has found potentially harmful microbes in every children's wading pool he has tested. "The chlorine goes so fast with all the kids whizzing in there," he said.

A Tale from the Crypto

On hot summer days no visit to the Minnesota Zoo was complete without stopping to enjoy the zoo's delightful fountain display. Built in 1994, the fountain sprayed jets of water one to six feet in the air. Although it was designed as a decorative fountain, it had soon become an interactive play area. Children enjoyed standing directly over the jets, letting the water soak them from head to toe. Among the zoo visitors getting a good soaking on June 29, 1997, were ten kids who had come for a birthday party. Within days, four developed diarrhea and abdominal cramps due to *Cryptosporidium*. When state health department officials checked with registered groups who had visited the zoo that weekend they found eleven additional cases, all in children who had played in the fountain.

On July 11 the fountain was closed and a public statement was issued. In all, 369 cases of intestinal disease associated with water from the fountain were then identified. In 20 percent *Cryptosporidium* infection was laboratory confirmed. Infected people ranged in age up to sixty-five years, but 95 percent were ten years of age or younger. Nearly all became infected within a three-day period, especially on Sunday, June 30. Exactly what happened is unknown. But investigators presume that a child wearing a soiled diaper contaminated the water while playing in the fountain (Centers for Disease Control and Prevention 1998d). The fountain's water drained into metal grates, passed through a sand filter, was chlorinated, and then recirculated. The zoo replaced the water on Mondays, Wednesdays, and Fridays, but no one flushed out the filter. After the incident, a fence was erected around the fountain and it was reopened for decorative display only.

Missed Opportunities for Vaccination

Another sign of deficiencies in the public health infrastructure is the reemergence of diseases that are easily preventable through immunization. Immunization is one of modern medicine's most effective interventions to prevent infectious diseases. Thanks to immunization programs, once-common childhood killers such as diphtheria, polio, and *Haemophilus influenzae* type b (Hib) have become extremely rare in most industrialized countries. In the United States, incidence rates for eight of the ten diseases covered on the routine vaccination schedule have fallen by more than 97 percent from their prevaccine peaks. While preventing suffering from disease, vaccines also save society money. As much as $29 is returned in health care savings for every dollar spent on immunization. When sufficient numbers of people are protected by vaccines, some diseases can even be eradicated.

Table 1. The Impact of Vaccination on Disease Incidence, United States

Disease	Peak Incidence	Year	1998 Incidence	% Decrease
Diphtheria	206,939	1921	1	100
Measles	894,134	1941	100	100
Mumps	152,209	1968	666	99.5
Whooping cough	265,269	1934	7,405	97.2
Polio (wild)	21,269	1952	0	100
Rubella	57,686	1969	364	99.4
Congenital rubella	20,000*	1964-5	7	100
Tetanus	1,560*	1948	41	97.4
Hib disease	20,000	1984	54	99.7

* These figures are estimates, as there was no national reporting in these years

Smallpox was driven to extinction worldwide through an active immunization campaign that culminated during the late 1970s. The last case in the United States was reported in 1949, about the time that public health visionaries called for its eradication across the globe. The eventual eradication of smallpox relieved the world of needless misery, but it made economic sense too. By the mid-1980s, the total American investment in stamping out smallpox was being recouped in medical cost savings every twenty-six days. Polio is next on the hit list. Only about five thousand children worldwide were stricken with the paralytic form of this disease during 1998, down 85 percent from 1988. Eradication efforts suffered a setback in 1999, when an epidemic in war-torn Angola claimed more than one thousand victims. Outbreaks were also reported in Afghanistan and Iraq. Some fifty countries still harbor the virus—all in southern Asia and Africa—but the end of polio is near. If current funding continues, and co-operation among nations is maintained, this crippling disease will vanish from the world by the end of 2001.

Until vaccine-preventable diseases are irreversibly eradicated, the unglamorous job of immunizing children must continue day after day. Complacency is an ever-present threat. As previously devastating diseases become rare and disappear from everyday experience, the public's memory of their seriousness fades. Uptake of vaccines falters, as completing the recommended immunization schedule takes a lower priority for parents and health professionals alike. "Our very success with infant and childhood vaccines during the past forty years has paradoxically proven to be one of our major liabilities," notes Samuel Katz (1999), a pediatric infectious disease specialist at Duke University. Young parents today have no recollection of the annual summertime horrors of polio in the 1950s or the massive surge in birth defects in the 1960s due to rubella infections during pregnancy. "These organisms have not disappeared, but have only receded into the background," Katz says.

Meanwhile, the infrequent, but sometimes serious, adverse events that follow immunization episodes have become more visible. Tragic stories of deaths or disability that occur shortly after vaccination have come to the forefront of public attention. Naturally, we feel compassion for the families involved, and on the surface their stories seem to suggest problems with vaccine safety. On further examination, however, there is usually no provable link to vaccination. But such incidents can feed the fears of those with reservations about vaccines, while bolstering the efforts of the small group of activists who fervently oppose immunization. In many countries where the dread of vaccine-preventable diseases has been lost, such individuals have become skilled at attracting media attention to their arguments. The result has been increased doubt and confusion about vaccines among parents who simply want honest information about the benefits and risks of immunization for their children. At some point, when sufficient numbers of parents lack confidence in vaccines, the viability of immunization programs to prevent childhood disease is undermined.

Without active promotion of immunization, the number of children susceptible to vaccine-preventable diseases will build toward a critical mass, able to sustain an epidemic chain-reaction. When that happens, long-forgotten pathogens return as the killers they once were. Measles, polio, and whooping cough provide good examples of diseases that can boomerang this way.

Measles

Measles is one of the most severe diseases of childhood. Complications such as pneumonia, diarrhea, and ear infections are common. Before vaccination began in 1963, measles killed about five hundred American children every year. Globally, the disease still accounts for about 10 percent of mortality in children under five years of age, or about nine hundred thousand deaths per year. The measles virus spreads by direct contact with the nose and throat secretions of infected people. It is among the most contagious infectious agents known, a fact that allows measles epidemics to spread with astonishing speed. In the first few months of 1875 nearly a quarter of Fiji's native population—forty thousand people—died from the disease. Today in industrialized countries, about 20 percent of people with measles end up in the hospital. About one in one thousand infections ends in death, and others lead to permanent brain damage. Given the harsh realities of measles, it is incredible that many people do not take this disease seriously. Some even consider it a normal part of growing up.

Such complacency led to a serious resurgence in measles in the United States, starting in 1989. That year, measles incidence increased to 18,193, a five-fold rise on the average rate in the previous eight years. In 1990, another 27,786 cases were reported. By the time the epidemic subsided in 1991, more than 11,000 people had been hospitalized and 120 had died. All age groups were affected, but the biggest increases were among preschool-aged children, especially in large urban centers. More than 80 percent of preschool-aged kids who caught the disease had never been vaccinated. Ninety percent of those who died in the epidemic were unvaccinated. Although a few cases were blamed on the failure of measles vaccine to protect against infection, the primary cause of the epidemic was the failure of society to offer the vaccine its most vulnerable members (Gindler, Atkinson, Markowitz 1992). Laws requiring immunization at school entry protected school-aged children, but vaccine coverage among younger children was chronically low. Importation of the virus from countries having high levels of measles activity then lit the powder keg. The same scenario caused a measles epidemic in New Zealand in 1997. Another epidemic was predicted in 1999 for Australia, where anti-immunization rhetoric is rife.

Polio

Polio, even on the brink of extinction, continues to prove it is a resilient foe. Polio viruses spread when microscopic amounts of feces from one person end up in the mouths of others, as inevitably happens when young children play. Infection in the digestive tract is often unnoticeable, but it can cause a mild illness marked by fever, fatigue, headache, nausea, and vomiting. In about one in two hundred cases, the virus escapes to the nervous system and causes paralysis, usually in the legs. When paralysis extends to the muscles involved in breathing, death is a common outcome. Before Jonas Salk introduced the first polio vaccine in 1955, upwards of thirteen thousand paralytic cases were reported in the United States each year. Infection of a young Franklin D. Roosevelt in 1921 showed that even future presidents were not spared. Thanks to immunization, wild polio virus has not circulated in the United States since 1979. Every case of polio paralysis reported since then has actually been due to the oral polio vaccine, which in very rare circumstances mutates in a way to cause paralytic disease. To eliminate the risk of vaccine-associated paralysis, however small, the CDC now recommends that children receive only the injected polio vaccine, an enhanced version of the original Salk vaccine.

The last cases of wild polio in the United States occurred among unvaccinated Amish people and others belonging to religious groups that do not accept immunization. Such "exemptors" from routine vaccination place themselves at greatly increased risk of all vaccine-preventable diseases. A recent study has shown they also increase the rates of disease for others living nearby, including those too young to receive vaccines and those in whom vaccination hadn't worked (Salmon, Haber, Gangarosa, et al. 1999). America's last wild polio cases could be linked to cases in the Netherlands. Dutch members of similar religious groups brought the virus across the Atlantic through contacts in Canada. In 1992, members of these sects in Holland suffered another epidemic; at least forty-one people were paralyzed and one died. The virus again turned up among their associates in Canada in 1993, but this time no one was paralyzed. It is clear from these episodes that until global eradication of polio is completed the potential for reintroduction of the virus to the United States is sizeable. If polio vaccination in the general population were stopped now, any accidental return of the virus would soon trigger epidemics on a large scale.

This was the case in several of the newly independent states of the former Soviet Union when a critical shortage of polio vaccine led to a rebound in paralytic polio there during the early 1990s (Sutter, Chudaiberdiev, Vaphakulov, et al. 1997). In the Samarkand region of Uzbekistan, polio vaccine was unavailable for ten months starting in November 1992. An outbreak of paralytic polio ensued, involving at least seventy-four cases. Nearly all the cases occurred in children under one year of age, children who would have been protected if the vaccine had been obtainable. During 1996, Albania also experi enced a large polio outbreak (Prevots, Ciofi degli Atti, Sallabanda, et al. 1998). After more than ten years without the disease, this small Balkan country suffered 138 paralytic cases, of which 16 were fatal. High rates of disease in young adults persuaded investigators that historic deficiencies in vaccine handling were partially to blame. It is likely that much of the oral polio vaccine that Albania used during its long period of authoritarian rule had been stored without refrigeration. This practice, sometimes seen even in the United States, causes temperature-sensitive vaccines to lose their potency. The opening of Albania's borders during the 1990s then allowed the reintroduction of the wild polio virus into a susceptible population.

Whooping Cough

Whooping cough, also called pertussis, is a disease that thrives on complacency and misinformation. Once common in childhood, incidence was reduced by vaccination to less than three thousand cases per year in the United States by the early 1980s. Since then, the number of reported cases has been increasing. Pertussis is a miserable illness characterized by an irritating cough that can last for months. Coughing fits often end in vomiting, which over time can result in weight loss. In young children, whooping cough can be complicated by seizures and inflammation of the brain. About one in two hundred infected children under one year of age die from the disease. Whooping cough is caused by a highly infectious bacterium, *Bordetella pertussis*, which is not easily treated with antibiotics. Prevention of the disease requires five doses of vaccine, including three doses during the first six months of life. The traditional whooping cough vaccine was a suspension of killed *B. pertussis* organisms, generally given as a component of a combination vaccine called DTP that also protects against diphtheria and tetanus. In recent years a costlier "acellular" pertussis vaccine, made from purified proteins of the bacteria, has been available. It too is given in a combination vaccine (DTaP).

No vaccine has stirred more controversy than the pertussis vaccine. It is well-known that DTP can cause unpleasant pain and swelling at the injection site. Fretfulness, drowsiness, low-grade fever, and a loss of appetite are also common short-term reactions that have been noted since the vaccine was introduced in the 1940s. But during the 1970s, anxiety that the vaccine might cause severe neurological reactions and lasting brain damage led to an abrupt decline in vaccine uptake in several countries. Japan and Sweden abandoned the vaccine altogether, although Japan went back in 1981, using an acellular vaccine. In the United Kingdom, pertussis immunization rates dropped from 81 percent to just 31 percent as unbalanced press reports kept alive fears about the vaccine's alleged dangers (Gangarosa, Galazka, Wolfe, et al. 1998). In each of these countries whooping cough deaths rebounded as immunization declined. By the early 1990s, rates of pertussis in Sweden exceeded those of neighboring Norway by one hundred to one. With more than ten thousand cases per year, Sweden's whooping cough incidence had become like that of many developing countries.

Confidence in pertussis vaccine in Australia remained strong in the 1970s, but has fallen away during the 1990s as the anti-immunization lobby has gained momentum. The crowning blow came in late 1996 when *Quantum*, a prestigious science program on the national TV network, openly questioned the value of immunization. The program highlighted the story of a child whose neurological disabilities appeared to follow pertussis vaccination. During the fifteen months after the program aired infant deaths from whooping cough in Australia climbed to nine. Sadly, health professionals down under have failed to speak in one voice with authoritative and scientifically sound advice about vaccine safety and effectiveness. The truth about pertussis vaccines is that if they do cause severe neurological reactions, including brain damage, the risk of such events is negligible compared to the risk of death and brain damage that accompanies the disease itself. In responding to the selective reporting of the *Quantum* program, Sandra Thompson, a medical researcher in Melbourne, compared the risks:

> If none of the children in a child care center of 150 children were immunized, and a whooping cough outbreak occurred, about 135 children would come down with the disease. On average, one child would get encephalitis (inflammation of the brain) as a result of the disease. If every child in the center was immunized correctly with [pertussis vaccine] possibly one child at the center every

170 years could get encephalitis as a result of immunization (Thompson 1997).

Wherever public and professional complacency about vaccines has developed, an articulate but ill-informed anti-immunization lobby has been able to fabricate myths about immunization that play upon the deep-seated emotions of some parents. Such myths propose that immunization is somehow "unnatural," or that vaccines actually suppress the immune system. They suggest that vaccines contain toxic additives, or that vaccines are contaminated with lethal viruses. These fanciful ideas, among others, can become an obstacle to achieving the levels of vaccine coverage required to prevent outbreaks. The myths of the anti-immunization lobby must be actively dispelled, or children will continue to suffer and die from preventable diseases. Until these diseases are completely eradicated, the work of immunizing children must never stop. Even if high immunization rates can be achieved, the pool of children susceptible to vaccine-preventable diseases will continue to grow every day. On a typical day 10,633 children are born in the United States. Each of them comes into the world unimmunized, but surely each deserves a fighting chance against the preventable diseases of childhood.

The Big Lie about MMR Vaccine

At the moment, childhood immunization rates in the United States are at record high levels. For now, public health professionals are winning the day against public apathy and antivaccine lobby groups. But this is not the case in every country, and no country can afford to rest on its laurels for long. Public opinion about immunization can be remarkably fickle, as recent slippage in vaccine coverage in the United Kingdom shows. The drop-off there began when a report by Andrew Wakefield and colleagues was published in *The Lancet*, a prestigious medical journal, in February 1998. The report described twelve children who had developed behavioral problems, particularly autism, in association with inflammatory bowel disease. Parents of eight of the twelve kids linked the onset of behavioral symptoms with receipt of the measles, mumps, and rubella vaccine (MMR) given in the second year of life. No scientific evidence was provided to back up any causal association with the vaccine, but the report electrified the British news media with the tantalizing notion that MMR might induce a raft of serious diseases of the brain and bowel.

In England, 92 percent of children had received MMR by their second birthday in 1996 and 1997. This is barely sufficient to prevent a buildup of susceptible children able to sustain a measles epidemic. After the Wakefield report hit the headlines, coverage fell to 88 percent. Similar downward trends have been noted in Wales and Scotland. In Wales, parents have begun to organize "measles parties," deliberately exposing their children to the virus in place of vaccination. Public health authorities say this is outrageous. "Wales is at a critical point with MMR vaccinations. We have gone from a high of 95 percent down to an average of 86 or 87 percent," says Meirion Evans (1999), a Welsh communicable disease consultant. "We're at the threshold of the disease coming back if we are not careful."

Larger, population-based studies have since demolished the hypothesis that MMR might cause autism or bowel disease. In a 1999 study that closely examined 498 children with autism in the North Thames region, Brent Taylor and colleagues found no link with MMR. There was no change in the incidence of autism after MMR was introduced in Britain in 1988; the age at diagnosis of autism had no relation to the time that MMR was received; and developmental regression was not more intense during the months after vaccination. It now seems certain that the onset of autism among some cases in the original report was coincidental with MMR, but unrelated to it (Taylor, Miller, Farrington, et al. 1999).

The new studies should lay the issue to rest, but don't count on it. In the same month that Taylor's report was released, another British study showed that the risk of inflammatory bowel disease was increased in those who had measles and mumps infections during the same year of life. This study only linked naturally acquired infections with bowel disease, and said nothing about receipt of the vaccine. But immediately the Fleet Street media jumped on the story as further evidence that MMR can cause long-term harm. It seems vaccine scares sell newspapers. But they're harsh on the daily task of keeping some of humanity's most dreaded diseases under control.

TB Returns to The Big Apple

Sometimes the most effective way to prevent infectious diseases is to offer free and accessible treatment to those in the community who are already infected. This explains why public health efforts to control sexually transmitted diseases focus primarily on providing free and confidential treatment at publicly subsidized sexual health clinics. Funding cutbacks for these clinics would have repercussions throughout the larger community, as untreated infections would spread unchecked. Similarly, modern approaches to tuberculosis control have centered on providing drug therapy for people with TB before their infections spread to others. Cutbacks in tuberculosis programs may offer governments short-term savings, but, as New York City found out after years of budget slashing, reduced treatment services can have disastrous consequences (Frieden, Fujiwara, Washko, et al 1995). In chapter 4, we have already seen how urban poverty, homelessness, and the HIV epidemic have created a global TB emergency. The other main factor behind the recent upsurge of TB is the failure of public health systems to cope with the disease. This dereliction has led to the emergence of multidrug-resistant (MDR) strains that threaten to make TB incurable. During the early 1990s, the breakdown in TB control was nowhere more apparent than in the most affluent metropolis in the world.

In 1960, New York City had a comprehensive TB treatment system, including hospitals and sanatoriums with more than twenty-four hundred beds. But as incidence of the disease declined, so did interest among policymakers in maintaining TB control programs. By the late 1980s, the city's Bureau of Tuberculosis Control was reduced to 140 workers, its hospitals were closed, and its outpatient clinics were cut from twenty-four to eight. While this occurred, the city was undergoing significant social upheaval, characterized by increased substance abuse, homelessness, a burgeoning HIV epidemic, over-crowded housing, and what sociologists call declining social cohesion. By 1992, the convergence of these factors led to a tripling of new TB cases, compared to the city's 1978 levels. In the city's most disadvantaged enclaves, such as central Harlem, the case rate exceeded that of many Third World countries. For the city's young black men, the rate of TB was almost forty-five times the United States average. Even worse, about one in five TB patients in New York City was infected with an MDR strain, more than double the rate seen in 1985. With only 3 percent of the United States population, the city had 15 percent of the country's TB cases and 61 percent of cases due to MDR strains.

The emergence of MDR-TB was especially alarming, as these strains are more difficult for doctors to treat. They are also far more expensive. Treatment of a single case of MDR-TB may cost as much as $250 thousand or about one hundred times the outlay required for nonresistant TB. These strains are also worrisome from a public health perspective, because patients with MDR-TB remain infectious for longer periods. The organisms they subsequently transmit to others are also resistant, so the epidemic is perpetuated. *Mycobacterium tuberculosis* has always been prone to developing antibiotic resistance. But uncoordinated management of cases between overburdened hospitals and understaffed outpatient programs was starting to magnify the problem by the late 1980s.

TB treatment is invariably an arduous process. Regimens may require half a dozen pills a day, to be taken over a period of six to nine months. After a few weeks of therapy, the debilitating symptoms of TB often diminish, although the bacteria remain in the lungs. Without close supervision, many patients, especially those living in disorganized surroundings, will abandon the therapy as soon as they feel better. This eventually results in relapses, while it creates conditions conducive to the development of drug resistance. A relapsing patient is five times more likely to carry a strain resistant to at least one drug than a patient with no previous treatment. Clearly, stop-start treatment regimens are worse than no treatment at all. But by 1989, that was the pattern in New York City. That year, fewer than 60 percent of people infected with TB completed the required therapy. At one major hospital only 11 percent of patients adhered to the full course of treatment. As MDR strains flourished in the city's streets, they inevitably turned up in New York's state prisons (Valway, Greifinger, Papania, et al. 1994). During 1990 and 1991, a total of 171 inmates were newly diagnosed with TB, of whom thirty-seven had MDR strains. Crowded living conditions and frequent inmate transfers between prisons facilitated the outbreak.

New York City has now turned the corner on its TB epidemic. After spending well over $1 billion on additional treatments and new infection control measures, new cases of TB dropped to 1,730 during 1997, compared with more than 3,800 cases in 1992. Rates of MDR-TB fell even faster, to just fifty-six cases in 1997. Unfortunately, the complacent attitudes and social disintegration that fostered the epidemic in New York City have since appeared in other places. While only thirteen states had reported MDR-TB in 1991, forty-five states hosted these strains between 1993 and 1998. Fortunately, MDR-TB now accounts for barely 1 percent of all TB cases in the United States, down from nearly 3 percent in 1993. But the global picture remains bleak. Worldwide, up to fifty million people are thought to be infected with drug-resistant TB. In countries that can barely afford the front-line drugs to treat ordinary TB, infection with resistant strains can amount to a death sentence. Hot spots for MDR-TB today include Argentina, the Dominican Republic, Côte d'Ivoire, Estonia, Latvia, and Russia. In Russia, MDR-TB has risen from 3 percent of total TB cases in 1991 to 6 percent today, as economic turmoil has made the completion of drug treatments increasingly difficult. Some 40 percent of TB in Russian prisons is now MDR.

War—The Ultimate Breakdown

Since 1945, the world has suffered more than one hundred wars, of which all but a few were fought in developing countries. In modern warfare, civilian casualties far outnumber those among military combatants. Increasingly, children are bearing the brunt of war-related deaths. The wide-ranging effects of modern military weaponry can put entire populations at risk, interrupting supplies of food and medicine, disturbing delicate ecosystems, and forcing mass evacuations of refugees. Civilian populations beset by war-related food shortages, lack of clean water, and scarce medical care are highly vulnerable to epidemic infectious diseases.

The main reason for Angola's recent epidemic of polio was the resumption of that impoverished country's twenty-five-year civil war in December 1998. When the fighting broke out, more than 1.5 million people were displaced and forced to live in crowded, unsanitary conditions around the capital and other cities. War may now be the largest impediment to the eradication of polio, as most of the remaining reservoirs of the virus are in regions plagued by armed conflict. "Ongoing civil conflicts in places like Angola and the Democratic Republic of the Congo are threatening the campaign against polio just as we approach the finish line," laments Carol Bellamy (1999), executive director of Unicef. The Angolan crisis in 1999 was all too familiar to international relief agencies working in Africa. Between July 14 and 17, 1994, nearly one million Rwandan men, women, and children crossed into Goma, Zaire, to flee civil war and mass genocide. Their presence quickly overwhelmed the local infrastructure and sparked fierce outbreaks of intestinal disease. During the first month of the crisis, more than forty-eight thousand bodies of deceased refugees were collected by trucks circulating through Goma's makeshift camps (Moore, Bloland, Zingeser, et al. 1995). Most people had died from cholera and dysentery due to a lack of safe drinking water and inadequate sanitation. Nine deaths out of ten occurred outside health facilities.

Since 1994, political strife in Rwanda and neighboring Burundi has continued to erode basic public health services, allowing diseases to spread. In fact, much of Africa today exists in a continuous state of war. In 1998 alone, protracted internal conflicts disrupted civilian life in Sudan, Sierra Leone, Guinea-Bissau, Liberia, and Lesotho. A rebellion against President Laurent Kabila in the Democratic Republic of the Congo threatened to pull several other African countries into an all-out war. Meanwhile, Nigeria and Cameroon were fighting over the oil-rich Bakassi peninsula, while Ethiopia and Eritrea went to war in a dispute over the Tigré province. In Zambia, Zimbabwe, and Kenya, tensions were heightened as democratic movements challenged autocratic rulers. Africa's combustible political environment has become the continent's single greatest threat to public health. State-sponsored tyranny, corruption, social instability, and senseless military conflicts all work together to divert scarce resources from primary health care, cripple the local public health infrastructure, discourage social investment, and supply fertile soil for epidemics.

Vector Control Out of Control

One last topic related to the decline in collective responsibility for protecting public health is vector control, the active elimination of insects, rats, and other vermin that transmit certain pathogens to humans. We have already seen how urbanization and international travel have helped dengue fever emerge as a serious threat to health in countless cities of the tropical world. Dengue also thrives because of failures to control *Aedes aegypti* mosquitoes. Elimination of urban breeding sites and selective applications of insecticide could substantially reduce the burden of dengue; but only a few countries, such as Singapore, are willing and able to maintain a consistent mosquito control program.

Yellow fever, another mosquito-borne viral disease, has also reemerged in the last two decades as vector control has lapsed. The World Health Organization estimates that two hundred thousand people are infected with yellow fever each year, including thirty thousand who die from the disease. Yellow fever gets its name from the jaundice it causes in some people. Symptoms of fever, muscle pains, headache, and nausea develop about three to six days after a person is bitten by an infected mosquito. Most patients improve in a few days, but about 15 percent rapidly turn jaundiced and begin to bleed profusely. At this point the kidneys may fail, which often leads to death. Yellow fever only occurs in equatorial regions of Africa and South America. Traditionally it was a disease of monkeys that were infected by wild forest-dwelling mosquitoes. Humans making forays into the jungle sometimes became accidental hosts. In recent years this jungle transmission cycle has spread into more populated areas of the African savanna, creating a new "zone of emergence" where human infections are more likely to occur.

More ominously, the disease has emerged in large African cities, carried by infected migrants arriving from the countryside. Here the vector for the yellow fever virus is the familiar *Aedes aegypti* mosquito, which spreads the disease from person to person in potentially explosive epidemics. Urban yellow fever was thought to be eliminated from the Americas during the first half of the twentieth century. While yellow fever remained a threat in South America's rainforests, the last cases transmitted in cities were reported in 1954. But recently, six cases of urban yellow fever have been documented in Santa Cruz, Bolivia, a city of nine hundred thousand people close to a known hot spot for forest transmission (Van der Stuyft, Gianella, Pirard, et al. 1999). As with the emergence of dengue fever, a key factor for the unwelcome return of urban yellow fever to Latin America is the inadequate control of *Aedes aegypti* mosquitoes. Infestations of *Aedes aegypti* were easy to find around Santa Cruz at the time of the outbreak. Unlike dengue, yellow fever can be prevented with a safe and highly effective vaccine. But for poor countries like Bolivia, and those saddled with urban yellow fever in Africa, money to buy enough vaccine for everyone at risk is difficult to find.

Malaria is another mosquito-borne disease advancing on the heels of diminished vector control activities. As we saw in chapter 2, malaria was once a common affliction in the southern United States, affecting up to half a million people each year. Starting in the mid-1930s, the federal government put thirty-six thousand men to work draining more than two million acres of mosquito-infested swamps. When the insecticide DDT joined the antimalaria campaign, it was possible to make the United States malaria-free by 1953. Two years later, the World Health Organization set out to eliminate malaria worldwide. The key strategy was applying DDT liberally to the interior walls of houses in malarial countries. Although this approach met with initial success, some mosquitoes soon developed resistance to DDT, especially in regions where the chemical was being used extensively in agriculture. Environmental concerns about DDT also appeared by the 1960s, and greater restrictions were put on its use. However, alternative insecticides are generally more toxic to humans and are much more expensive to purchase. If a global ban on DDT is imposed, poor countries, especially in Africa, may have to give up most of their mosquito control programs. Even in the United States, mosquito control has fallen on hard times; *Anopheles* mosquitoes capable of transmitting malaria are now common during the summer in all forty-eight contiguous states.

The malaise affecting mosquito control efforts was evident when West Nile encephalitis came to New York City in 1999. The city had one of the least aggressive mosquito control programs in its region, after budget cuts in 1993 had slashed spending for mosquito abatement to just $120 thousand per year. With only two full-time staff devoted to mosquito control, the city had no system to monitor mosquito populations and implement controls before the insects could spread diseases to residents. By contrast, nearby Suffolk County employed thirty-three people to control mosquitoes on an annual budget of $2 million. "If you aren't monitoring mosquitoes for something you end up using people as a surveillance tool," says Robert Novak (1999), a medical entomologist at the University of Illinois. "That is what happened in New York." City officials pointed out that mosquito-borne disease had rarely been a problem in their built-up environment. That meant the city wasn't eligible for state funds to

---

Wrestling with Rabies

People love to pet animals, especially kids. Cute and cuddly animals can be too irresistible not to reach out and touch. So it is no surprise that petting zoos and tourist-oriented farms that encourage direct contact with animals are popular. Unfortunately, these enterprises are not well regulated and they create easy opportunities to spread animal diseases to humans. This was the case in Iowa in August 1999, when a black bear cub at a petting zoo was found to be infected with rabies (Centers for Disease Control and Prevention 1999f). Visitors to the zoo had been permitted to feed the bear and even wrestle with it. In this way, several people may have been nipped. That month, the bear had also been taken to a barn-warming, where it had reportedly nipped some of the guests. In all, approximately four hundred people from ten states and Australia had contact with the bear during the time it could have transmitted the rabies virus. Needless to say it was a big job for public health authorities to locate those people and determine their need for treatment.

Health officials were also busy in Wales when at least seventeen people developed *E. coli* O157:H7 infection after visiting an open farm in June 1999. Six visitors had to be hospitalized. Several animals at the farm were found to carry the same bacterial strain as the people infected in the outbreak. An educational petting farm in Michigan was the setting for an outbreak of *Cryptosporidium* infection in 1996. At least twenty-three children and three adults became ill after visiting the farm. Most had not washed their hands after petting the animals. That year at least thirty-nine people in Colorado became ill with *Salmonella enteritidis* (SE) after visiting a traveling exhibit of Komodo dragons at a local zoo. No one was allowed to touch the giant lizards, but a wooden barrier surrounding the dragon pen was contaminated with SE and spread the infection to visitors.

---

combat mosquitoes. Such excuses didn't impress public health experts who bemoaned the city's vulnerability to mosquito-borne diseases. "You can't get complacent just because things haven't happened in the past," noted Kellogg Schwab (1999), an environmental microbiologist at Johns Hopkins University.

Rodent control is another neglected public health function today. Budget cutbacks have forced many American communities to abandon routine rat poisoning programs in recent years. Before the 1980s, cities and states received federal money earmarked specifically for rodent abatement. But during the Reagan years, strings dictating how states spent their grants were removed. That was a mistake, says John Beck (1993), a rodent control expert based in Phoenix. "The money goes where the squeakiest wheel lobbies for it. Rats are a thing that most politicians would prefer to ignore," he says. "There's very little glamour associated with rodent control, so politicians steer away from it as much as possible." Eventually rat numbers can become so high that politicians are forced to take action. In 1999, officials in Dearborn, Michigan, more than doubled the city's budget for rodent control to $250 thousand after a rat explosion swept the Detroit area. Warm winters and lax enforcement of trash containment laws were among the reasons for the crisis, according to officials in nearby Hamtramck.

In some communities stray cats are also poorly controlled. Young cats can transmit the bacterium *Bartonella henselae* when they scratch, or sometimes bite or lick, an unsuspecting human. Not surprisingly, the resulting disease is called cat-scratch disease. It affects about twenty-two thousand people each year in the United States, causing enlarged lymph glands that persist for months. Occasionally more serious problems develop, including encephalitis. In 1994, three children from Broward County, Florida, developed encephalitis attributed to cat-scratch disease within a twenty-six-hour period. Each child had seizures, became comatose, and required artificial respiration. Two additional cases with encephalitis occurred in nearby Palm Beach County the following month. All of the infected children had handled stray cats.

Like most core public health activities, controlling human diseases spread by animals as large as bears or as small as mosquitoes isn't glamorous work. No one who pursues a public health career does it for recognition, especially because recognition comes only when something goes wrong. The public's indifference to infectious threats surely makes the job of preventing diseases more difficult, but it makes the job no less important. Complacency about traditional disease-control measures is not likely to end soon, but there is hope it will decline as people realize the value of public health in their lives. Until then, apathy will inevitably bring about infectious consequences. One day it might even aid the cause of those who would intentionally infect others with harmful microbes. The next chapter considers the risks when biological agents are used for terrorist objectives.

What You Can Do to Help Control Vaccine-Preventable Diseases

We have seen how public complacency about vaccine-preventable childhood infections can allow long-forgotten diseases to stage surprise comebacks. As grandparents who can remember the bad old days of the prevaccine era are starting to die away, it will become even more important in the years ahead to keep alive the necessity of vaccinating children on time. Otherwise epidemics will continue to catch us off-guard. Another trend of our time is a growing distrust of science, medicine, government, and authority figures of all kinds. In some places this postmodern perspective is giving rise to a movement that openly questions immunization. If you are confronted with claims that vaccines are "unnatural" or cause more harm than good, stop and consider this:

- No medicine given to literally billions of people is 100 percent safe or effective. However, the benefits of vaccination to the individual far outweigh the risk of serious health effects.

- There is no reliable evidence that vaccines cause any chronic illness.

- Minor reactions, such as redness and swelling at the injection site, are common. More severe reactions occur very rarely, if at all.

- People who seek to boost the immune system with "natural" substances are allowing children to battle serious diseases without the help of antibodies that could have developed through vaccination.

- If vaccination were stopped, uncontrollable epidemics of serious diseases would soon return. Death and disability in childhood would be common.

Chapter 11

Biological Terrorism

Biological weapons, whether wielded by the military forces of nations or by terrorists, will continue to pose a serious threat to international security for the foreseeable future.

—Raymond A. Zilinskas,
Center for Public Issues in
Biotechnology, University of Maryland

Up to this point we have considered ways that serious infectious diseases might emerge as the unintended consequences of various precipitating factors. We have assumed that when new infections arise they do so inadvertently, as unforeseen outcomes of changing human activities or natural processes. This chapter examines the possibility that epidemics in the future might also arise from willful acts, that infectious agents might be used purposefully as instruments of terror or war. The few incidents thus far in which biological weapons have played a part suggest that we need to take the threat of biological aggression seriously. An epidemic of anthrax, plague, or smallpox begun as a terrorist act could represent an unprecedented global crisis. The idea of such an attack is so morally repugnant that we may naturally feel reluctant even to think about it: surely in a civilized society such barbaric weapons are not a relevant cause for concern. But such denial is not helpful. It plays into the hands of the few who would pervert science in this way to bring civil society to its knees. It is time to look the evil in the eye.

Biological agents are the ultimate antipersonnel weapons. They promise to achieve the catastrophic effects alleged for the infamous "neutron bomb" during the 1980s: killing people but leaving property untouched. They accomplish their savage objectives by invading the bodies of their victims, multiplying there, and destroying them from within. Certain agents can even spread from person to person, so the ruinous effects of the initial attack can be amplified across a larger population. Compared to conventional weapons, which can kill hundreds or thousands in a single explosion, bioweapons have much greater killing potential. The death toll from a properly executed attack could reach hundreds of thousands, even millions. Biological weapons can be produced and deployed at relatively low cost and with little scientific knowledge. Raw materials and production equipment are easily acquired from unregulated commercial sources and are easy to hide. Moreover, most communities are completely unprepared to counter the risk. A metropolitan area targeted by a determined Unabomber-style anarchist or a malicious terrorist organization might well be indefensible against such loathsome weapons.

Although the idea of biological warfare is not new, Western attention to the risk of biological attacks on vulnerable civilian targets has never been greater. A number of recent events have heightened the concern. First, the break-up of the USSR revealed that the Soviet military had flagrantly violated international conventions during the Cold War, developing a ghoulish bioweapon program of enormous proportions. Many former Soviet scientists and technicians cannot be accounted for today, and are presumed to be selling their expertise overseas. Secondly, United Nations inspections have shown that Iraq has developed ominous capabilities to produce a diverse repertoire of biological warfare agents. Iraq, a known sponsor of international terrorism, appeared ready to use its ample stockpiles of bioweapons during the 1991 Persian Gulf War. Largely because President Saddam Hussein appeared willing to deploy these weapons again, American and British warships and bombers pounded suspected Iraqi military targets for four nights in December 1998, a mission that was named Operation Desert Fox.

Finally, extremist groups bent on violence have been on the rise worldwide during the 1990s. Such groups, and even certain disgruntled individuals, might be attracted to biological weapons to vent their grievances and further their causes. Recent bombings of New York's World Trade Center and the Oklahoma City Federal Building have brought home to Americans the growing threat to society posed by the desperate and deranged. Weaponized biological agents could magnify that risk, while offering police few chances for early detection. Such weapons present what defense experts call an "asymmetrical threat," a way for those wishing to demolish the societal order to achieve their ends without directly engaging our military or police forces. For years, the nihilistic cult Aum Shinrikyo enjoyed unconstrained movement in Japanese society without arousing suspicion of its doomsday objectives; only after the cult attacked Tokyo's subway system with a fatal nerve gas was it found to be actively engaged in bioweapon research and testing.

At a time when the world has finally stepped back from the brink of nuclear holocaust, biological weapons have emerged as nasty new hazards capable of mass destruction on a similar scale. In 1999, the British Medical Association warned that biological weapons are just as deadly as nuclear warheads, but are easier to acquire. D. A. Henderson (1998) agrees. He led the global campaign for the eradication of smallpox from 1966 to 1977. Now he directs the Johns Hopkins Center for Civilian Biodefense Studies, a think tank that aims to educate the public and policy-makers about the bioterrorist threat. "The specter of biological weapons use is an ugly one, every bit as grim and foreboding as that of a nuclear winter," he says. Henderson feels American communities today are ill-prepared to anticipate a biological attack, to detect an attack once it has begun, or to manage the potentially devastating consequences. A report published in 1999 by the Institute of Medicine suggested that one such incident "could result in civilian mortality and morbidity that have not been seen in natural disasters or infectious outbreaks in the United States since the influenza epidemic of 1918-1919."

As awareness of the danger of biological terrorism has grown, civil defense planners have begun to consider ways to meet the threat. The first step in preparing an effective response is to give up the attitude that "it couldn't happen here." No community can pretend it is not at risk. No city can afford not to reflect on its response. "The chilling truth is that biological weapons are a threat to people in every land, however secure or remote it might seem," says John Holum (1996), director of the United States Arms Control and Disarmament Agency. To appreciate the abhorrent nature of the bioweapon threat, a good place to start is Sverdlovsk, a bleak industrial city in Russia's vast heartland. From piecemeal accounts of a mysterious disease outbreak there twenty years ago, we can begin to understand the enormity of the hazards we face.

A Cruel April in Sverdlovsk

On Monday, April 2, 1979, the 1.2 million residents of Sverdlovsk awoke to a chilly spring morning with a brisk northerly wind. A cold front had passed over the city during the night, and temperatures at the start of the day hovered around twelve degrees Fahrenheit. But the morning sun shone brightly in the cloudless sky as Sverdlovsk's wide boulevards filled with workers on their way to the city's many factories. It seemed like an unremarkable day in this rather unremarkable city on the eastern edge of the Ural Mountains, nine hundred miles east of Moscow. Here, where Europe gives way to Asia, the last Russian czar, Nicholas II, had been executed with his family and attendants on the night of July 16, 1918. At that time, the city was called Ekaterinburg, in honor of the eighteenth-century czarina, Catherine I. But under the Communists, the city had been renamed for a Bolshevik revolutionary.

After the revolution, Sverdlovsk remained a provincial backwater, servicing the local mining and farming interests. Then, with the German advance on Stalingrad during World War II, it was transformed almost overnight into a leading center for arms production. After the war, the city continued to be a major producer of armaments and was thought to be a focal point for Soviet military research. The KGB ensured that Sverdlovsk was closed to nearly all foreign visitors during the Cold War, but United States satellite reconnaissance confirmed a substantial military presence in the city. Of particular interest was a military microbiology laboratory, part of a group of buildings known as Compound 19 in the southern sector of the city. Besides the lab, the installation included accommodation for workers and their families; bland, four- and five-story apartments that housed about five thousand people. Further south lay the Chkalovskiy *rayon*, or neighborhood, a mixed residential and light industrial area with a population density of about twenty-five thousand per square mile. Here and elsewhere in Sverdlovsk, shopkeepers and other small business owners knew the local economy depended on income from military jobs. Few people even thought to question the military's activities in 1979, least of all the relatively unknown chief of the local Communist Party, Boris Yeltsin.

But as news of a deadly outbreak that spring reached the West, medical and military observers around the world had plenty of questions about what was going on in Sverdlovsk (Wade 1980). The outbreak began on April 4 when hospital emergency clinics in the city started seeing patients complaining of fever, muscle aches, a cough, and general weakness. The initial symptoms suggested the flu and caused no alarm. But within days the patients unexpectedly deteriorated. Suddenly they had difficulty breathing, and would sweat profusely. They lost color, and most of them died within twenty-four hours as their lungs filled with fluids. Many patients also developed a strange kind of meningitis, marked by a profuse bleeding into the clear fluid that normally surrounds the brain and spinal cord. At first doctors were at a loss to explain the bizarre epidemic. Then, as Faina Abramova performed an autopsy on one of the first victims, she recalled a specimen she had seen years before at her medical school's pathology museum (Abramova, Grinberg, Yampolskaya, et al. 1993). That specimen was the preserved brain of a patient with hemorrhagic meningitis. It was labeled "a cardinal's cap," because the brain was so completely covered in blood that it resembled the crimson head-wear of a Catholic cardinal. Now here was a patient with the same finding. When bacterial cultures on the bloody fluid were examined the next day, Abramova's worst fears were confirmed. The patient had died from anthrax.

Anthrax is a bacterial disease of sheep, cattle, horses, goats, and other herbivores that is occasionally transmitted to humans. The causative agent, *Bacillus anthracis*, is extremely resistant to adverse environmental conditions, able to survive for years in soils and other substrates as a spore. Human infection generally occurs when people handle infected animals or their fleeces. In fact, skin infections account for more than 90 percent of human anthrax cases worldwide. Usually these unpleasant sores can be treated with antibiotics, and the infection is contained. A more serious form of the disease, some-times called "wool sorter's disease," results from inhaling dust parti-cles containing spores of anthrax. To trigger the disease, the particles must be very small—less than five micrometers in diameter—so they can drift into the deep recesses of the lungs. The pulmonary form of anthrax was first recognized in 1847 among workers in the worsted industry at Bradford, England. They had inhaled spores buried in imported goat hair and alpaca wool. Inhalational anthrax emerged again during the first decade of the twentieth century, this time among eighty-nine peasant women in the Povolzhye region of south-western Russia. The women contracted the disease as they worked at home with infected animal fibers during the cold months of the year.

Inhalational anthrax is almost always fatal, unless appropriate antibiotics are given early. Spores that settle in the lungs are trans-ported to nearby lymph nodes where they germinate, multiply, and produce powerful toxins. From there the activated bacteria can dis-seminate throughout the body, infecting the meninges surrounding the brain and other tissues. Death results from overwhelming blood poisoning. Fortunately, anthrax is not spread from person to person. The inhalational variety is extremely rare, with only eighteen cases reported in the United States between 1900 and 1980. A single case would sound a public health alarm. In Sverdlovsk, there were eight fatal cases in just the first few days of the outbreak. To the amazement of local doctors, all of the cases were in young, previously healthy people.

Predictably, the discovery of so much human anthrax prompted an immediate public health response. By April 10, an emergency commission was appointed, led by the USSR deputy minister of health. Care for patients having suspected anthrax was centralized at one hospital. Bodies of those who died were treated with chlorinated lime and buried in a designated area of the city cemetery. Medical teams moved from house to house wherever cases occurred, administering antibiotics to other householders and disinfecting sickrooms. In the Chkalovskiy *rayon*, where the largest number of patients resided, fire brigades hosed down building exteriors and trees. Police shot stray dogs, and unpaved roads were covered in asphalt. In mid-April, a vaccine against anthrax was offered to all healthy residents of the *rayon* between eighteen and fifty-five years of age. About forty-seven people accepted the offer, roughly 80 percent of those who were eligible. By May 19, the epidemic was over, after at least sixty-six people had died. The real toll may have been much higher.

Bad Meat or a Mishap of Germ Warfare?

From the beginning, Soviet authorities denied that the Sverdlovsk outbreak was due to inhalational anthrax. They maintained that the outbreak resulted from consumption of contaminated meat, which had been supplied by "private butchers" operating south of the city. Residents were warned to avoid eating uninspected meat, and certain shipments of meat entering the city were seized and destroyed. At the same time, the KGB confiscated all hospital records, epidemiological summaries, and autopsy reports related to the outbreak. Nine years later, a delegation of Soviet physicians visiting the United States held fast to the official version of events (Marshall 1988). That delegation, which included the deputy health minister who had directed the emergency response, maintained that certain cattle on private farms south of the city had been infected with anthrax after they had consumed contaminated meat-and-bone meal produced at a nearby factory. The outbreak spread to humans after the sickest animals were slaughtered and sold for meat on the black market, they said.

Western public health authorities and arms control experts were unconvinced by the Soviet explanation of the Sverdlovsk outbreak. Human anthrax acquired from food is exceedingly rare, if it occurs at all. A much more plausible explanation was that an aerosol of anthrax spores had been accidentally released from the microbiological research facility in Compound 19. People living and working downwind from the installation became ill after they inhaled the spores. This was a serious allegation, as it implied that the USSR was secretly involved in developing an agent of biological warfare. Such activity was expressly forbidden in the Biological Weapons Convention of 1972, a treaty signed by the USSR, the United States, and more than one hundred other governments, which banned the development, production, and stockpiling of all bacteriological weapons.

Throughout the 1980s, American officials demanded the opportunity to inspect the site of the catastrophe and examine the evidence for themselves. Then in 1990, as *glasnost* allowed greater freedom of speech, articles began to appear in the Russian press questioning the official Soviet rationale for the outbreak. The following year, Boris Yeltsin, by then the president of Russia, ordered an official inquiry. At about that time, Abramova and other pathologists who conducted the autopsies at Sverdlovsk unveiled some microscopic slides and notes they had hidden from the KGB in 1979. An international review of this material proved that the victims had died from inhalational anthrax. In May 1992, Yeltsin reported that according to the KGB "our military developments were the cause" of the outbreak.

That year, and again in 1993, an international team led by Matthew Meselson of Harvard University visited Sverdlovsk, which by then had returned to its prerevolutionary name of Ekaterinburg. Although hospital and public health records had long been destroyed, Meselson's team was able to retrieve a list of names and addresses of outbreak victims, including all but one of the sixty-six confirmed deaths. This list led them to the relatives and friends of most of those who died, and eventually to some survivors. They found that all but six of their patients could definitely be placed during the week of April 2 in a narrow geographical band pointing south and slightly east from the microbiology lab at Compound 19, predominantly in the Chkalovskiy *rayon*. Moreover, veterinary records showed that anthrax deaths in farm animals south of the city also fell neatly on the same axis, up to thirty miles away. This striking distribution provided convincing evidence that the outbreak resulted from the wind-borne spread of an anthrax aerosol emanating from the laboratory. The direction of the plume corresponded with northerly winds seen only on Monday, April 2, according to weather records from Sverdlovsk airport. The best directional fit was recorded at 10 A.M., a time when gusts exceeded fifteen feet per second.

Given the narrowness of the high-risk zone, and the fact that it pointed in a direction rarely paralleled by winds that spring,

Meselson's team concluded that the escape of anthrax spores had occurred that Monday during a very brief interval. The fact that some cases of the disease erupted within days while others lay dormant for many weeks merely attests to the variable incubation period of inhalational anthrax, they said. The team was unable to say how the accident at Compound 19 actually occurred. Perhaps an anthrax culture container broke, or an animal exposure chamber was mistakenly vented to the air outside. Perhaps an experimental weapon went astray. A recent book by Ken Abilek (1999), a Soviet bioweapon designer who defected to the United States in 1992, blames the accident on a failure to replace an air filter that had been removed during a maintenance check. Such filters prevented stray anthrax spores inside the busy bioweapons facility from seeping through exhaust pipes into the air outside. Abilek believes the accident occurred on the previous Friday, when workers who were anxious to get home or have a drink at a nearby bar neglected to replace the critical filter.

Thanks to the thoroughness of the KGB's efforts to conceal the truth, we may never know exactly what happened at Compound 19 or know exactly when the invisible cloud of anthrax spores escaped from the plant. But Meselson's team was able to judge the total weight of the spores released in the mishap by using estimates of lethal doses determined from experiments on nonhuman primates. They concluded that the dose released into the outside air was tiny, ranging from only a few milligrams to nearly one gram. A gram of powdered anthrax spores would not begin to fill an ordinary thimble.

The Inglorious History of Germ Warfare

The deliberate use of harmful microbes to achieve military ends is not a recent idea. Mongol warriors attacking the Black Sea port of Caffa in 1348 catapulted the dead bodies of plague victims over the city's walls. In the 1760s, British forces in Western Pennsylvania furnished blankets contaminated with smallpox to the Native American tribes they wished to subdue. Germany attempted to spread anthrax among some of the livestock exported to allied countries during World War I. Moral indignation over the deployment of poison gas during the war led to the 1925 Geneva Protocol, the first diplomatic attempt to prohibit the use of both chemical and biological weapons. It declared that such weapons are "justly condemned by the general opinion of the civilized world."

Unfortunately, the Geneva treaty was weak. It did not prevent research, production, or possession of biological weapons, only their use. In 1932, Japan began a massive bioweapon program, employing more than three thousand scientists at its largest facility. Testimony obtained for war crime prosecutions after World War II revealed that Japan had attacked at least eleven Chinese cities with biological weapons, including bubonic plague. As many as fifteen million fleas infected with plague were dumped from aircraft to start epidemics. Chinese researchers have claimed that by 1945 such attacks caused ninety-four thousand deaths in their country, but the Japanese government has never acknowledged that its army conducted germ warfare. Great Britain, France, Italy, Canada, and the USSR were also engaged in bioweapon research by the start of World War II. The United States program began in 1942, but it was beset with problems until Japanese scientists in American custody after the war provided useful information about developing biological weapons in exchange for immunity from war crime indictments.

For the next twenty-five years the United States amassed a substantial biological arsenal, including numerous bacterial pathogens, toxins, and fungal plant pathogens. The antiplant weapons were intended to annihilate an enemy's food supplies. Between 1949 and 1968 military researchers carried out numerous covert experiments in New York, San Francisco, and other American cities, simulating the means by which pathogenic agents could be dispersed as aerosols in the atmosphere (Christopher, Cieslak, Pavlin, et al. 1997). Shortly before the American public became aware of these tests, biological weapons lost favor with military planners. Aside from obvious ethical concerns, President Richard Nixon's advisers worried that in the battlefield such weapons would be too unpredictable and might put American soldiers at risk. They felt that the United States had more to gain by outlawing these relatively inexpensive weapons of mass destruction before they proliferated.

On the basis of such reasoning, Nixon terminated the United States bioweapon program in 1970, and threw American support behind a British proposal for a more effective international treaty banning biological warfare. That proposal led to the 1972 pact, and by 1973 all United States stockpiles of weaponized biological agents were destroyed. During the remaining years of the Cold War, accusations of ongoing bioweapon research and development surfaced occasionally on both sides of the East-West conflict, especially after the Sverdlovsk incident. But during the 1980s any unfounded suspicions about biological weapon development seemed far less threatening to global security than the escalating nuclear arms race.

After Sverdlovsk

If knowing the true cause of Sverdlovsk outbreak has taught us anything, it is that biological agents can make powerful and insidious weapons. Aerosolized anthrax is clearly a potent, albeit secretive, killer. If a gram or less of anthrax spores could strike down more than sixty people after a momentary release, how much more harm might occur if a larger dose were dispersed intentionally on an unsuspecting public? In 1993, the United States Office of Technology Assessment (OTA) suggested that the harm could be enormous. The OTA estimated that on a clear, calm night a single light plane fitted with a modified crop sprayer could deliver a fatal dose of anthrax spores to three million people during a short flight over Washington, D.C. A mere 220 pounds of powdered anthrax spores would be required. The plane might be seen on radar, but its deadly payload would be invisible, odorless, and tasteless. There would be no evidence that an attack had even occurred until the first cases of disease appeared in hospitals days later. By that time the bioterrorists would have vanished without a trace.

Meanwhile, on the ground in Washington or any major city hit by an anthrax attack, panic over the fatal epidemic would quickly descend into chaos. Within days the need for tons of antibiotics would exhaust all existing stockpiles. As the death toll mounted, civil disorder in the streets might make the city ungovernable without martial law. In time, the turmoil could threaten the supremacy of the state, undermine investor confidence in world markets, and ultimately plunge the global economy into ruin. Even after the immediate effects had passed, the targeted city might remain uninhabitable for decades. Scotland's Gruinard Island remained off-limits for more than forty years because of viable anthrax spores left over from bioweapon tests in the 1940s. The island was reopened in the late 1980s, but only after an expensive decontamination effort. If the Allies had weaponized anthrax during World War II, parts of Europe and Japan might still be contaminated today.

Perhaps the most disturbing aspect of such apocalyptic scenarios is how relatively simple the production of a biological weapon would be. Techniques to grow bacteria like *B. anthracis* are taught on every university campus. Low-tech recipes for biological weapons can be downloaded from the Internet. A small vial of organisms, obtained from a legitimate research facility or isolated from natural sources in the wild, could be developed into a significant arsenal in a matter of days. Only the barest knowledge of culture methods would be required, along with some fairly conventional laboratory equipment. According to Leonard Cole (1996), a bioweapons policy expert at Rutgers University, "One can cultivate trillions of bacteria at relatively little risk to one's self with gear no more sophisticated than a beer fermenter and a protein-based culture, a gas mask, and a plastic overgarment."

Cole estimates that a covert bioweapons lab could be set up for a paltry $10 thousand. This shop of horrors would occupy a room barely twelve feet across. It is no wonder that biological weapons are sometimes called "the poor man's atom bomb." Probably the most challenging part of developing a weapon would be transforming the chosen agent into a powder suitable for efficient air-borne dissemination. Both the technical know-how needed to produce high-quality aerosols and the expensive milling equipment required to grind up an extremely fine powder are currently out of reach for most domestic terrorist groups. But cruder preparations can be made using equipment readily available today in the biotech industry. Moreover, reckless backyard terrorists might settle for low-technology weapons that lack precise targeting and dispersion capabilities, but would still cause serious havoc. Such was the case when a religious cult unleashed an epidemic of *Salmonella* on a small Oregon community in 1984.

The Widening Circle of Biological Terror

Initially the only country suspected to be breaching the 1972 Biological Weapons Convention was the USSR. But by 1995, at least seventeen countries had active biological weapon programs, according to the OTA. Even the Soviet program turned out to be far more extensive than anyone in the West had imagined. Before the ink dried on the 1972 agreement, the Soviet Politburo set out to create a new bioweapons agency known as Biopreparat, to join the Ministry of Defense in designing offensive biological weapons. Soon the new organization would employ at least fifty thousand people, including many of Russia's top biologists, to oversee research, development, testing, and production of what became an enormous biological armory (Davis 1999). Behind a facade of civilian biotechnology research, Biopreparat established some forty major facilities across the USSR to generate a host of potent new bioweapons, including those that could be mounted on intercontinental ballistic missiles aimed at the United States and other targets. Biopreparat's scientists

Self-Service Salmonella

Wasco County is home to twenty-one thousand people on Oregon's side of the scenic Columbia River Valley. Centered on the small riverside city known as The Dalles, the county is best known locally for its plentiful fruit orchards and large wheat farms. In 1981, Wasco County gained international notoriety when it became the headquarters of the Indian-born guru Bhagwan Shree Rajneesh. The guru's utopian commune, built on one of the county's remote ranches, was controversial from the start. As his "City of Rajneeshpuram" attracted hundreds of disciples from around the world, it quickly encountered stiff opposition from local residents. Elected county commissioners repeatedly turned down the guru's somewhat grandiose land-use plans, and by 1984 tensions in this otherwise quiet rural area threatened to boil over.

In mid-September that year, doctors in The Dalles noted a sudden increase in diarrhea due to *Salmonella* (Torok, Tauxe, Wise, et al. 1997). All the cases, which eventually numbered more than 750, were due to the same species, *S. typhimurium*. When a public health investigation showed that most people who became sick had eaten food from self-serve salad bars during the previous week, all eleven salad bars in the town were promptly shut down. The outbreak ended, but the cause of the ailment remained a mystery. The implicated food items differed among the affected restaurants, and there were no obvious breaches of hygienic food handling anywhere. As none of the usual explanations for such outbreaks panned out, investigators considered the awful possibility that the salad bar foods had been contaminated intentionally. But nothing could be proven at first.

Only months later, when the FBI was investigating the cult on other charges, was it shown that Rajneeshpuram commune members had deliberately prepared cultures of *S. typhimurium* in a clandestine laboratory and secretly poured them on salad bar foods all over the town. A strain of *S. typhimurium* uncovered at the commune's lab was identical to the outbreak strain. Apparently commune members had spiked the salad bar foods to test a plan to incapacitate voters in the county's upcoming local election and influence the outcome of balloting.

Stricter public health regulations may not be sufficient to prevent outbreaks like the one in The Dalles. Salad bars and other sources of self-service foods are especially vulnerable to this amateurish type of bioterrorism. Fortunately, intentional food poisonings are rare events. In the 1960s, several outbreaks of typhoid fever and dysentery in Japan were eventually linked to the deliberate contamination of foods by a malevolent bacteriologist. Four Canadian students became ill in 1970 after their food had been intentionally tainted with the eggs of a large ringworm that normally infects pigs. In 1996, muffins and doughnuts maliciously infected with an unusual variant of *Shigella dysenteriae* were offered anonymously to laboratory workers at a Texas hospital (Kolavic, Kimura, Simons, et al. 1997). All twelve workers who ate the pastries became ill, and four had to be admitted to the hospital for treatment. The source of the pathogen was the laboratory's own freezer.

conducted endless experiments to optimize the dispersion of biological aerosols, and they even used genetic engineering to create modified pathogens of inconceivable virulence.

By 1990, the Soviets could produce two tons of weapon-grade anthrax per day. But Biopreparat remained one of Moscow's most closely guarded secrets and its existence could never be proven until the eve of the Soviet collapse. By contrast, there was no secret about Iraq's nefarious chemical attacks during its war with Iran from 1983 to 1988. The world watched in silence as thousands of innocent civilians fell victim to an extensive barrage of chemical agents. "Fear of an Iranian victory stifled serious outcries against a form of weaponry that had been universally condemned," Cole recalled. As Iraq showed that it could use chemical weapons with impunity, and do so with apparent success in the battlefield, the taboo against hoarding other weapons of mass destruction started to crumble. Using materials imported from the West, Iraq launched its biological weapon program in earnest in 1985 (Zilinskas 1997). Other rogue governments soon followed, unable to pass up the killing power available at comparatively low cost.

At the end of the Persian Gulf War, in 1991, Iraq was ordered to destroy its stockpiles of biological warfare agents. By that time Iraqi scientists had investigated the weapon potential of at least five bacteria, five viruses, and one fungus. Iraq's secret bio-weapon facilities had produced about two thousand gallons of concentrated anthrax solution and five thousand gallons of botulinum toxin, among other projects. Botulinum toxin is a nerve poison formed by the bacteria *Clostridium botulinum*. The toxin, which causes botulism disease when ingested, is thought to be at least one hundred thousand times more toxic than the sarin nerve gas used in the Tokyo subway attack. In all, Iraq put two hundred bombs and twenty-five ballistic missiles loaded with biological agents on stand-by during the 1991 war, but none was used. The Iraqis claim that they terminated their bioweapon program in 1991, but weapon inspectors with the United Nations Special Commission (UNSCOM) have questioned this.

After the war, UNSCOM inspectors supervised the destruction of much of Iraq's nuclear and chemical weapon capacity, although by the time of Operation Desert Fox they had encountered increasing difficulty gaining access to suspected research and production facilities. By contrast, on the eve of the December 1998 air strikes, Iraq's biotechnology infrastructure was still largely intact. Iraq had more than eighty biotech facilities that could easily be converted to military uses, while maintaining their medical or other civilian appearances. With its cadre of dedicated military scientists, it was thought that

Iraq could probably reconstitute a significant bioweapon arsenal in a matter of months. In January 1998, the British foreign secretary had alleged that Iraq was producing enough anthrax spores to fill two missile warheads every week. The cessation of UN inspections has heightened concerns that such production is continuing now, but with no chance of detection. As a precaution, the United States Department of Defense has ordered all 1.5 million Americans serving in the military to be immunized against anthrax. The vaccine requires a primary course of six injections, followed by annual booster doses to maintain immunity. For the moment, United States vaccine supplies are limited to military use.

Home-Grown Bioterrorists

As dangerous as tyrants like Saddam Hussein may seem, recent concerns over biological aggression have been focusing more on groups at the fringes of society, those having no claims of legitimacy to restrain their murderous acts. Recently Richard Butler (1998), the chief UN weapons inspector in Iraq, noted, "Everyone wonders what kinds of delivery systems Iraq may have for biological weapons, but it seems to me that the best delivery system would be a suitcase left on a Washington subway." Most governments, or armed opposition groups with straightforward political agendas, realize that staging a bioweapons attack would jeopardize their public credibility. However, splinter groups or disenchanted individuals guided by less comprehensible aims would have much less to lose in a biological Armageddon. Their indifference to the public's revulsion against their crimes make them that much more dangerous. They are also more difficult for law enforcement agencies to monitor and impede, as the atrocities they may wish to commit are fairly unpredictable.

Religious extremists, particularly those led by charismatic leaders who isolate their followers from mainstream society, may pose the greatest risk, says Jessica Stern (1999). She is a fellow at the Council on Foreign Relations in Washington. "They are unconstrained by fear of government or public backlash, since their actions are carried out to please God and themselves, not to impress a secular constituency, " Stern writes. "Their ultimate objective is to create so much fear and chaos that the government's legitimacy is destroyed. Their victims are often viewed as subhuman since they are outside the group's religion or race." Religious or not, terrorists today seem to be less restrained about committing large-scale murder. "Terrorism has changed," says Brad Roberts in a 1998 interview with *New Scientist*. He is a bioweapons expert at the Institute for Defense Analyses in Virginia. "Traditional terrorists wanted political concessions. But now, some groups say their main aim is mass casualties. That makes biological weapons appealing."

As the prospects for domestic bioterrorism have grown, the FBI and other legal authorities have recently put high-risk groups and individuals under increased scrutiny. In February 1998, two men were arrested in Las Vegas with a cache of anthrax spores in the trunk of their car. One, a microbiologist by training, reportedly had ties to a white supremacist group. He had once told *US News and World Report* that "in this world there are two types of people: the people of God and the Luciferians, and there is no demilitarized zone" (Kaplan 1997). At the time of his arrest he was on probation for wire fraud, after purchasing isolates of *Yersinia pestis*, the bacteria that cause bubonic plague, from a commercial supplier. He had nearly succeeded in acquiring three vials of the bacteria through the mail using nothing but a credit card and a phony letterhead. Publicity around the Las Vegas arrest soon triggered a flood of anthrax-related hoaxes and intimidation. Bioterrorist threats reported to the FBI increased from 75 in 1997 to 150 in 1998. More than 240 threats were reported in just the first four months of 1999. So far such incidents have not caused any injuries or illness, but they can cost up to $100 thousand to investigate and have caused widespread alarm.

Once upon a time it would have seemed impossible that skilled scientists could be recruited into a band of terrorists. But Japan's Aum Shinrikyo religious cult has shattered such delusions. The forty thousand-member sect included many young Japanese biologists, chemists, and other qualified scientists among its rank and file. Under the guidance of a megalomaniac guru, Aum Shinrikyo spent untold millions equipping clandestine laboratories with sophisticated scientific gear. Although sarin gas was chosen for the Tokyo subway assault, the sect's preferred weapons for apocalyptic warfare may have been biological. Before the subway attack, cult members had tried unsuccessfully to release biological agents on the Japanese public on multiple occasions. Police raids on Aum Shinrikyo's facilities in 1995 uncovered a deadly arsenal of botulinum toxin and two radio-controlled drone aircraft equipped with spray tanks. During 1993, some sixteen doctors and nurses belonging to the cult traveled to Zaire on what they called a "medical mission." But the real aim of the trip was to learn all they could about Ebola hemorrhagic fever, and, if possible, bring home samples of the deadly virus (Olsen 1999).

Smallpox: An Endangered Species No More

Aside from anthrax, the most likely agent to be released in a well-orchestrated biological attack today is smallpox. Smallpox has the sinister advantage of spreading readily from person to person, a feature that could vastly enlarge the impact of a single, localized release. There is still no curative treatment for smallpox, and up to 30 percent of cases in an outbreak today would end in a painful death. What's more, many survivors would be blinded or seriously scarred for life. The only defense against smallpox is vaccination, but virtually no one has been vaccinated against the disease since 1980. As protection from the vaccine declines after ten years, only a small fraction of people on Earth now have residual immunity against the disease. The United States stockpile of smallpox vaccine has declined to about six million doses, not nearly enough to protect a population of 271 million. No one anywhere makes the vaccine any more, and even a crash program to redevelop adequate manufacturing capacity would require three years of intensive work.

But wait, you ask, wasn't the smallpox virus eradicated from the world through a multinational effort in the 1970s? Hasn't the World Health Organization declared the planet smallpox free? Surely smallpox couldn't be converted into a biological weapon. Surely this most dreaded virus couldn't stage a comeback now and undo the single greatest public health achievement of the twentieth century. The notion sounds more like a Hollywood movie fantasy than a matter for serious public health concern. Unfortunately, weaponized smallpox is not a figment of screenwriters' imaginations. It now seems certain that the smallpox virus was not contained in the two high-security laboratories where it was imprisoned after eradication. There is convincing evidence that Soviet scientists were developing an arsenal of smallpox weapons, and that clandestine stocks of the virus may exist elsewhere today. For this reason, the WHO has postponed its plan to incinerate the last declared repositories of the virus, on the assumption that retaining the virus could help in the development of new drugs and vaccines.

To imagine the potential havoc resulting from even a minor smallpox release, it is worth considering the outbreak that rocked Yugoslavia in 1972. That year, a pilgrim returning home from Mecca introduced the virus into the country's relatively well-vaccinated population for the first time since 1927. Before doctors correctly diagnosed the disease, 150 people had become infected and could have soon passed the virus to countless others. To limit further spread, Yugoslavia's autocratic government had no choice but to bring normal life to a sudden halt. Military police sealed off villages, set up roadblocks, and converted hotels and apartment buildings into isolation wards. Some ten thousand people who may have been exposed to the virus were kept in quarantine for two weeks or more, while more than twenty million people were revaccinated against the disease. For a time, Yugoslavia's borders with the outside world were completely sealed.

The Yugoslav outbreak was controlled, but would a similar incident in a more open society like ours be contained as successfully? With so little immunity in the population, and such rapid movement of people across borders, an outbreak of smallpox anywhere in the world today would constitute a global emergency. How would we cope? Replenishing vaccine supplies seems a sensible first step. As the editors of the medical journal *The Lancet* (Anonymous 1999) note, the return of smallpox may only be a matter of time. "The threat of smallpox persists, and the world is unprotected and unprepared. Declaring a disease eradicated does not consign it to history," they write.

Responding to the Menace of Biological Weapons

As public policy-makers have recently begun to accept the reality of the bioweapon threat, they have started to weigh society's best options for confronting biological aggression. Preventing attacks before they occur would be ideal, but this may not be possible in every case. For this reason, some analysts stress the importance of early detection and prompt treatment in the event of an attack. "While prevention measures must continue to be pursued, the greatest payoff in fighting biological warfare terrorism lies in improving our response to an incident," says Jeffrey Simon (1997), a California-based terrorism expert. Other specialists emphasize the need for a firm moral stand, backed up by diplomatic maneuvers to strengthen the 1972 Biological Weapons Convention. Perhaps a dual strategy offers the best hope. This approach would combine an unwavering commitment to prevention with improvements in our readiness to manage the consequences of an attack if it occurs.

Preparing for an attack of unknown size in an unknown place from an unknown agent is a daunting exercise, but certain steps in devising an adequate response are obvious. Most importantly, health care professionals must be trained to recognize the signs and symptoms of likely agents, and be ready to report suspected cases to local and national civil defense coordinators. Doctors and nurses will be the first people to realize that a biological attack has occurred. Their rapid assessment of the situation could spell the difference between thousands or tens of thousands of casualties. But as D.A. Henderson (1998) points out, few emergency room personnel today know what to look for. "Few have ever seen so much as a single case of smallpox, plague, or anthrax, or, for that matter, would recall the characteristics of such cases," he says. "Few, if any, diagnostic laboratories are prepared to confirm promptly such diagnoses." Similarly, many local public health departments are ill equipped to distinguish a bioterrorist attack from a natural occurrence. They will need training to investigate the likely sources of unusual disease outbreaks and to communicate critical information to the public through the media in the event of an attack.

The carnage following an act of biological terrorism will probably evoke strong psychological responses in survivors, including panic and demoralization. Medical teams, police and fire departments, and other "first responders" should be trained to deal with the mass hysteria that is likely to arise from even a small incident. Hospitals need to develop biological disaster management plans, much as they now prepare for earthquakes or airline crashes. It will be especially important for hospitals to ensure that they can quickly obtain adequate supplies of suitable antibiotics, antitoxins, and vaccines. Likewise, there must be access to appropriate personal protective gear, such as biosuits and gas masks, and specialized laboratory tests must be available at a moment's notice. Most vital of all, communication links among emergency response agencies must be well tested and effective under all conditions. Strategic planning for civilian bioterrorism isn't a simple exercise. But as Henderson notes, "To remain unprepared is to invite disaster."

Recent progress gives hope that disaster can be averted. In his 1998 State of the Union message, President Bill Clinton said, "We must act to prevent the use of disease as a weapon of war and terror." That year his administration asked Congress to fund a $294 million initiative to improve American readiness for domestic incidents that involve either chemical or biological weapons. The Clinton package, which received additional money in 1999, aims to train and equip specialist health and rescue workers in twenty-five major cities; upgrade local and regional laboratory capacity for identifying suspicious pathogens; expand research on vaccines, diagnostic tests, and therapies effective against likely agents; and build for the first time a civilian stockpile of antibiotics and other medicines ready for deployment as needed. Although some critics suggest the plan does not go far enough, the infusion of cash is welcome news for those seeking to strengthen the country's public health infrastructure, even if acts of biological terrorism never materialize. As President Clinton noted in his speech to the National Academy of Sciences in 1998: "These cutting edge efforts will address not only the threat of weapons of mass destruction, but also the equally serious danger of emerging infectious diseases."

Beyond planning for ways to mitigate the effects of bioweapon offensives, policy-makers must also act collectively to prevent attacks from occurring in the first place. Signatories to the 1972 convention should push for more stringent verification procedures under the pact, including on-site inspections of suspected violators. Controls on the diffusion of biotechnology could be tightened to reduce the chances that essential equipment or deadly organisms fall into the wrong hands. Such measures are bound to help, but they will never be effective by themselves. The cornerstone of preventing the proliferation and use of biological weapons must be to develop a global consensus that affirms that these and other weapons of mass destruction have no place in civilized society. If we, the potential victims of a terrorist act, can express with one voice our moral revulsion to biological weapons, we may yet stay the hand of their savagery. "There is no technical solution to the problem of biological weapons," says Joshua Lederberg (1998), the Nobel biologist who has advised the United States government on emerging infections and biological weapon control (see chapter 1). He says: "It needs an ethical, human, and moral solution if it's going to happen at all. Don't ask me what the odds are for an ethical solution, but there is no other solution."

What You Can Do to Prevent the Spread of Emerging Infections

By now it should be obvious there are limits to what people can do on their own to fight emerging infections. All of the measures cited in the previous boxes at the end of each chapter are worthwhile, but they are not enough by themselves. The threat of disease from acts of terrorism or war exposes the futility of purely individual approaches to emerging infections. No steps we can take as individuals—that is, acting alone—will diminish the growing traffic in microbes resulting from globalized trade. As individuals we cannot stop the emergence of diseases through ecological degradation, climate change, or technological advances in food processing or hospital care. None of us can prevent antigenic shifts in flu viruses or avert the development of antibiotic resistance due to the overuse of these drugs in agribusiness. Safe drinking water, adequate sewage disposal, and protection against the intentional use of biological agents cannot be delegated as individual responsibilities. No one can fight infectious diseases alone.

Our best hope for limiting the spread of emerging infections involves collective action, collaboration that goes beyond what any individuals can achieve in isolation. Just as cities protect themselves from the threat of fire by equipping and training a professional fire department, society's best option for fending off new disease threats will depend on equipping and training a professional public health service. So what can one person do? Certainly it is important to practice good personal hygiene, to prepare your foods safely, to immunize your kids, and be responsible about your sexual behavior. But ultimately the best thing anyone can do to address the problem of emerging infections is to stay aware of the risks and press for a stronger, more skilled, and more responsive public health infrastructure that serves us all. The next chapter looks at ways this can be achieved.

Chapter 12

Responding to the Threats

Microbes were here, learning every trick for survival, two billion years before humans arrived, and it is likely that they will be here two billion years after we depart.

—Richard M. Krause,
National Institutes of Health

When the residents of Venice were threatened with the emergence of bubonic plague during the fourteenth century, their strategy to cope with the problem was fairly straightforward. Starting in 1377, all ships seeking to drop anchor at Venice were required to remain off-shore for a period of forty days, an interval that came to be called *la quarantena*, or quarantine. During such a period of isolation, plague or other infectious diseases that might be incubating aboard incoming ships could be recognized at a safe distance, before they spread to susceptible contacts on shore. The quarantine created a sanitary boundary around the city, and the model was soon adopted throughout the world to prevent the entry of new and dangerous diseases.

Quarantine laws remain on the books in most countries to this day, but in the modern world of high-speed travel and competitive global commerce they are difficult to enforce, if at all. Even if it were possible to detain all new arrivals as Venice once did, diseases with long silent periods of infectivity, such as AIDS and hepatitis C, would still slip through the most austere border controls. These days, the containment of emerging infections is far more complicated than the doges of Venice would have ever imagined. Today no city or country can simply hoist up the gangways that link it to the outside world in the barren hope that its people will escape future pandemics. The challenges that confront us from the microbial world now are too numerous and too immediate to pin all of society's hopes on such simplistic and archaic disease control models as quarantine. Today's challenges call for the best responses humanity can muster. They demand our concerted attention, our most clever thinking, and our most sincere commitment. There will be no quick fix in today's life-and-death struggle with infectious diseases.

"The problems we face in devising strategies to cope with new or emerging infections are as complex as the threats posed by the agents themselves," says D. A. Henderson (1994), director of the bioweapons think tank at Johns Hopkins University. "I cannot visualize a single 'magic bullet' or a simple straightforward blueprint as an adequate approach." Henderson, who once led the global campaign to eradicate smallpox, knows how difficult it is to mobilize the diverse members of the human family to beat back a microbial foe. Addressing the problem of emerging infections in the twenty-first century is not going to be easy: "It demands a great deal more than an augmented research grants portfolio, a few training programs, a laboratory or two, or mild international interest," he says.

The first step in confronting emerging infections is to increase public awareness of the real threats. As we have seen in this book, the hazards of emerging diseases are not theoretical, nor are they far off in the future. We are not talking about the collision of the Earth with an asteroid, or the hypothetical dangers posed by eating genetically modified foods. We are talking about real events that are already happening, events that are already touching our homes and neighborhoods to some degree. Chances are high that you, or someone you know, has been infected with an emerging pathogen, or one that was resistant to drugs that were once effective. If anyone in America is still taking for granted humanity's subjugation of infectious diseases, it is time to discard such delusive thoughts. Moreover, it is time to bring into the open the truth about the new microbial threats to human health and get people from all walks of life to talk together about what can be done.

On the other hand, it is all too easy to overstate the dangers. There is already a vague, free-floating anxiety in the public about unseen armies of malevolent infectious agents that seem to arise inexplicably from the abyss. Dramatic news media coverage of plagues like Ebola hemorrhagic fever and mad cow disease, sensational new science-fiction books, and blockbuster movies based on infectious disease themes have all played on such fears. The distorted pictures of emerging infections portrayed on television screens, in novels, and in cinema halls have raised the public profile of the problem, but they may not be contributing to constructive solutions. It would be far more empowering for people to understand the real dangers we face from the microbial world, and to recognize the ways that human activities are contributing to emerging infections today. This book is aimed at encouraging that understanding.

Building a Better Defense against Emerging Infections

Once health professionals and the public at large recognize the significance of the infectious disease threat, they begin to see what a tenuous hold the current public health system has on preventing potentially devastating epidemics. Constructive action to prevent a crisis from emerging diseases clearly requires a renewed commitment to many of the traditional activities of public health that have recently lost their luster. It also requires greater use of new tools and technologies, such as electronic communications and innovations in molecular biology, to identify and track dangerous pathogens. Finally, it requires partnership and collaboration, a joining of hands across the community to prepare for the unexpected and promote a healthier future. Partners in the combat against emerging infections must include health departments, health care providers, research institutions, private industry, international governments, and non-governmental organizations. But the partnership shouldn't stop there. At a local level, we must also involve schools, faith communities, the media, and families. Everyone in an informed and motivated public has a vital role to play.

Fortunately, the world's two foremost public health agencies are rising to the challenge of infectious disease, and have recently laid the groundwork for leading a new offensive against microbial emergence in the new millennium. In 1998, the CDC launched a multifaceted strategy under the slogan "watch, learn, prepare, act." This plan, titled *Preventing Emerging Infectious Diseases: A Strategy for the Twenty-First Century*, was an update of the agency's first blueprint on preventing new infections released in 1994. In 1999, the World Health Organization (WHO) outlined its strategy in a document titled *Removing Obstacles to Healthy Development*. Both approaches call for a redoubling of public health efforts to increase our watchfulness for microbial threats, to improve our knowledge about how and why diseases emerge, and to build up the global capacity to investigate disease outbreaks and implement prevention and control programs.

The new strategies will cost money. Luckily the tax-paying public now seems predisposed to restoring the public-health muscle needed to control infectious hazards, according to two telephone surveys (Centers for Disease Control and Prevention 1998f). One survey, conducted by Louis Harris and Associates on one thousand randomly selected adults, found that "preventing the spread of infectious diseases" was ranked as a "very important" public health service by 93 percent of respondents. No other public health service attracted so many high rankings. The other survey, conducted by the Field Institute, surveyed a representative sample of forty-eight hundred Californians. It found that "ensuring safe drinking water" and "ensuring that foods are free from contamination," were the two public health services considered to be "top priority" by the most respondents (84 percent and 77 percent, respectively). In contrast, only one-third of the respondents thought the public health system was "very effective" at delivering those services at present.

How then should we act? There are three crucial elements in the CDC and WHO strategies: surveillance, applied research, and the upgrading of the public health infrastructure with improved training and equipment. Let's consider each of these briefly.

Surveillance

The cornerstone of an effective public health response to emerging infections is the ability to detect diseases as they occur and sound the alarm for action. Like early warning systems that detect military threats to national security, disease surveillance systems function like radar for tracking new and unusual infections in the population. Early detection of emerging diseases is important because it buys time to implement appropriate responses, before epidemics become out of control. It tells you where a threat is emerging, how it is moving, and who is at risk. It provides early evidence of how new diseases arise, how they spread, and how they can be stopped. Surveillance may never be perfect enough to intercept all emerging infections before they erupt in serious epidemics. For instance, it would have been hard to anticipate the emergence of HIV even if the best network of laboratories and epidemiologists had been on fulltime alert for new diseases. But it is a safe bet that improved monitoring of trends in disease diagnosis, vector distribution, hospital infections, antibiotic resistance, and vaccine coverage would go a long way toward early identification of most potential new threats.

If the proposed strategies are implemented, new technologies will be at the heart of tomorrow's surveillance systems. Disease reports that are now stored in a myriad of electronic databases in laboratories, hospitals, and health departments will be integrated at a state or national level to give a clearer overall picture of changing trends. Recently developed molecular techniques, such as DNA fingerprinting, will also play a larger role. These techniques can rapidly distinguish subtle differences among various strains of the same infectious organisms. With access to this technology, public health departments can begin to identify outbreaks scattered over wide geographic areas, outbreaks that might otherwise have gone undetected. This is especially important for controlling food-borne diseases. As we saw in chapter 6, high output technologies have created a new outbreak scenario in which widely distributed foods are contaminated at relatively low levels. Since 1998, a national network of laboratories has begun to share the DNA fingerprints of bacteria they have isolated from patients and contaminated foods. When fingerprints submitted by two participating labs match up, a computer alerts health departments nearby that an outbreak may be underway.

Applied Research

Most of the stories recounted in this book are drawn from the published results of applied research into new and resurgent diseases. Much has been learned about the factors related to the emergence of these diseases, but much more remains to be discovered. Without understanding the behaviors, environments, and genetic factors that create opportunities for new infections to emerge and spread, there is little chance that we will prevent or control them. Research needs are particularly acute for new clinical tests that can offer accurate, fast, and inexpensive diagnoses. For some diseases it is not yet possible to distinguish past infection from current infection. For others the available tests are too expensive or too unreliable for routine use. Research is also needed to develop new vaccines, new antibiotics, and new strategies to reduce insect vectors and control animal reservoirs of disease. Public health interventions like food irradiation, new treatments for drinking water, sexual health counseling, and promotion of childhood immunization all need rigorous testing and evaluation to optimize best practice. New, more effective interventions must be devised when past solutions are no longer working.

Infrastructure and Training

Sizeable investments are needed to train and equip the local, state, and federal public health workforce to protect us from emerging infections. Momentous changes in disease incidence and advances in disease control methods demand that public health professionals routinely receive in-service training to keep up to date. In every large community we need well-trained people who can investigate outbreaks of disease, test the safety of our food and water, and educate the public about reducing infection risks. Advanced training for laboratory scientists and field-oriented epidemiologists is particularly important. Professional career opportunities in public health must be given a higher profile in high schools, colleges, and schools of medicine, nursing, dentistry, and veterinary medicine.

Beyond this, we need to build more clinical laboratories, equipped with the latest technologies to detect and characterize agents of disease. Specialized tests need not be available at every laboratory, but such services must be readily accessible anywhere in the country through larger regional laboratories. We need more investment in hardware and software to build new computer networks, and we need the know-how to use them. Only with such networks in place can we maximize the benefits of new integrated surveillance systems and speed up communication among those charged with monitoring disease patterns. We need well-trained staff and adequate supplies in every community to control mosquitoes, rodents, and other carriers of disease. Finally, we need an unequivocal commitment from the government to provide effective health care services for people with tuberculosis, sexually transmitted diseases, and dependence on drugs. The health and well-being of the population in the twenty-first century will depend on our commitment to rejuvenate America's public health infrastructure today.

"Submerging" Diseases

Not all the news about infectious diseases is doom and gloom. Well-coordinated public health efforts today are successfully preventing small outbreaks of emerging diseases from becoming much larger. Nearly all of the recent outbreaks cited in this book could have spread much further than they did but for rapid public health action. Local lessons learned in controlling new diseases are now incorporated quickly into public health practice throughout the United States and around the world. For example, when evidence showed that zidovudine treatment of HIV-positive pregnant women reduced the risk of transmitting the virus to their babies by 66 percent, HIV counseling and voluntary testing of all pregnant women immediately became a standard practice. Since then, the United States incidence of pediatric AIDS has been reduced by more than 40 percent.

Today many once-common infections are coming under control thanks to the dedicated work of international public health partnerships. Such diseases aren't emerging; they are "submerging," and one day they may disappear completely. We have already discussed the global eradication of smallpox and the near-eradication of polio. Other diseases that are rapidly reaching the end of the line because of ongoing public health efforts include:

Guinea-Worm Disease

Guinea-worm disease, also known as dracunculiasis, is an infection of the skin and deeper tissues caused by a large worm. Although dracunculiasis was once common in more than one hundred countries, the incidence of the disease has dropped by 95 percent since 1986 due to an active campaign of containing cases and providing safe drinking water to reduce exposure. Today the disease persists in only a few African countries where war and social upheaval have prevented complete eradication.

Leprosy

This much-feared and stigmatizing disease has disappeared from all but 28 of the 122 countries where it was still prevalent in the 1980s. Almost ten million people have been cured in the past fifteen years, bringing the number infected worldwide to under one million in 1998. However, more than half a million new cases still occur each year, mostly in India. Public health efforts to eliminate leprosy transmission must continue.

Neonatal Tetanus

Neonatal Tetanus is a fatal disease of newborn babies that has been eliminated in more than one hundred countries. But as we saw in chapter 5, it continues to kill almost three hundred thousand babies each year in nearly fifty countries. Complete control of neonatal tetanus will require continued outreach to immunize women during pregnancy and ensure they have access to safe maternity and newborn services.

Among the other diseases we have discussed in this book, those succumbing to public health offensives today are onchocerciasis, Chagas disease, and measles. More than 90 percent of children in the western hemisphere are now immunized against measles, and global momentum is building for the total eradication of this disease in the next few years. Today, for the first time, it now seems conceivable that the measles virus —perhaps a bigger killer of children than any other single microbe—will one day go the way of smallpox.

Learning More and Taking the Lead

Our understanding of emerging infectious diseases is constantly changing. New infections appear in new places, and new advances in knowledge are gained from every new attempt to control them. Just when it seems nothing could surprise you any more, an African virus shows up on the streets of New York City. The microbial world is full of new surprises, and maybe that's why the study of emerging diseases is so fascinating. No book can stay at the cutting edge of such a dynamic field. Fortunately there are plenty of readily available sources of information that can carry on where this book leaves off. Surveillance data, reports on outbreak investigations, and results of applied research are obtainable by anyone with an interest who knows where to look. Increasingly, the World Wide Web is a rich source of up-to-date public health intelligence from disease control agencies throughout the world. The World Health Organization, the Centers for Disease Control and Prevention, and numerous other state and local public health departments now maintain user-friendly Web sites packed with useful information. A list of key Web sites relevant to infectious disease control can be found in the appendix.

Another important source of late-breaking information is the International Program for Monitoring Emerging Infectious Diseases (ProMED). ProMED operates a computerized network that distributes numerous electronic postings each day on infectious disease occurrences from around the globe. The service, established in 1994 by the Federation of American Scientists, is available free of charge to anyone with an Internet connection. ProMED now has more than fifteen thousand subscribers from more than 140 countries. Details on subscribing are given in the appendix.

As we learn more about emerging diseases and join the movement advocating for a stronger, more flexible public health system, we are bound to cross boundaries. Emerging disease is not simply a health problem, and solutions cannot be limited to the health sector. Economic and social policies have as much to contribute to the prevention of new and resurgent infections as strategies arising from the traditional domains concerned with health. In fact, new initiatives in employment, education, and housing may do more to reduce the burden of infectious diseases than any purely medical approaches, however well-intentioned. Public health practitioners and others concerned about infectious diseases also need to interact more with environmental scientists to tackle the infectious disease risks emerging from degradation of the physical environment.

Similarly, emerging disease is not just an American problem. Solutions cannot be limited to any one region, one state, or one country. Our public health interests in the United States are intrinsically connected to people across the world whom we will never see, in places we have never heard of. Just as our perspective must be broadened to see beyond the traditional boundaries of public health, so must our perspective be broadened to remain alert to the emergence of diseases in countries far beyond our shores. We must be prepared to collaborate with people overseas to monitor disease occurrence and to contribute quickly to outbreak investigations and control activities. International networks like ProMED are good beginnings. More bridge building is needed. Americans have everything to gain from taking a lead in the international battle against infectious diseases, just as the United States has taken the lead economically and politically during the past century. The need for resolute leadership has never been greater.

Already the topic of emerging infections is on the agenda of high-level international bodies, such as the Group of Eight Industrialized Nations (G8) and the forum for Asia-Pacific Economic Cooperation (APEC). In the end, the worldwide spread of infectious diseases may do more to draw together people of different races, religions, nationalities, and language groups than all the international treaties, alliances, and common markets thus far attempted. To microbial pathogens, all humans are essentially the same, regardless of skin color, faith, birthplace, or tongue. In the swarm of human pathogens arrayed against us—both agents known and unknown—humanity has a common enemy. Differences that divide us only work to the enemy's advantage. The competitive model that drives so many human relations today may in the end defeat us, unless we seize the opportunity now to work together for the good of all.

Appendix

On-line Resources in Emerging Infectious Diseases

Federal Government Sites

Centers for Disease Control and Prevention
   http://www.cdc.gov
Department of Health and Human Services
   http://os.dhhs.gov
Environmental Protection Agency
   http://www.epa.gov
Food and Drug Administration
   http://www.fda.gov
Food Safety and Inspection Service, Department of Agriculture
   http://www.fsis.usda.gov
National Institutes of Health
   http://www.nih.gov
National Library of Medicine
   http://www.nlm.nih.gov

Selected State Health Department Sites

California Department of Health Services
   http://www.dhs.cahwnet.gov

Florida Department of Health
http://www.doh.state.fl.us

Illinois Department of Public Health
http://www.idph.state.il.us

Massachusetts Department of Public Health
http://www.state.ma.us/dph/dphhome.htm

Minnesota Department of Health
http://www.health.state.mn.us

New York State Department of Health
http://www.health.state.ny.us

Ohio Department of Health
http://www.odh.state.oh.us

Pennsylvania Department of Health
http://www.health.state.pa.us

Washington State Department of Health
http://www.doh.wa.gov

For other states, go to the Centers for Disease Control and Prevention site above.

International Sites

World Health Organization

WHO Communicable Disease Surveillance and Response
http://www.who.int/emc/

WHO Disease Outbreak News
http://www.who.int/emc/outbreak_news/index.html

WHO Initiative on HIV/AIDS and STDs
http://www.who.int/asd/

WHO National Influenza Centres (FluNet)
http://oms.b3e.jussieu.fr/flunet/

International Government/Organization Sites

Australian National Centre for Disease Control
http://www.health.gov.au/pubhlth/cdi/cdihtml.htm

French Ministry of Health ("Sentiweb" in English)
http://www.b3e.jussieu.fr/sentiweb/en
Health Canada
http://www.hc-sc.gc.ca
Hong Kong Department of Health
http://www.info.gov.hk/dh
Israeli Ministry of Health
http://www.health.gov.il/welcome.html
Japanese Infectious Disease Surveillance Center
http://idsc.nih.go.jp
Malaysian Department of Public Health
http://dph.gov.my
Mexican Secretariat of Health (Secretaria de Salud)
http://cenids.ssa.gob.mx
New Zealand Ministry of Health
http://www.moh.govt.nz
Pan American Health Organization
http://www.paho.org
Singapore Ministry of Health
http://www.gov.sg/moh
Taiwan Department of Health
http://www.doh.gov.tw/english
United Kingdom Department of Health
http://www.doh.gov.uk/dhhome.htm
United Kingdom Public Health Laboratory Service
http://www.phls.co.uk

International Travel Information

Centers for Disease Control and Prevention
http://www.cdc.gov/travel
International Society of Travel Medicine
http://www.istm.org
Medical College of Wisconsin International Travelers Clinic
http://www.intmed.mcw.edu/travel.html
Travel Health Online
http://www.tripprep.com
United Kingdom Department of Health
http://www.doh.gov.uk/hat/hatcvr.htm

WHO International Travel and Health
http://www.who.int/ith/index.html

Electronic Journals Related to Emerging Infections

American Journal of Public Health
http://www.apha.org/news/publications/journal/AJPH2.html

Australian Communicable Disease Intelligence (CDI)
http://www.health.gov.au/pubhealth/cdi/cdihtml.htm

BMJ (Journal of the British Medical Association)
http://www.bmj.com

Canadian Communicable Disease Report (CCDR)
http://www.hc-sc.gc.ca/hpb/lcdc/publicat/ccdr

Emerging Infectious Diseases, CDC
http://www.cdc.gov/ncidod/eid/index.htm

Eurosurveillance Weekly
http://www.eurosurv.org/update

JAMA (Journal of the American Medical Association)
http://www.jama.com

Journal of Infectious Diseases
http://www.journals.uchicago.edu/JID

Lancet
http://www.thelancet.com

MMWR (Morbidity and Mortality Report)
http://www2.cdc.gov/mmwr

Nature
http://www.nature.com

New England Journal of Medicine
http://www.nejm.org

New Scientist
http://www.newscientist.com

Science
http://sciencemag.org

Scientific American
http://www.sciam.com

UK Communicable Disease Report (CDR)
http://www.phls.co.uk/publications/cdr.htm

WHO Weekly Epidemiological Record
http://www.who.int/wer/index.html

Other Online Resources

Alliance for the Prudent Use of Antibiotics
http://www.healthsci.tufts.edu.apua

American Association of Blood Banks
http://www.aabb.org

American Public Health Association
http://www.apha.org

American Society for Microbiology
http://www.asmusa.org

Council of State and Territorial Epidemiologists (CSTE)
http://www.cste.org

Emerging Infections Information Network, Yale University
http://info.med.yale.edu/EIINet

Johns Hopkins Infectious Diseases
http://hopkins-id.edu

Global Health Network
http://www.pitt.edu/HOME/GHNet

Infectious Diseases Society of America (IDSA)
http://www.idsociety.org

Medscape
http://www.medscape.com

Outbreak
http://www.outbreak.org

ProMED
http://www.healthnet.org/programs/promed.html#archives

Subscribing to ProMED

ProMED is an electronic mail conference that provides subscribers
with daily messages on emerging infectious disease topics. A panel of
experts moderates the discussions so that only suitable messages are
posted. There is no fee for the service.

To subscribe, simply go to the ProMED Web site listed above, or
send an e-mail message to majordomo@usa.healthnet.org and type
the message "subscribe promed."

Glossary of acronyms

AIDS	acquired immunodeficiency syndrome
APEC	Asia-Pacific Economic Cooperation
BPF	Brazilian purpuric fever
BSE	bovine spongiform encephalopathy
CDC	Centers for Disease Control and Prevention
CJD	Creutzfeldt-Jakob disease
CMV	cytomegalovirus
DDT	1,1,1-trichloro-2,2-bis(p-chlorophenyl)ethane
DEET	N,N-diethyl-metatoluamide
DHF	dengue hemorrhagic fever
DNA	deoxyribonucleic acid
DTP	diphtheria toxoid, tetanus toxoid, pertussis vaccine
DTaP	diphtheria toxoid, tetanus toxoid, acellular pertussis vaccine
ENSO	El Niño Southern Oscillation
EPA	Environmental Protection Agency
EU	European Union
EV7	1enterovirus 71
FBI	Federal Bureau of Investigation
FDA	Food and Drug Administration
FSE	feline spongiform encephalopathy
G8	Group of Eight Industrialized Nations
GATT	General Agreement on Tariffs and Trade
GDP	gross domestic product
GISA	glycopeptide intermediate-resistant *Staphylococcus aureus*

HFMD	hand, foot, and mouth disease
Hib	*Haemophilus influenzae* type b
HIV	human immunodeficiency virus
HPS	hantavirus pulmonary syndrome
HPV	human papillomavirus
HSV-2	herpes simplex virus type 2
HUS	hemolytic uremic syndrome
IDU	injecting drug user
IOM	Institute of Medicine
JRA	juvenile rheumatoid arthritis
KGB	Committee of State Security, USSR
MBM	meat-and-bone meal
MDR-TB	multidrug-resistant tuberculosis
MMR	measles, mumps, rubella vaccine
MRSA	methicillin-resistant *Staphylococcus aureus*
MWW	Milwaukee Water Works
NTU	nephelometric turbidity units
OTA	Office of Technology Assessment
PID	pelvic inflammatory disease
PPNG	penicillinase-producing *Neisseria gonorrhoeae*
ProMED	Program for Monitoring Emerging Infectious Diseases
PRSP	penicillin-resistant *Streptococcus pneumoniae*
RhIG	Rh$_o$D immune globulin
RNA	ribonucleic acid
SE	*Salmonella enteritidis*
SLE	St. Louis encephalitis
STD	sexually transmitted disease
TSS	toxic shock syndrome
UNSCOM	United Nations Special Commission
vCJD	variant Creutzfeldt-Jakob disease
VRE	vancomycin-resistant enterococci
WHO	World Health Organization

Bibliography

Aaskov J. G, J. U. Mataika, G. W. Lawrence, et al. 1981. An epidemic of Ross River virus infection in Fiji, 1979. *American Journal of Tropical Medicine and Hygiene* 30: 1053-9.

Abbasi, K. 1999. The World Bank and world health: healthcare strategy. *BMJ* 318: 933-6.

Abilek K. and S. Handelman. 1999. *Biohazard: The Chilling True Story of the Largest Covert Biological Weapons Program in the World—Told from the Inside by the Man Who Ran it.* New York: Random House.

Abramova F.A., L. M. Grinberg, O. V. Yampolskaya, et al. 1993. Pathology of inhalational anthrax in 42 cases from the Sverdlovsk outbreak of 1979. *Proceedings of the National Academy of Sciences of the United States of America* 90: 2291-4.

Agerton T., S. Valway, B. Gore, et al. 1997. Transmission of a highly drug-resistant strain (strain W1) of Mycobacterium tuberculosis. *JAMA* 278: 1073-7.

Aiyar S. 1998. Dengue–Thailand. ProMED-mail post, 6 January.

Alexander J. L. 1998. Plague, pet prairie dogs – USA (Texas). ProMED-mail post, 10 July.

Almond J. and J. Pattison. 1997. Human BSE. *Nature* 389: 437-8.

Almond J. Cited by BBC World Television. 1996. The great British beef fiasco. Panorama, September.

Altekruse S. F., N. J. Stern, P. I. Fields, et al. 1999. *Campylobacter jejuni*–an emerging foodborne pathogen. *Emerging Infectious Diseases* 5: 28-35.

American Meat Institute. 1996. *Putting the food-handling issue on the table: the pressing need for food safety education.* Washington: American Meat Institute.

American Society for Microbiology. 1996. *Americans get caught dirty handed.* Washington: American Society for Microbiology.

Anonymous. 1999. Is smallpox history? *The Lancet* 353: 1539.

Anonymous. Cited by A. J. Bollet. 1987. *Plagues & Poxes: The Rise and Fall of Epidemic Disease.* New York: Demos Publications.

Arias J. R., P. S. Monteiro, F. Zicker. 1996. The reemergence of visceral leishmaniasis in Brazil. *Emerging Infectious Diseases* 2: 145-6.

Barnes P. F., Z. Yang, J. M. Pogoda, et al. 1999. Foci of tuberculosis transmission in central Los Angeles. *American Journal of Respiratory and Critical Care Medicine* 159: 1081-6.

Barrett-Connor E. 1979. Infectious and chronic disease epidemiology: separate and unequal? *American Journal of Epidemiology* 109: 245-9.

Bartlett J.G. 1997. Infectious diseases. *JAMA* 277: 1865-6.

Bauchner H., S. I. Pelton, J. O. Klein. 1999. Parents, physicians, and antibiotic use. *Pediatrics* 103: 395-401.

BBC World Television. 1996. The great British beef fiasco. Panorama, September.

Beck J. Cited by T. Johnson. 1993. Rodent-borne virus is a killer, but control lags. *Pest Control*, August, 24-7.

Bell B. P., M. Goldoft, P. M. Griffin, et al. 1994. A multistate outbreak of *Escherichia coli* O157:H7 - associated bloody diarrhea and hemolytic uremic syndrome from hamburgers: the Washington experience. *JAMA* 272: 1349-53.

Bellamy C. Cited by J. Wise. 1999. Unicef warns of polio risk in conflict regions. *BMJ* 319: 214.

Bollet A .J. 1987. *Plagues and Poxes: The Rise and Fall of Epidemic Disease.* New York: Demos Publications.

Bouma M. J., C. Dye. 1997. Cycles of malaria associated with El Niño in Venezuela. *JAMA* 278: 1772-4.

Bouma M. J., H. J. van der Kaay. 1996. The El Niño Southern Oscillation and the historic malaria epidemics in the Indian subcontinent and Sri Lanka: an early warning system for future epidemics? *Tropical Medicine and International Health* 1: 86-96.

Brazilian Purpuric Fever Study Group. 1987. Brazilian purpurpic fever: epidemic purpura fulminans associated with antecedent purulent conjunctivitis. *The Lancet* 2: 757-63.

Breiman R. F. 1996. Impact of technology on the emergence of infectious diseases. *Epidemiologic Reviews* 18: 4-9.

Breman J. 1995. From 1976 to 1995: an alumnus' perspective on Ebola. *EIS Bulletin*, Fall, 8-9.

British Medical Association. Cited by W. Barnaby. 1999. Blood on their hands. *New Scientist*, 30 January, 45.

Broder S. 1988. Pathogenic human retroviruses. *New England Journal of Medicine* 318: 243-5.

Brown P. 1992. Parasites move in when forests are cleared. *New Scientist*, 10 October, 5.

Brundtland G. H., speaking at World Federation of Public Health Associations, October 1997. Cited by N. Unwin, G. Alberti, T. Aspray, et al. 1998. Economic globalisation and its effects on health: some diseases could be eradicated for the cost of a couple of fighter planes. *BMJ* 316: 1401-2.

Buller R. S., M. Arens, S. P. Hmiel, et al. 1999. *Ehrlichia ewingii,* a newly recognized agent of human ehrlichiosis. *New England Journal of Medicine* 341: 148-55.

Burnet M. 1953. *The Natural History of Infectious Disease,* 2nd ed. Cambridge: Cambridge University Press. Cited by S. Lang. 1998. Infectious diseases. *New Ethicals Journal* 1: 17-18.

Burstein G. R., C. A. Gaydos, M. Diener-West, et al. 1998. Incident *Chlamydia trachomatis* infections among inner-city adolescent females. *JAMA* 280: 521-6.

Butler R. Cited by R. Preston. 1998. The bioweaponeers. *The New Yorker,* 9 March, 52-65.

Carlton J. T. and J. B. Geller. 1993. Ecological roulette: the global transport of nonindigenous marine organisms. *Science* 261: 78-82.

Centers for Disease Control. 1985. Fatal degenerative neurologic disease in patients who received pituitary derived human growth hormone. *MMWR* 34: 359-66.

Centers for Disease Control. 1986. Hepatitis B associated with jet gun injection – California. *MMWR* 35: 373-6.

Centers for Disease Control and Prevention. 1993. Imported cholera associated with a newly described toxigenic *Vibrio cholerae* O139 strain – California, 1993. *MMWR* 42: 516-7.

Centers for Disease Control and Prevention. 1997a. Outbreaks of leptospirosis among white-water rafters – Costa Rica, 1996. *MMWR* 46: 577-9.

Centers for Disease Control and Prevention. 1997b. Nosocomial hepatitis B virus infection associated with reusable fingerstick blood sampling devices – Ohio and New York City, 1996. *MMWR* 46: 217-21.

Centers for Disease Control and Prevention. 1998a. Trends in sexual risk behaviors among high school students – United States, 1991-1997. *MMWR* 47: 749-52.

Centers for Disease Control and Prevention. 1998b. Nosocomial *Burkholderia cepacia* infection and colonization associated with intrinsically contaminated mouthwash – Arizona, 1998. *MMWR* 47: 926-8.

Centers for Disease Control and Prevention. 1998c. Deaths among children during an outbreak of hand, foot, and mouth disease – Taiwan, Republic of China, April-July 1998. *MMWR* 47: 629-32.

Centers for Disease Control and Prevention. 1998d. Outbreak of cryptosporidiosis associated with a water sprinkler fountain. Minnesota, 1997. *MMWR* 47: 856:60.

Centers for Disease Control and Prevention. 1998e. *Preventing Emerging Infectious Diseases: a Strategy for the 21st Century.* Atlanta: Centers for Disease Control and Prevention.

Centers for Disease Control and Prevention. 1998f. Public opinion about public health – California and the United States, 1996. *MMWR* 47: 69-73.

Centers for Disease Control and Prevention. 1999. *National Center for HIV, STD, and TB Prevention News and Notes* 1:14.

Centers for Disease Control and Prevention. 1999a. Outbreaks of *Shigella son-nei* infection associated with eating fresh parsley – United States and Canada, July-August 1998. *MMWR* 48: 285-9.

Centers for Disease Control and Prevention. 1999b. Trichinellosis outbreaks – Northrhine-Westfalia, Germany, 1998-1999. *MMWR* 48: 488-92.

Centers for Disease Control and Prevention. 1999c. Outbreaks of gastrointestinal illness of unknown etiology associated with eating burritos – United States, October 1997-October 1998. *MMWR* 48: 210-3.

Centers for Disease Control and Prevention. 1999d. Four pediatric deaths from community-acquired methicillin-resistant *Staphylococcus aureus* – Minnesota and North Dakota, 1997-1999. *MMWR* 48: 707-10.

Centers for Disease Control and Prevention. 1999e. Outbreak of *Escherichia coli* O157:H7 and *Campylobacter* among attendees of the Washington County fair – New York, 1999. *MMWR* 48: 803.

Centers for Disease Control and Prevention. 1999f. Multiple human exposures to a rabid bear cub at a petting zoo and barnwarming – Iowa, August 1999. *MMWR* 48: 761.

Chanteau S., L. Ratsifasoamanana, B. Rasoamanana, et al. 1998. Plague, a ree-merging disease in Madagascar. *Emerging Infectious Diseases* 4: 101-4.

Chen L. C. 1994. New diseases: the human factor. *Annals of the New York Academy of Sciences* 740: 319-24.

Childs J. Cited by H. Saul. 1996. Year of the rat. *New Scientist*, 5 October, 32-7.

Christopher G. W., T. J. Cieslak, Pavlin J. A., et al. 1997. Biological warfare: a historical perspective. *JAMA* 278: 412-7.

Cohen M. S. 1998. Sexually transmitted diseases enhance HIV transmission: no longer a hypothesis. *The Lancet* 351: (Suppl III) 5-7.

Cole L. A. 1996. The specter of biological weapons. *Scientific American*, December, 30-5.

Collinge J. 1999. Variant Creutzfeldt-Jakob disease. *The Lancet* 354: 317-23.

Collins J. E. 1997. Impact of changing consumer lifestyles on the emergence/reemergence of food-borne pathogens. *Emerging Infectious Diseases* 3: 471-9.

Colwell R. R. 1996. Global climate and infectious disease: the cholera paradigm. *Science* 274: 2025-31.

Cope, S. E., et al. 1993. Status of *Aedes aegypti* in the Republic of Djibouti. *Proceedings of the Meeting of the American Mosquito Control Association*.

Curtis C. F., G. B. White. 1984. *Plasmodium falciparum* transmission in England: entomological and epidemiological data relative to cases in 1983. *Journal of Tropical Medicine and Hygiene* 87: 101-14.

Davey R. Cited by S. Gottlieb. 1999. U.S. considers ban on British blood. *BMJ* 318: 1574.

Davis C. J. 1999. Nuclear blindness: an overview of the biological weapons programs of the former Soviet Union and Iraq. *Emerging Infectious Diseases* 5: 509-12.

De Souza Lopes O., L. de Abreu Sacchetta, D. B. Francy, et al. 1981. Emergence of a new arbovirus disease in Brazil. III Isolation of rocio virus from

Psorophora ferox (Humboldt, 1819). *American Journal of Epidemiology* 113: 122-5.

Detwiler L. Cited by S. Gottlieb. 1999. U.S. considers ban on British blood. *BMJ* 318: 1574.

Dickson N., C. Paul, P. Herbison, et al. 1996. The lifetime occurrence of sexually transmitted diseases among a cohort aged 21. *New Zealand Medical Journal* 109: 308-12.

Diermayer M., K. Hedberg, F. Hoesly, et al. 1999. Epidemic serogroup B meningococcal disease in Oregon: the evolving epidemiology of the ET-5 strain. *JAMA* 281: 1493-7.

Duchin J. S., F. T. Koster F.T., C. J. Peters, et al. 1994. Hantavirus pulmonary syndrome: a clinical description of 17 patients with a newly recognized disease. *New England Journal of Medicine* 330: 949-55.

Dunne E. F., M. Weidmann, D. Morse, et al. 1999. A multistate outbreak of listeriosis traced to processed meats, August 1998-February 1999. Late-breaking report, 48th Annual Epidemic Intelligence Service Conference, Atlanta.

Easton A. 1997. El Niño causes diarrhoea outbreaks. *BMJ* 315: 1485.

Easton A. 1999. Leptospirosis in Philippine floods. *BMJ* 319: 212.

Engelthaler D. M., D. G. Mosley, J. E. Cheek, et al. 1999. Climatic and environmental patterns associated with hantavirus pulmonary syndrome, Four Corners region, United States. *Emerging Infectious Diseases* 5: 87-94.

Engelthaler D. M., T. M. Fink, C. E. Levy, et al. 1997. The reemergence of *Aedes aegypti* in Arizona. *Emerging Infectious Diseases* 3: 241-2.

English R. and G. Foster. 1997. *Living with Hepatitis C*. London: Robinson. Cited by D. Walford and N. Noah. 1999. Emerging infectious diseases – United Kingdom. *Emerging Infectious Diseases* 5: 189-94.

Epstein P. 1998. Weeds bring disease to the east African waterways. *The Lancet* 351: 577.

Epstein P. R. Cited by C. Ezzell C. 1999. It came from the deep. *Scientific American*, June, 18-19.

Evans M. 1999. Cited in Measles, deliberate exposures–UK (Wales). ProMED-mail post, 7 September.

Faruque S. M. and J. Albert. 1992. Genetic relation between *Vibrio cholerae* 01 strains in Ecuador and Bangladesh. *The Lancet* 339: 740-1.

Fleming D. T., G. M. McQuillan, R. E. Johnson, et al. 1997. Herpes simplex virus type 2 in the United States, 1976 to 1994. *New England Journal of Medicine* 337: 1105-11.

Ford T. Cited by V. Kiernan. 1996. Wealthy nations face drinking water crisis. *New Scientist*, 1 June, 10.

Frieden T. R., P. I. Fujiwara, R. M. Washko, et al. 1995. Tuberculosis in New York City—turning the tide. *New England Journal of Medicine* 333: 229-33.

Fukuda K. 1997. Cited by *Hong Kong Standard and Electronic Telegraph*, 11 December 1997. Cited by www.outbreak.org. H5N1 flu strain chronology, part 2.

Gangarosa E. J., A. M. Galazka, C. R. Wolfe, et al. 1998. Impact of anti-vaccine movements on pertussis control: the untold story. *The Lancet* 351: 356-61.

Gao F., E. Bailes, D. L. Robertson, et al. 1999. Origin of HIV-1 in the chimpanzee *Pan troglodytes troglodytes*. *Nature* 397: 436-41.

Gardner H., K. Kerry, M. Riddle, et al. 1997. Poultry virus infection in Antarctic penguins. *Nature* 387: 245.

Gaydos C. A., M. R. Howell, B. Pare, et al. 1998. Chlamydia trachomatis infections in female military recruits. *New England Journal of Medicine* 339: 739-44.

Gerba C. P. Cited by C. Murphy. 1997. Something in the water: one man's pursuit of microbial mayhem. *The Atlantic Monthly*, September, 27-28.

Gerbase A. C., J. T. Rowley, T. E. Mertens. 1998. Global epidemiology of sexually transmitted diseases. *The Lancet* 351: (Suppl III) 2-4.

Gindler J. S., W. L. Atkinson, L. E. Markowitz. 1992. Update–the United States measles epidemic, 1989-1990. *Epidemiologic Reviews* 14: 270-6.

Gladwell M. 1997. The dead zone. *The New Yorker*, 29 September, 52-65.

Glynn M. K., C. Bopp, W. DeWitt, et al. 1998. Emergence of multidrug-resistant *Salmonella enterica* serotype typhimurium DT104 infections in the United States. *New England Journal of Medicine* 338: 1333-8.

Goh K. T. 1997. Dengue–a reemerging infectious disease in Singapore. *Annals of the Academy of Medicine of Singapore* 26: 664-70.

Gonzales R., J. F. Steiner, M. A. Sande, et al. 1997. Antibiotic prescribing for adults with colds, upper respiratory tract infections, and bronchitis by ambulatory care physicians. *JAMA* 278: 901-4.

Grattan L. M., D. Oldach, T. M. Perl, et al. 1998. Learning and memory difficulties after environmental exposure to waterways containing toxin-producing *Pfiesteria* or *Pfiesteria*-like dinoflagellates. *The Lancet* 352: 532-9.

Groopman J. 1998. The shadow epidemic. *The New Yorker*, 11 May, 48-60.

Gustafson R., B. Svenungsson, M. Forsgren, et al. 1992. Two-year survey of the incidence of Lyme borreliosis and tick-borne encephalitis in a high-risk population in Sweden. *European Journal of Clinical Microbiology and Infectious Diseases* 11: 894-900.

Haile R.W., J. S. Witte, M. Gold, et al. 1999. The health effects of swimming in ocean water contaminated by storm drain runoff. *Epidemiology* 10: 355-63.

Hales S., P. Weinstein, A. Woodward. 1996. Dengue fever epidemics in the South Pacific: driven by El Niño Southern Oscillation? *The Lancet* 348: 1664-5.

Handsfield H. H., P. F. Sparling. 1995. *Neisseria gonorrhoeae*. In *Principles and Practice of Infectious Diseases*, 4th ed, edited by G. L. Mandell, J. E. Bennett, and R. Dolin. New York: Churchill Livingstone.

Hardy I.R.B., S. Dittmann, R. W. Sutter. 1996. Current situation and control strategies for resurgence of diphtheria in the newly independent states of the former Soviet Union. *The Lancet* 347: 1739-44.

Harpaz R., L. Von Seidlein, F. M. Averhoff, et al. 1996. Transmission of hepatitis B virus to multiple patients from a surgeon without evidence of inadequate infection control. *New England Journal of Medicine* 334: 549-54.

Hart C.A. 1998. Antibiotic resistance: an increasing problem? *BMJ* 316: 1255-6.

Henderson D. A. 1994. Role of the United States in the global response to emerging infections. *Journal of Infectious Diseases* 170: 284-5.

Henderson D. A. 1998. Bioterrorism as a public health threat. *Emerging Infectious Diseases* 4: 488-92.

Hennessy T. W., C. W. Hedberg, L. Slutsker, et al. 1996. A national outbreak of *Salmonella enteritidis* infections from ice cream. *New England Journal of Medicine* 334: 1281-6.

Herold B. C., L. C. Immergluck, M. C. Maranan, et al. 1998. Community-acquired methicillin-resistant *Staphylococcus aureus* in children with no identified predisposing risk. *JAMA* 279: 593-8.

Herrera-Basto E., D. R. Prevots, M. A. L. Zarate, et al. 1992. First reported outbreak of classical dengue fever at 1,700 meters above sea level in Guerrero state, Mexico, June 1988. *American Journal of Tropical Medicine and Hygiene* 46: 649-53.

Herwaldt B. L., M. L. Ackers, and the *Cyclospora* Working Group. 1997. An outbreak in 1996 of cyclosporiasis associated with imported raspberries. *New England Journal of Medicine* 336: 1548-56.

Hiramatsu K. 1998. The emergence of *Staphylococcus aureus* with reduced susceptibility to vancomycin in Japan. *American Journal of Medicine* 104: 7S-10S.

Hiramatsu K., H. Hanaki, T. Ino, et al. 1997. Methicillin-resistant *Staphylococcus aureus* clinical strain with reduced vancomycin susceptibility. *Journal of Antimicrobial Chemotherapy* 40: 135-6.

Hlady W. G., J. V. Bennett, A. R. Samadi, et al. 1992. Neonatal tetanus in rural Bangladesh: risk factors and toxoid efficacy. *American Journal of Public Health* 82: 1365-9.

Hoge C. W., D. R. Shlim, R. Rajah, et al. 1993. Epidemiology of diarrhoeal illness associated with coccidian-like organism among travellers and foreign residents in Nepal. *The Lancet* 341: 1175-9.

Holmes A., J. Govan, R. Goldstein. 1998. Agricultural use of *Burkolderia (Pseudomonas) cepacia*: a threat to human health? *Emerging Infectious Diseases* 4: 221-7.

Holum J. D. 1996. Speech to the 4th Review Conference of the Biological Weapons Convention, Geneva, Switzerland, 26 November 1996. Cited at www.acda.gov.

Homewood B. 1996. Pneumonia runs riot in Brazil's creches. *New Scientist*, 26 October, 7.

Hotez P. J., F. Zheng, L. Xu, et al. 1997. Emerging and reemerging helminthiases and the public health of China. *Emerging Infectious Diseases* 3: 303-10.

Institute of Medicine. 1992. Lederberg J., R. E. Shope, S. C. Oaks, eds. *Emerging Infections: Microbial Threats to Health in the United States.* Washington: National Academy Press.

Institute of Medicine. 1997. T. R. Eng and W. T. Butler, eds. *The Hidden Epidemic: Confronting Sexually Transmitted Diseases.* Washington: National Academy Press.

Institute of Medicine. 1999. *Chemical and Biological Terrorism: Research and Development to Improve Civilian Medical Response.* Washington: National Academy Press.

Jackson L. A., D. H. Spach. 1996. Emergence of *Bartonella quintana* infection among homeless persons. *Emerging Infectious Diseases* 2: 141-3.

Jahrling P. Cited by J. Cohen. 1997. Is an old virus up to new tricks? *Science* 277: 312-3.

Jarvis W. Cited by J. Stephenson. 1997a. Worry grows as antibiotic-resistant bacteria continue to gain ground. *JAMA* 278: 2049-50.

Jarvis W. 1997b. Cited by the Associated Press, 21 August 1997. Cited by www.outbreak.org. Vancomycin-resistant staph in the U.S.

Jerrigan D. B., J. Hofmann, M. S. Cetron, et al. 1996. Outbreak of legionnaires' disease among cruise ship passengers exposed to a contaminated whirlpool spa. *The Lancet* 347: 494-9.

Joffe G. P., B. Foxman, A. J. Schmidt, et al. 1992. Multiple partners and partner choice as risk factors for sexually transmitted disease among female college students. *Sexually Transmitted Diseases* 19: 272-8.

Jones C. G., R. S. Ostfeld, M. P. Richard, et al. 1998. Chain reactions linking acorns to gypsy moth outbreaks and Lyme disease risk. *Science* 279: 1023-6.

Jouan A., B. LeGuenno, J. P. Digoutte, et al. 1988. A RVF epidemic in southern Mauritania. *Annales de l'Institut Pasteur, Virology* 139: 307-8.

Kafka F. Cited by E. A. Belongia and B. Schwartz. 1998. Strategies for promoting judicious use of antibiotics by doctors and patients. *BMJ* 317: 668-71.

Kaminski, J. C. 1994. *Cryptosporidium* and the public water supply. *New England Journal of Medicine* 331: 1529-30.

Kaplan D. E. 1997. Interview with "…" *US News and World Report*, September 2 electronic version.

Kasse M. Cited by E. R. Shell. 1997. Resurgence of a deadly disease. *The Atlantic Monthly*, August, 45-60.

Katz, S. L. 1999. Today's vaccine paradox: our success in immunization has become a major liability. *Needle Tips: Bulletin of the Immunization Action Coalition*, Spring/Summer, 3.

Kenyon G. 1999. Scientists try new strategy to eradicate dengue fever. *BMJ* 318: 555.

Kenyon T. A., S. E. Valway, W. W. Ihle, et al. 1996. Transmission of multidrug-resistant *Mycobacterium tuberculosis* during a long airplane flight. *New England Journal of Medicine* 334: 933-8.

Khan A. Cited by J. Cohen. 1997. Is an old virus up to new tricks? *Science* 277: 312-3.

Khodakevich L., Z. Jezek, D. Messinger. 1988. Monkeypox virus: ecology and public health significance. *Bulletin of the World Health Organization* 66: 747-52.

Kilbourne E. D. 1990. New viral diseases. A real and potential problem without boundaries. *JAMA* 264: 68-70.

King M. 1990. Health is a sustainable state. *The Lancet* 336: 664-7.

Kitron U., J. Swanson, M. Crandell, et al. 1998. Introduction of *Aedes albopictus* into a La Crosse virus-enzootic site in Illinois. *Emerging Infectious Diseases* 4: 627-30.

Klein J. O. 1986. Infectious diseases and day care. *Reviews of Infectious Diseases* 8: 521-6.

Knapp J. S., K. K. Fox, D. L. Trees, et al. 1997. Fluoroquinolone resistance in *Neisseria gonorrhoeae. Emerging Infectious Diseases* 3: 33-9.

Koch R. Cited by J. J. Ellner, A. R. Hinman, S. W. Dooley, et al. 1993. Tuberculosis symposium: emerging problems and promise. *Journal of Infectious Diseases* 168: 537-51.

Kohl K. S., D. Wendell, T. Farley. Sexual risk behavior in men who have sex with men: statewide gay bar surveys, Louisiana, 1995-1998. *Abstracts of the 48th Annual Epidemic Intelligence Service Conference 1999.* Atlanta: Centers for Disease Control and Prevention.

Kolavic S. A., A. Kimura, S. L. Simons, et al. 1997. An outbreak of *Shigella dysenteriae* type 2 among laboratory workers due to intentional food contamination. *JAMA* 278: 396-8.

Krag E. 1998. Cited by K. Abbasi. Facing the microbial threat. *BMJ* 317: 620.

Krause R. M. 1994. Dynamics of emergence. *Journal of Infectious Diseases* 170: 265-71.

Krause R. M. 1994. Dynamics of emergence. *Journal of Infectious Diseases* 170: 265-71.

Lanchester J. 1996. A new kind of contagion. *The New Yorker,* 2 December, 70-81.

Lattimer G.L. and R. A. Ormsbee. 1981. *Legionnaires' Disease.* New York: Marcel Dekker.

Laumann E. O., J. H. Gagnon, R. T. Michael, et al. 1994. *The Social Organization of Sexuality: Sexual Practices in the United States.* Chicago: University of Chicago Press.

Laver W. G., N. Bischofberger, R. G. Webster. 1999. Disarming flu viruses. *Scientific American,* January, 56-65.

Layton M. C. 1997. *Cyclospora*: clinical and epidemiological aspects of an emerging parasitic disease. 35th Annual Meeting of the Infectious Diseases Society of America, San Francisco.

Le Maitre A. and D. D. Chadee. 1983. Arthropods collected from aircraft at Piarco International Airport, Trinidad, West Indies. *Mosquito News* 43: 21-3.

LeChevallier M.W., W. D. Norton, R. G. Lee. 1991. Occurrence of *Giardia* and *Cryptosporidium* spp. in surface water supplies. *Applied and Environmental Microbiology* 57: 2610-6.

Lederberg J. 1988. Medical science, infectious disease and the unity of humankind. *JAMA* 260: 684-5.

Lederberg J. Cited by B. J. Culliton. 1990. Emerging viruses, emerging threat. *Science* 247: 279-80.

Lederberg J. Cited by R. Preston. 1998. The bioweaponeers. *The New Yorker*, 9 March, 52-65.

Lee S. H., S. T. Lai, J. Y. Lai, et al. 1996. Resurgence of cholera in Hong Kong. *Epidemiology and Infection* 117: 43-9.

Levins R. 1994. The challenge of new diseases. *Annals of the New York Academy of Sciences* 740: xvii-xix.

Levy S. B. 1998. The challenge of antibiotic resistance. *Scientific American*, March, 46-53.

Lopez N., P. Padula, C. Rossi, et al. 1996. Genetic identification of a new hantavirus causing severe pulmonary syndrome in Argentina. *Virology* 220: 223-6.

Lord Soulsby. 1998. Cited by K. Abbasi. Report calls for action on antibiotic resistance. *BMJ* 316: 1261.

Mac Kenzie W. R., N. J. Hoxie, M. E. Proctor, et al. 1994. A massive outbreak in Milwaukee of *Cryptosporidium* infection transmitted through the public water supply. *New England Journal of Medicine* 331: 161-7.

Mantel C. F., C. Klose, S. Scheurer, et al. 1995. *Plasmodium falciparum* malaria acquired in Berlin, Germany. *The Lancet* 346: 320-1.

Marshall B. J., J. R. Warren. 1984. Unidentified curved bacilli in the stomach of patients with gastritis and peptic ulceration. *The Lancet* 1: 1311-5.

Marshall E. 1988. Sverdlovsk: anthrax capital? *Science* 240: 383-5.

Mattei J. F. Cited by D. D. de Bousingen. 1999. Europe supports moratorium on xenotransplantation. *The Lancet* 353: 476.

McMinn P., I. Stratov, G. Dowse. 1999. Enterovirus 71 outbreak in Western Australia associated with acute flaccid paralysis: preliminary report. *Communicable Disease Intelligence* 23: 199.

McMurray L. M., M. Oethinger, S. B. Levy. 1998. Triclosan targets lipid synthesis. *Nature* 394: 531-2.

Mead P. S. and P. M. Griffin. 1998. *Escherichia coli* O157:H7. *The Lancet* 352: 1207-12.

Medical Device Technologies. Cited by Anonymous. 1997. Virus transfer ungloved as infections spread. *New Zealand GP Weekly*. 2 April, 12.

Mekalanos J. J. Cited by P. Brown. 1996. Cholera's deadly hitchhiker. *New Scientist*, 6 July, 14.

Melnick J. L. 1984. Enterovirus type 71 infections: a varied clinical pattern sometimes mimicking paralytic poliomyelitis. *Reviews of Infectious Diseases* 6(Suppl 2): S387-90.

Meltzer M. I., N. J. Cox, K. Fukuda. 1999. The economic impact of pandemic influenza in the United States: priorities for intervention. *Emerging Infectious Diseases* 5: 659-71.

Merritt T. 1998. Climate change and human health in the Asia-Pacific region. *Snow's Field: The Newsletter of the Australasian Faculty of Public Health Medicine*, March 1998, pp.1-2.

Meselson M., J. Guillemin, M. Hugh-Jones, et al. 1994. The Sverdlovsk anthrax outbreak of 1979. *Science* 266: 1202-8.

Michele T. M., W. A. Cronin, N. M. H. Graham, et al. 1997. Transmission of *Mycobacterium tuberculosis* by a fiberoptic bronchoscope. *JAMA* 278: 1093-5.

Mindel A. 1998. Genital herpes—how much of a public health problem? *The Lancet* 351: (SIII) 16-18.

Ministries of Agriculture, Fisheries, and Food. 1989. *Report on the Working Party on Bovine Spongiform Encephalopathy*. Surrey, England.

Monath T. P. 1993. Arthropod-borne viruses. In *Emerging Viruses*, edited by S. S. Morse. New York: Oxford University Press.

Moore C. G., C. J. Mitchell. 1997. *Aedes albopictus* in the United States: ten-year presence and public health implications. *Emerging Infectious Diseases* 3: 329-34.

Moore J. M., P. Bloland, J. Zingeser. 1995. Mortality surveillance among Rwandan refugees in Zaire, 1994. *Abstracts of the 44th Annual Epidemic Intelligence Service Conference 1995*. Atlanta: Centers for Disease Control and Prevention.

Morse S. S. 1991. Emerging viruses: defining the rules for viral traffic. *Perspectives in Biology and Medicine* 34: 387-409.

Morse S. S. Cited by B. J. Culliton. 1990. Emerging viruses, emerging threat. *Science* 247: 279-80.

Moser M. R., T. R. Bender, H. S. Margolis, et al. 1979. An outbreak of influenza aboard a commercial airliner. *American Journal of Epidemiology* 110: 1-6.

Mott K. E., I. Nuttall, P. Desjeux, et al. 1995. New geographical approaches to control of some parasitic zoonoses. *Bulletin of the World Health Organization* 73: 247-57.

Mott K. E., P. Desjeux, A. Moncayo, et al. 1990. Parasitic diseases and urban development. *Bulletin of the World Health Organization* 68: 691-8.

N'Goran E. K., S. Diabate, J. Utzinger, et al. 1997. Changes in human schistosomiasis levels after the construction of two large hydroelectric dams in central Côte d'Ivoire. *Bulletin of the World Health Organization* 75: 541-5.

National Center for Infectious Diseases, Centers for Disease Control and Prevention. 1999. Rabies Section, Viral and Rickettsial Zoonoses, Branch Division of Viral and Rickettsial Diseases.

Navajo chief. Cited by P. R. Epstein. 1995. Emerging diseases and ecosystem instability: new threats to public health. *American Journal of Public Health* 85: 168-72.

New York City Board of Health. Annual Report, 1915. Cited by R. Coker. 1998. Lessons from New York's tuberculosis epidemic. *BMJ* 317: 616.

New York Times. 1918. Documents taken from German prisoners indicate they are having a hard time with the new influenza. Cited by A. J. Bollet. 1987. *Plagues and Poxes: The Rise and Fall of Epidemic Disease.* New York: Demos Publications.

Nicholls N. 1993. El Niño-Southern Oscillation and vector-borne disease. *The Lancet* 342: 1284-5.

Noah D. L., C. L. Drenzek, J. S. Smith, et al. 1998. Epidemiology of human rabies in the United States, 1980 to 1996. *Annals of Internal Medicine* 128: 922-30.

Noble W. C., Z. Virani, R. G. Cree. 1992. Co-transfer of vancomycin and other resistance genes from *Enterococcus faecalis* NCTC 12201 to *Staphylococcus aureus*. *FEMS Microbiology Letters* 72: 195-8.

Novak R. Cited by J. Steinhauer. 1999. Lax monitoring led to encephalitis, experts suggest. *New York Times*, 19 September.

Nyquist A. C., R. Gonzales, J. F. Steiner, et al. 1998. Antibiotic prescribing for children with colds, upper respiratory tract infections, and bronchitis. *JAMA* 279: 875-7.

O'Brien T. Cited by M. Day. 1997. Phew, what a sickwave. *New Scientist*, 23 August, 4.

Office of Technology Assessment. 1993. Cited by R. Taylor. 1996. All fall down. *New Scientist*, 11 May, 32-7.

Olsen K.B. 1999. Aum Shinrikyo: once and future threat? *Emerging Infectious Diseases* 5: 513-6.

Osterholm M. 1997a. Cited by J. Wise. Global food markets increase risk of infectious disease. *BMJ* 314: 1645.

Osterholm M. 1997b. Emerging infectious diseases: fact or fiction? 35th Annual Meeting of the Infectious Diseases Society of America, San Francisco.

Osterholm M. 1999. Lessons learned again: cyclosporiasis and raspberries. *Annals of Internal Medicine* 130: 233-4.

Ostroff S. M. 1999. Continuing challenge of pneumococcal disease. *The Lancet* 353: 1201-2.

Ostrowski S. R., M. J. Leslie, T. Parrott, et al. 1998. B-virus from pet macaque monkeys: an emerging threat in the United States? *Emerging Infectious Diseases* 4: 117-20.

Passaro D. J., L. Waring, R. Armstrong, et al. 1997. Postoperative *Serratia marcescens* wound infections traced to an out-of-hospital source. *Journal of Infectious Diseases* 175: 992-5.

Patz J. A., P. R. Epstein, T. A. Burke, et al. 1996. Global climate change and emerging infectious diseases. *JAMA* 275: 217-23.

Paul C., J. Fitzjohn, J. E. Eberhart-Phillips, et al. 1999. Twenty-one year olds who have not had sexual intercourse: the importance of religion. (Unpublished).

Payment P., J. Siemiatycki, L. Richardson, et al. 1997. A prospective epidemiological study of gastrointestinal health effects due to the consumption of drinking water. *International Journal of Environmental Health Research* 7: 5-31.

Pearce F. 1999. Shining clean: if you fancy a swim in the sea, you'd better time it carefully. *New Scientist*, 14 August, 20.

Pittet D., R. P. Wenzel. 1995. Nosocomial bloodstream infections: secular trends in rates, mortality, and contribution to total hospital deaths. *Archives of Internal Medicine* 155: 1177-84.

Plotkin B. J., A. M. Kimball. 1997. Designing an international policy and legal framework for the control of emerging infectious diseases: First steps. *Emerging Infectious Diseases* 3: 1-9.

Prevots D. R., M. L. Ciofi degli Atti, A. Sallabanda, et al. 1998. Outbreak of paralytic poliomyelitis in Albania, 1996: high attack rate among adults and apparent interruption of transmission following nationwide mass vaccination. *Clinical Infectious Diseases* 26: 419-25.

Prusiner S. B. 1995. The prion diseases. *Scientific American*, January, 30-7.

Rahman A. 1999. Cited in CJD–Risk from blood. ProMED-mail post, 20 April.

Rao K. S., R. D. Pilli, A. S. Rao, et al. 1999. Sexual lifestyle of long distance lorry drivers in India: questionnaire survey. *BMJ* 318: 162-3.

Reid A. H., T. G. Fanning, J. V. Hultin, et al. 1999. Origin and evolution of the 1918 "Spanish" influenza virus hemagglutinin gene. *Proceedings of the National Academy of Sciences of the United States of America* 96: 1651-6.

Riley L. W., R. S. Remis, S. D. Helgerson, et al. 1983. Hemorrhagic colitis associated with a rare *Escherichia coli* serotype. *New England Journal of Medicine* 308: 681-5.

Roberts B. Cited by D. MacKenzie. 1998. Bioarmageddon. *New Scientist*, 19 September, 42-6.

Rodier G. R., J. P. Parra, M. Kamil, et al. 1995. Recurrence and emergence of infectious diseases in Djibouti city. *Bulletin of the World Health Organization* 73: 755-9.

Rogers D. J. and M. J. Packer. 1993. Vector-borne diseases, models and global change. *The Lancet* 342: 1282-4.

Rosatte R. 1999. Rabies, raccoon – Canada (Ontario). ProMED-mail post, 24 July.

Roy E., J. F. Boivin, N. Haley, et al. 1998. Mortality among street youth. *The Lancet* 352: 32.

Rupprecht C. E., J. S. Smith, M. Fekadu, et al. 1995. The ascension of wildlife rabies: a cause for public health concern or intervention? *Emerging Infectious Diseases* 1: 107-14.

Russell R. C. 1987. Survival of insects in the wheel bays of a Boeing 747B aircraft on flights between tropical and temperate airports. *Bulletin of the World Health Organization* 65: 659-62.

Salmon D. A., M. Haber, E. J. Gangarosa, et al. 1999. Health consequences of religious and philosophical exemptions from immunization laws: individual and societal risk of measles. *JAMA* 282: 47-53.

Sang T. H. 1998. Guest editorial. *Pacific Health Dialog* 5: 4-5.

Schlech W.F., K. N. Shands, A. L. Reingold, et al. 1982. Risk factors for development of toxic shock syndrome: association with a tampon brand. *JAMA* 248: 835-9.

Schneider E., R. A. Hajjeh, R. A. Spiegel, et al. 1997. A coccidioidomycosis outbreak following the Northridge, Calif., earthquake. *JAMA* 277: 904-8.

Schwab K. Cited by J. Steinhauer. 1999. Lax monitoring led to encephalitis, experts suggest. *New York Times*, 19 September.

Schwartz B. Cited by S. Ostroff and J. Hughes. 1998. New ways to tackle influenza highlighted at ICAAC. *The Lancet* 352: 1123.

Sehgal R. 1997. Dengue fever and El Niño. *The Lancet* 349: 729-30.

Selden S. M. and A. S. Cameron. 1996. Changing epidemiology of Ross River virus disease in South Australia. *Medical Journal of Australia* 165: 313-7.

Shell E. R. 1997. Resurgence of a deadly disease. *The Atlantic Monthly*, August 1997, pp. 45-60.

Shell E. R. 1998. Could mad cow disease happen here? *The Atlantic Monthly*, September, 92-106.

Shilts R. 1987. *And the Band Played On*. New York: St. Martin's Press.

Sibley R. 1996. Cited by J. Lanchester. A new kind of contagion. *The New Yorker*, 2 December, 70-81.

Sieradzki K., Roberts R. B., Haber S. W., et al. 1999. The development of vancomycin resistance in a patient with methicillin-resistant *Staphylococcus aureus* infection. *New England Journal of Medicine* 340: 517-23.

Simon J.D. 1997. Biological terrorism: preparing to meet the threat. *JAMA* 278: 428-30.

Smith K. E., J. M. Besser, C. W. Hedberg, et al. 1999. Quinolone-resistant *Campylobacter jejuni* infections in Minnesota, 1992-1998. *New England Journal of Medicine* 340: 1525-32.

Smith T. L., M. L. Pearson, K. R. Wilcox, et al. 1999. Emergence of vancomycin resistance in *Staphylococcus aureus*. *New England Journal of Medicine* 340: 493-501.

Sobsey M. Cited by A. Coghlan. 1997. Jet-setters send festering faeces round the world. *New Scientist*, 17 May, 7.

St. John R. 1996. Emerging infectious disease: repeat of an old challenge. *Canadian Journal of Public Health* 87: 365-6.

Stanecki K. A. and P. O. Way. 1999. Focusing on HIV/AIDS in the developing world. In *World Population Profile: 1998*, edited by T. M. McDevitt. Washington: U.S. Census Bureau.

Steere A.C., S. E. Malawista, D. R. Syndman, et al. 1977. Lyme arthritis: an epidemic of oligoarticular arthritis in children and adults in three Connecticut communities. *Arthritis and Rheumatism* 20: 7-17.

Stern J. 1999. The prospect of domestic bioterrorism. *Emerging Infectious Diseases* 5: 517-22.

Suarez L., E. Swayne, R. Castaneda, et al. 1995. A role for funerals in transmission of cholera in the Peruvian Andes, 1994. *Abstracts of the 44th Annual Epidemic Intelligence Service Conference 1995*. Atlanta: Centers for Disease Control and Prevention.

Sutter R. W., Y. K. Chudaiberdiev, S. H. Vaphakulov, et al. 1997. A large outbreak of poliomyelitis following temporary cessation of vaccination in
Samarkand, Uzbekistan, 1993-1994. *Journal of Infectious Diseases* 175(Suppl
1): S82-5.

Swafford S. 1997. Invasive devices increase risk of infection. *BMJ* 314: 1503.

Swerdlow D. 1998. Food-borne diseases in the global village. In *Emerging
Infections 2*, edited by W. M. Scheld, W. A. Craig, and J. M. Hughes. Washington: American Society for Microbiology.

Tallis G. and J. Gregory. 1997. An outbreak of hepatitis A associated with a
spa pool. *Communicable Diseases Intelligence* 21: 353-4.

Tan P. Cited by W. W. Gibbs. 1999. Trailing a virus. *Scientific American*,
August, 65-71.

Taubenberger J. K. 1997. Cited by M. Gladwell. The dead zone. *The New
Yorker*, 29 September, 52-65.

Tauxe R. V. 1997. Emerging foodborne diseases: an evolving public health
challenge. *Emerging Infectious Diseases* 3: 425-34.

Taylor B., E. Miller, C. P. Farrington, et al. 1999. Autism and measles,
mumps, and rubella vaccine: no epidemiological evidence for a causal
association. *The Lancet* 353: 2026-9.

Teoh Y. L., K. T. Goh, K. S. Neo, et al. 1997. A nationwide outbreak of
coconut-associated paratyphoid A fever in Singapore. *Annals of the Academy of Medicine of Singapore* 26: 544-8.

Thompson S. 1997. Vaccination: protection at what price? *Australian and New
Zealand Journal of Public Health* 21: 1-8.

Torok T.J., R. V. Tauxe, R. P. Wise, et al. 1997. A large community outbreak
of salmonellosis caused by intentional contamination of restaurant salad
bars. *JAMA* 278: 389-95.

Townes J. M., C. Landrigan, S. Monroe, et al. 1995. Outbreak of Norwalk
virus gastroenteritis associated with eating raw imported limpets.
Abstracts of the 44th Annual Epidemic Intelligence Service Conference 1995.
Atlanta: Centers for Disease Control and Prevention.

United States Bureau of Labor Statistics. Cited by Peth-Pierce R. 1998. The
National Institute of Child Health and Human Development Study of
Early Child Care. Bethesda: National Institute of Child Health and Human
Development.

United States Custom Service. Cited by American Association of Port
Authorities. 1999. Port facts and statistics. www.aapa-ports.org/port-
facts/portfact.html.

United States Department of Agriculture. 1996. Take out foods – handle with
care. *The Food Safety Educator* 1: 2.

United States Fish and Wildlife Service News Release. 1998. Federal agents
target illegal bird trade. May 29.

Valway S. E., R. B. Greifinger, M. Papania, et al. 1994. Multidrug-resistant
tuberculosis in the New York state prison system, 1990-1991. *Journal of
Infectious Diseases* 170: 151-6.

Van der Stuyft P., A. Gianella, M. Pirard, et al. 1999. Urbanisation of yellow fever in Santa Cruz, Bolivia. *The Lancet* 353: 1558-62.

Venczel L.V., M. Desai, B. Bell, et al. 1998. The role of child-care in a community-wide outbreak of hepatitis A, Maricopa County, Arizona, 1997. *Abstracts of the 47th Annual Epidemic Intelligence Service Conference 1998.* Atlanta: Centers for Disease Control and Prevention.

Wade N. 1980. Death at Sverdlovsk: a critical diagnosis. *Science* 209: 1501-2.

Wakefield A. J., S. H. Murch, A. Anthony, et al. 1998. Ileal-lymphoid-nodular hyperplasia, non-specific colitis, and pervasive developmental disorder in children. *The Lancet* 351: 637-41.

Waldor M. K., J. J. Mekalanos. 1996. Lysogenic conversion by a filamentous phage encoding cholera toxin. *Science* 272: 1910-4.

Waldvogel F.A. 1999. New resistance in *Staphylococcus aureus*. *New England Journal of Medicine* 340: 556-7.

Walker J. 1997. Malaria in the 1990s: plus ça change, plus ça même chose. *Australian and New Zealand Journal of Public Health* 21: 244-6.

Waterman S. H., G. Juarez, S. J. Carr, et al. 1990. *Salmonella arizona* infections in Latinos associated with rattlesnake folk medicine. *American Journal of Public Health* 80: 286-9.

Watts J. 1997. Japan's just crazy about cleanliness. *The Lancet* 350: 574.

Webster J., D. Macdonald. Cited by H. Saul. 1996. Year of the rat. *New Scientist*, 5 October, 32-7.

Webster R. G. 1993. Influenza. In *Emerging Viruses*, edited by S. S. Morse. New York: Oxford University Press.

Webster R. G., Y. Kawaoka, W. J. Bean. 1986. Molecular changes in A/chicken/Pennsylvania/83 (H5N2) influenza virus associated with virulence. *Virology* 149: 165-73.

Wegener H. C., F. M. Aarestrup, L. B. Jensen, et al. 1999. Use of antimicrobial growth promoters in food animals and *Enterococcus faecium* resistance to therapeutic antimicrobial drugs in Europe. *Emerging Infectious Diseases* 5: 329-35.

Wenzel R. P., M. B. Edmond. 1997. Tuberculosis infection after bronchoscopy. *JAMA* 278: 111.

Williams A. E., R. A. Thomson, G. B. Schreiber, et al. 1997. Estimates of infectious disease risk factors in US blood donors. *JAMA* 277: 967-72.

Willocks L., A. Crampin, L. Milne, et al. 1998. A large outbreak of cryptosporidiosis associated with a public water supply from a deep chalk borehole. *Communicable Disease and Public Health* 1: 239-43.

Winslow C. E. A. 1943. *The Conquest of Epidemic Disease*. Princeton: Princeton University Press.

World Health Organization. 1993. TB: a global emergency. *World Health*.4:3.

World Health Organization. 1995. *World Health Report 1995*. Geneva: World Health Organization.

World Health Organization. 1998a. Global Tuberculosis Program. Fact Sheet 104: Tuberculosis. February.

World Health Organization. 1998b. An outbreak of rift valley fever, eastern Africa, 1997-1998. *Weekly Epidemiological Record* 73: 105-9.

World Health Organization. 1999. *Removing Obstacles to Healthy Development.* Geneva: World Health Organization.

Wrage S. 1996. Watering to endanger. *The Atlantic Monthly*, June, 41-2.

Yasuno M., R. J. Tonn. 1970. A study of biting habits of *Aedes aegypti* in Bangkok, Thailand. *Bulletin of the World Health Organization* 43: 319-25.

Zhu T., B. T. Korber, A. J. Nahmias, et al. 1998. An African HIV-1 sequence from 1959 and implications for the origin of the epidemic. *Nature* 391: 594-7.

Zilinskas R. A. 1997. Iraq's biological weapons: the past as future? *JAMA* 278: 418-24.

Zilinskas R. A. 1998. Bioethics and biological weapons. *Science* 279: 635.

Zinsser H. 1934. *Rats, Lice and History.* Boston: Little, Brown and Company.

Index

More New Harbinger Titles

Some Other New Harbinger Self-Help Titles

Multiple Chemical Sensitivity: A Survival Guide, $16.95
Dancing Naked, $14.95
Why Are We Still Fighting, $15.95
From Sabotage to Success, $14.95
Parkinson's Disease and the Art of Moving, $15.95
A Survivor's Guide to Breast Cancer, $13.95
Men, Women, and Prostate Cancer, $15.95
Make Every Session Count: Getting the Most Out of Your Brief Therapy, $10.95
Virtual Addiction, $12.95
After the Breakup, $13.95
Why Can't I Be the Parent I Want to Be?, $12.95
The Secret Message of Shame, $13.95
The OCD Workbook, $18.95
Tapping Your Inner Strength, $13.95
Binge No More, $14.95
When to Forgive, $12.95
Practical Dreaming, $12.95
Healthy Baby, Toxic World, $15.95
Making Hope Happen, $14.95
I'll Take Care of You, $12.95
Survivor Guilt, $14.95
Children Changed by Trauma, $13.95
Understanding Your Child's Sexual Behavior, $12.95
The Self-Esteem Companion, $10.95
The Gay and Lesbian Self-Esteem Book, $13.95
Making the Big Move, $13.95
How to Survive and Thrive in an Empty Nest, $13.95
Living Well with a Hidden Disability, $15.95
Overcoming Repetitive Motion Injuries the Rossiter Way, $15.95
What to Tell the Kids About Your Divorce, $13.95
The Divorce Book, Second Edition, $15.95
Claiming Your Creative Self: True Stories from the Everyday Lives of Women, $15.95
Six Keys to Creating the Life You Desire, $19.95
Taking Control of TMJ, $13.95
What You Need to Know About Alzheimer's, $15.95
Winning Against Relapse: A Workbook of Action Plans for Recurring Health and Emotional Problems, $14.95
Facing 30: Women Talk About Constructing a Real Life and Other Scary Rites of Passage, $12.95
The Worry Control Workbook, $15.95
Wanting What You Have: A Self-Discovery Workbook, $18.95
When Perfect Isn't Good Enough: Strategies for Coping with Perfectionism, $13.95
Earning Your Own Respect: A Handbook of Personal Responsibility, $12.95
High on Stress: A Woman's Guide to Optimizing the Stress in Her Life, $13.95
Infidelity: A Survival Guide, $13.95
Stop Walking on Eggshells, $14.95
Consumer's Guide to Psychiatric Drugs, $16.95
The Fibromyalgia Advocate: Getting the Support You Need to Cope with Fibromyalgia and Myofascial Pain, $18.95
Healing Fear: New Approaches to Overcoming Anxiety, $16.95
Working Anger: Preventing and Resolving Conflict on the Job, $12.95
Sex Smart: How Your Childhood Shaped Your Sexual Life and What to Do About It, $14.95
You Can Free Yourself From Alcohol & Drugs, $13.95
Amongst Ourselves: A Self-Help Guide to Living with Dissociative Identity Disorder, $14.95
Healthy Living with Diabetes, $13.95
Dr. Carl Robinson's Basic Baby Care, $10.95
Better Boundries: Owning and Treasuring Your Life, $13.95
Goodbye Good Girl, $12.95
Fibromyalgia & Chronic Myofascial Pain Syndrome, $19.95
The Depression Workbook: Living With Depression and Manic Depression, $17.95
Self-Esteem, Second Edition, $13.95
Angry All the Time: An Emergency Guide to Anger Control, $12.95
When Anger Hurts, $13.95
Perimenopause, $16.95
The Relaxation & Stress Reduction Workbook, Fourth Edition, $17.95
The Anxiety & Phobia Workbook, Second Edition, $18.95
I Can't Get Over It, A Handbook for Trauma Survivors, Second Edition, $16.95
Messages: The Communication Skills Workbook, Second Edition, $15.95
Thoughts & Feelings, Second Edition, $18.95
Depression: How It Happens, How It's Healed, $14.95
The Deadly Diet, Second Edition, $14.95
The Power of Two, $15.95

Call **toll free, 1-800-748-6273,** or log on to our online bookstore at **www.newharbinger.com** to order. Have your Visa or Mastercard number ready. Or send a check for the titles you want to New Harbinger Publications, Inc., 5674 Shattuck Ave., Oakland, CA 94609. Include $3.80 for the first book and 75¢ for each additional book, to cover shipping and handling. (California residents please include appropriate sales tax.) Allow two to five weeks for delivery.

Prices subject to change without notice.